Machine Learning and Deep Learning Techniques for Medical Image Recognition

Machine Learning and Deep Learning Techniques for Medical Image Recognition comprehensively reviews deep learning-based algorithms in medical image analysis problems including medical image processing. It includes a detailed review of deep learning approaches for semantic object detection and segmentation in medical image computing and large-scale radiology database mining. A particular focus is placed on the application of convolutional neural networks with the theory and varied selection of techniques for semantic segmentation using deep learning principles in medical imaging supported by practical examples.

Features:

- Offers important key aspects in the development and implementation of machine learning and deep learning approaches toward developing prediction tools and models and improving medical diagnosis
- Teaches how machine learning and deep learning algorithms are applied to a broad range of application areas, including chest X-ray, breast computer-aided detection, lung and chest, microscopy, and pathology
- Covers common research problems in medical image analysis and their challenges
- Focuses on aspects of deep learning and machine learning for combating COVID-19
- Includes pertinent case studies

This book is aimed at researchers and graduate students in computer engineering, artificial intelligence and machine learning, and biomedical imaging.

Advances in Smart Healthcare Technologies

Editors: Chinmay Chakraborty *and* **Joel J. P. C. Rodrigues**

This book series focus on recent advances and different research areas in smart healthcare technologies including Internet of Medical Things (IoMedT), e-Health, personalized medicine, sensing, Big Data, telemedicine, etc. under the healthcare informatics umbrella. Overall focus is on bringing together the latest industrial and academic progress, research, and development efforts within the rapidly maturing health informatics ecosystem. It aims to offer valuable perceptions to researchers and engineers on how to design and develop novel healthcare systems and how to improve patient's information delivery care remotely. The potential for making faster advances in many scientific disciplines and improving the profitability and success of different enterprises is to be investigated.

Blockchain Technology in Healthcare Applications
Social, Economic and Technological Implications

Bharat Bhushan, Nitin Rakesh, Yousef Farhaoui, Parma Nand Astya and Bhuvan Unhelkar

Digital Health Transformation with Blockchain and Artificial Intelligence
Chinmay Chakraborty

Smart and Secure Internet of Healthcare Things
Nitin Gupta, Jagdeep Singh, Chinmay Chakraborty, Mamoun Alazab and Dinh-Thuan Do

Practical Artificial Intelligence for Internet of Medical Things
Emerging Trends, Issues, and Challenges

Edited by Ben Othman Soufiene, Chinmay Chakraborty, and Faris A. Almalki

Intelligent Internet of Things for Smart Healthcare Systems
Edited by Durgesh Srivastava, Neha Sharma, Deepak Sinwar, Jabar H. Yousif, and Hari Prabhat Gupta

Future Health Scenarios
AI and Digital Technologies in Global Healthcare Systems

Edited by Maria Jose Sousa, Francisco Guilherme Nunes, Generosa do Nascimento and Chinmay Chakraborty

Machine Learning and Deep Learning Techniques for Medical Image Recognition
Edited by Ben Othman Soufiene and Chinmay Chakraborty

For more information about this series, please visit: www.routledge.com/Advances-in-Smart-Healthcare-Technologies/book-series/CRCASHT

Machine Learning and Deep Learning Techniques for Medical Image Recognition

Edited by
Ben Othman Soufiene
and Chinmay Chakraborty

CRC Press
Taylor & Francis Group
Boca Raton London New York

CRC Press is an imprint of the
Taylor & Francis Group, an **informa** business

First edition published 2024
by CRC Press
2385 NW Executive Center Drive, Suite 320, Boca Raton FL 33431

and by CRC Press
4 Park Square, Milton Park, Abingdon, Oxon, OX14 4RN

CRC Press is an imprint of Taylor & Francis Group, LLC

© 2024 selection and editorial matter, Ben Othman Soufiene and Chinmay Chakraborty; individual chapters, the contributors

ISBN: 9781032416168 (hbk)
ISBN: 9781032432212 (pbk)
ISBN: 9781003366249 (ebk)

DOI: 10.1201/9781003366249

Typeset in Times
by Deanta Global Publishing Services, Chennai, India

Contents

Preface

With the booming growth of artificial intelligence (AI), especially the recent advancements of deep learning, utilizing advanced deep learning–based methods for medical image analysis has become an active research area both in the medical industry and academia. Many image diagnosis tasks require an initial search to identify abnormalities and quantify measurements and changes over time. Automated image analysis tools based on machine learning algorithms are the key enablers to improve the quality of image diagnosis and interpretation by facilitating efficient identification of findings.

Deep learning is an extensively applied technique that provides state-of-the-art accuracy. It opened new doors in medical image analysis. Applications of deep learning in healthcare cover a broad range of problems ranging from cancer screening and disease monitoring to personalized treatment suggestions. These developments have a huge potential for medical imaging technology, medical data analysis, medical diagnostics, and healthcare, in general, slowly being realized.

Deep learning is providing exciting solutions for medical image analysis problems and is seen as a key method for future applications. This book gives a clear understanding of the principles and methods of neural networks and deep learning concepts, showing how the algorithms that integrate deep learning as a core component have been applied to medical image detection, segmentation and registration, and computer-aided analysis, using a wide variety of application areas.

About the Editors

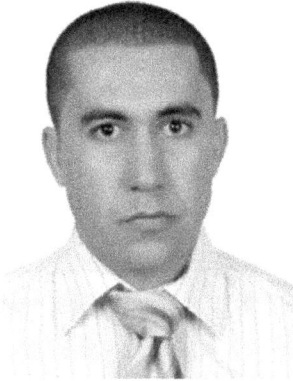

Ben Othman Soufiene was Assistant Professor of computer science at the University of Gabes, Tunisia, from 2016 to 2021. He received his PhD in computer science from Manouba University in 2016 for his dissertation on secure data aggregation in wireless sensor networks. He also earned an MS from Monastir University in 2012. His research interests focus on the Internet of Medical Things, wireless body sensor networks, wireless networks, artificial intelligence, machine learning, and big data.

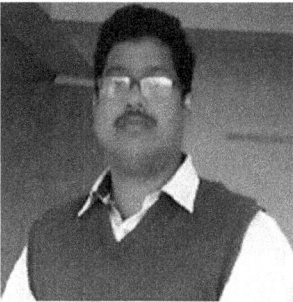

Chinmay Chakraborty is Assistant Professor in the Department of Electronics and Communication Engineering, BIT Mesra, India, and a Postdoctoral Fellow of the Federal University of Piauí, Brazil. His primary areas of research include wireless body area networks, Internet of Medical Things (IoMT), point-of-care diagnosis, mHealth/e-health, and medical imaging. Chakraborty is the co-editor of many books on smart IoMT, healthcare technology, and sensor data analytics.

Contributors

Aayush
School of Sciences
Christ (Deemed to be University), Delhi
Delhi, India

D Ajitha
Vellore Institute of Technology
Tamil Nadu, India

Harishchander Anandaram
Centre for Excellence in Computational
   Engineering and Networking
Coimbatore, India

M Arun Anoop
Department of Computer Science and
   Engineering, Alva's Institute of
   Engineering and Technology
Karnataka, India

Rajesh P Barnwal
CSIR-Central Mechanical Engineering
   Research Institute
Durgapur, India

Bassem Ben Salah
Tunisia Polytechnic School
University of Carthage
La Marsa, Tunisia

Manivasagan C
School of Computer Studies (UG)
Rathnavel Subramaniam College of
   Arts & Science
Coimbatore, India

Chinmay Chakraborty
Electronics and Communication
   Engineering
Birla Institute of Technology, Mesra
Jharkhand, India

Arvind Choubey
Indian Institute of Information
   Technology Bhagalpur
Bihar, India

S Devaraju
School of Computing Science and
   Engineering (SCSE)
VIT Bhopal University
Bhopal, India

P Divyashree
Indian Institute of Information
   Technology (IIIT), Sri City, Chittoor
Sri City, India

Priyanka Dwivedi
Indian Institute of Information
   Technology (IIIT), Sri City, Chittoor
Sri City, India

Iheb Elghaieb
National Engineering
   School of Gabes
Gabes University
Gabes, Tunisia

Chaker Esiid
Tunisia Polytechnic School
University of Carthage
La Marsa, Tunisia

Tharuni Gelli
Sreenidhi Institute of Science and
   Technology
Hyderabad, India

Haifa Ghabri
National Engineering School of Gabes
Gabes University
Gabes, Tunisia

Biswadev Goswami
Roy Engineering College
Durgapur, India

Challa Sri Gouri
Sreenidhi Institute of Science and
    Technology
Hyderabad, India

Mohamed Hamroun
3IL–XLIM
University of Limoges
Limoges, France

Sujith Jayaprakash
BlueCrest University College
Accra, Ghana

Chandan Kumar Jha
Indian Institute of Information
    Technology Bhagalpur
Bihar, India

Nehru Kandasamy
Madanapalle Institute of Technology
    and Science
Madanapalle, India

Maheshkumar H Kolekar
Indian Institute of Technology, Patna
Bihar, India

Tapas Pal
CSIR-CMERI Campus
Durgapur, India

Karthikeyan Pathinettampadian
Velammal College of Engineering and
    Technology
Viraganoor, Madurai, Tamil Nadu,
    India

Kumar Raja D R
REVA University
Bangalore, India

Hedi Sakli
EITA Consulting
Montesson, France

Marwen Sakli
Tunisia Polytechnic School
University of Carthage
La Marsa, Tunisia

Poonkuntran Shanmugam
VIT Bhopal University
Bhopal, India

Ben Othman Soufiene
PRINCE Laboratory Research
ISITcom
University of Sousse
Sousse, Tunisia

Abdelbaki Souid
National Engineering
    School of Gabes
Gabes University
Gabes, Tunisia

Jawahar Sundaram
School of Sciences
Christ (Deemed to be
    University), Delhi
Delhi, India

Rabiaa Tbibe
National Engineering School of Gabes
Gabes University
Gabes, Tunisia

Nagarjuna Telagam
GITAM University
Bangalore, India

Ahmed Zouinkhi
MACS Research Laboratory
    RL16ES22, National Engineering
    School of Gabes, Gabes University
Gabes 6029, Tunisia

1 Medical Image Detection and Recognition Using Machine Learning and Deep Learning

M Arun Anoop, P Karthikeyan, and S Poonkuntran

1.1 INTRODUCTION

Digital image authenticity is a challenging task, especially for digital camera-based images. The advancements of digital cameras and the internet have made it simple for anybody to capture digital images and digital image manipulation tools are available to modify and circulate the images around the world. For marketing strategies, there are many reasons for manipulated image creation. Some people prefer manipulation for improving brightness; others use brightness to hide important features, or they add new regions to the original ones, falsifying an image and spreading false data. A lot of research has been done on the detection and localization or recognition of image manipulations, but authenticity and integrity are issues. As the main forgeries include copying and moving desired image regions, combining two or more images in one, merging images, and resizing images and their regions, multimedia manipulation detection is a very broad task.

1.1.1 TYPES OF IMAGE FORGERY ATTACKS

1.1.1.1 Copy–Move Forgery Attack

This attack involves copying a part of an image and pasting it onto another part of the same image. Some people add to the interested region or improve the image quality, falsifying the image. Some may remove the interested region from an image to falsify medical payment claims.

1.1.1.2 Photomontage or Splicing of Image Forgery Attack

A photomontage or splicing is combining two or more images to make others. It is very easy to do because of the freely available image manipulation tools. If this happens in an medical image, it may negatively affect a patient's life.

DOI: 10.1201/9781003366249-1

1.1.1.3   Resizing of Images or Region Image Forgery Attack

Resizing an image or an image shifting from left to right is a part of data augmentation. But in this image forgery attack, resizing does not mean resizing the entire image, instead, it applies to a particular region of the image.

1.1.1.4   Photomontage

The photomontage is a kind of image manipulation that combines two images. Normally researchers use this method to compare the original image with the image output.

1.1.1.5   Colorized Images

Color-based manipulations can also be done with the help of freely available image manipulation tools.

1.1.1.6   Camera-Based Image Forgery Attack

With the advancement of the digital image processing software and editing tools, a digital image can be easily manipulated.

1.1.1.7   Format-Based Image Forgery Attack

Anyone can consider one image type, falsify it, and change it to another format. It sometimes may hide the clues regarding manipulation. See Table 1.1.

The proposed decision tree is shown in Figure 1.1. The proposed flow of the digital forgery detection is in Figure 1.2; the algorithm pseudocode was later added. In today's digital era, many people use different image-improving tools to improve the quality of their digital images. In most cases, those seeing the manipulated image may not have any idea regarding the original, especially if the original is not readily available for comparison. Due to the availability of image editing application software, especially for operating systems like Windows or Android-based tools, the authenticity of a given image is always a big task in the research field and it is a question of integrity.

In this chapter, we present a forgery detection method that applies to different forgery cases. The proposed transform domain technique relies on both second-order statistical methods (gray level co-occurrence matrix [GLCM], gray level difference matrix [GLDM], gray level run length matrix [GLRLM]) and local binary pattern variants. Feature scaling methods for redundant and irrelevant features were used from the feature dataset. Lexicographic sorting and the Euclidian distance method were used for single- and multiple-image forgery localization. And finally, 16 supervised machine learning (ML) methods, deep learning methods, model stacking, and voting methods were applied to predicting genuine and forged images.

The rest of the chapter is arranged as follows. Section 1.2 presents a survey of the related work. This is followed by the presentation of the problem definition and proposed method in Sections 1.3 and 1.4. Section 1.5 discusses the extreme learning machines, and Sections 1.6 and 1.7 deal with the experimental results and performance evaluation of advanced local binary pattern and gray level (ALBPVG) based on different machine learning methods and deep learning, respectively. Section 1.8 concludes the chapter.

TABLE 1.1
Different ML classifiers

CatBoost	CatBoost is a high-performance open-source library for gradient boosting on decision trees (pip install catboost) and CatBoostClassifier() function from catboost with some options used for the evaluation process.
Naïve Bayes	We need to find the probability that an image is genuine. The probability of finding a genuine in the total images is P(Genuine). The probability of finding a forged image in the total images is P(Forged). The probability of finding a forged image among the genuine images is $P\left(Forged\,/\,Genuine\right)$. The Naïve Bayes equation of the problem is $$P\left(\frac{Genuine}{Forged}\right) = \frac{P\left(Forged\,/\,Genuine\right) * P\left(Forged\right)}{P\left(Genuine\right)}$$
Decision trees	The tuning parameters mainly are information gain, Gini index, and chi square. Entropy is a metric for impurity measuring. Entropy reduction is measured by information gain. The Gini index is the measure of both purity and impurity. It is always used in CART decision trees.
XGBoost	XGBoost consists of bias, variance, bagging, and boosting concepts. XGBoost stands for Extreme Gradient Boosting, which consists of the combination of the results of many models. Also, it is a regularization method to reduce overfitting issues. It involves tree pruning and built-in cross-validation steps. XGBoost prunes the tree backward and stops the process if no positive gains. Import XGBoost and use the XGBRegressor() function.
AdaBoost	It combines multiple classifiers for better accuracy. Can call "sklearn-ensemble" and use the AdaBoostClassifier() function for results.
Bagging classifier	It is an ensemble machine learning method for improving the accuracy of predictions used by a supervised learning algorithm. Can call "sklearn-ensemble" and use the BaggingClassifier() function for results displaying.
Extra tree classifier [49]	Can call "sklearn-tree" and use the ExtraTreeClassifier() function for prediction process.
Bernoulli Naïve Bayes [48]	Can call "sklearn-naïve_bayes" and process BernoulliNB() for results.
Passive aggressive classifier [47]	Can call "sklearn.linear_model" and process it based on the PassiveAggressiveClassifier() method.
Support vector machine [46]	Can call "sklearn.svm" and process the code based on the LinearSVC() function.
K-neighbors classifier [45]	Can use "sklearn.neighbors" and process KNeighborsClassifier() for results.
Logistic regression [42]	It is another linear model and it can be processed by the LogisticRegression() function.
Random forest classifier [34]	It is in ensemble and it can be processed by using the RandomForestClassifier() function.
Gradient boosting classifier [31]	It is also in ensemble and it can be processed by using the GradientBoostingClassifier() method.
Linear discriminant analysis [30]	It is from "sklearn.discriminant_analysis" and can retrieve it from the LinearDiscriminantAnalysis() function.
Extreme learning machine [36]	ELM is a single hidden layer supporting a feed forward neural network. ELM supports single/different layers of hidden nodes. Hidden nodes are not fixed by any values. It can be checked with trial-and-error values as per the instruction mentioned in that algorithm. One of the benefits of ELM is it is effective in feature learning and grouping. It is a quick learning calculation. A few variants of ELM are TELM and MLELM.

Is an image authentic?

Region of image == No changes

Yes   No

No alterations?   More than one alteration

Yes   No   Yes   No

Genuine   Forged   Forged   Genuine

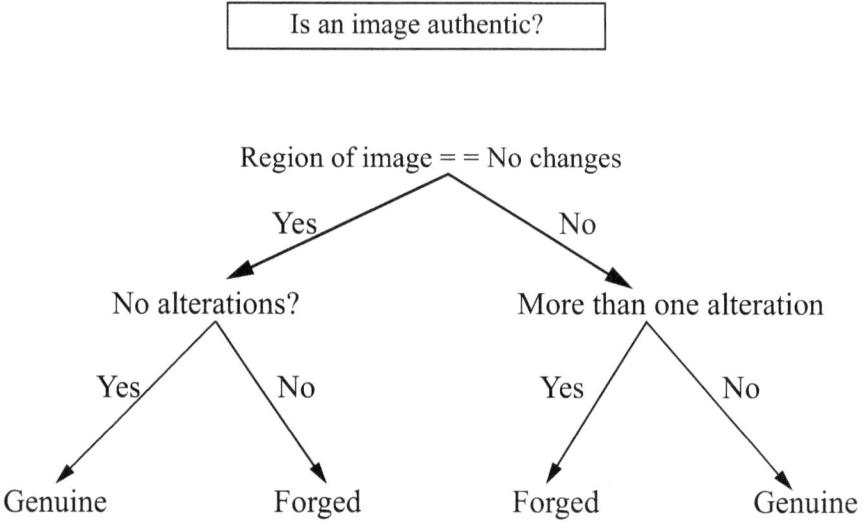

FIGURE 1.1   Decision tree.

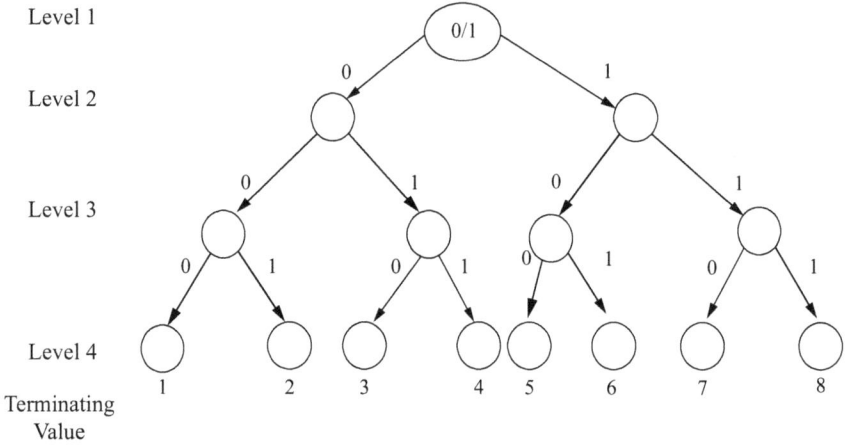

Level 1   0/1

                    0   1
Level 2

            0   1   0   1
Level 3

        0   1   0   1   0   1   0   1

Level 4

        1   2   3   4   5   6   7   8
Terminating
Value

FIGURE 1.2   Modified ELM for this work and its working mechanism.

1.2   RELATED WORKS

See Table 1.2.

TABLE 1.2
Comparison evaluation

Algorithm	Reference
Gray level co-occurrence matrix (GLCM)	[9] used for biofilm.
Gray level difference matrix (GLDM)	[12] used for iris tissue recognition.
Gray level run length matrix (GLRLM)	[13] for ultrasound medical image classification.
Improved LTP (ILTP)	[6] for intuitionistic logic.
Robust LBP (RLBP)	[3] for classification, detection and recognition.
Significant LBP (SLBP)	[4] used for face detection.
Local binary pattern (LBP)	[8] used for medical image categorization.
Local ternary pattern (LTP)	[7] used for named entity recognition.
Improved LBP (ILBP)	[10] used for texture and face recognition.
Median binary pattern (MBP)	[5] used for face recognition.

Short runs emphasis (SRE), gray level non-uniformity (GLN), run percentage (RP), long runs emphasis (LRE), run length non-uniformity (RLN), low gray level runs emphasis (LGLRE), high gray level runs emphasis (HGLRE) – [13] used to classify ultrasound medical images and [14] used for acute lymphoblastic leukemia (ALL) detection.

[43] referenced about later and before postprocessing clue removal strategies considering histogram of oriented gradients (HOG) calculation.

[24] proposed a strategy to identify real image falsification for smart healthcare. In their exploratory outcomes, they determined the precision of regular and mammogram medical images.

[2] surveyed and clearly explained image forgery detection and methods.

[38] proposed a forgery detection method based on hybrid features using SIFT and KAZE. The creators assessed accuracy and review in light of posthandling changes in SIFT, SURF, Zernike Minutes, and Bravo with their proposed combination approach.

[39] proposed another methodology in light of LBP and methods like SVD and they carried out precise recognition of falsified pictures. Furthermore, they contrasted their outcomes with SVD alone and both SVD and DCT.

[44] referenced LBP histogram Fourier elements for picture altering identification. In their future they may focus on identifying the numerous falsifications present in pictures and recognition of precise imitation in high locales. They failed to do high locale recognition.

[26] proposed a technique of contactless procurement of palm feature extraction.

[41] proposed a binomial circulation of the likelihood of right responses with the assistance of relative recurrence and irregular likelihood in the field of radiographic picture brightness forgery recognition. They grouped the right and wrong responses by picture set.

[16, 40] proposed a strategy to distinguish video outline fabrication in light of LBP and cell automata. In their future work, they will plan new techniques to identify video copy–move forgery where just a piece of a casing is reordered to an alternate edge in a similar grouping.

[23] examined picture control, apparatuses, and their recognition. In the future they will study if there is a genuine requirement for a stricter strategy or measures that recover, bar, or keep away from the deceitful use of computerized radiographs in dentistry.

(Continued)

TABLE 1.2 CONTINUED
Comparison evaluation

[27] proposed a recognition framework and this technique utilizes multipart LBP with pyramid structure and assessed the precision of noisy pictures.

[11] proposed exposing image forgeries by detecting inconsistencies in the geometry of cast shadows.

[20] proposed DNA chaos blend to secure medical privacy.

[21] proposed a joint spatial and discrete cosine transform.

[22] proposed recolored image detection via a deep discriminative model.

[32] proposed performance evaluation based on previous copy–move forgery methods under conditions of plain copy–move forgery as well as postprocessing conditions like brightness changes, contrast adjustments, color reduction, and blurring.

[15] proposed efficient copy–move forgery detection method with an automatic threshold selection.

1.3   PROBLEM DEFINITION

The principal issue we noted is a change in the size of a tumor; the size predicts the stage of cancer. So, changing the size may lead to a wrong diagnosis. Many articles have concluded that the removal of a breast sample is needed to test for breast cancer using a breast biopsy. A pathologist usually removes a tumor section to identify if a patient has breast cancer and at what stage. Other ways suggested are needle biopsy, ultrasound, or MRI guidance, which are commonly used for prediction. If a portion of the tumor is removed and pasted onto a normal region, then it may lead to a wrong diagnosis. If a small region is altered to a large region or a large region to a small region may also lead to a wrong diagnosis. Based on studies, it is clear that doctors can identify breast cancer by removing a tumor section, but there is a chance of digital image forgery. To save a patient's life, every medical system requires an authenticity measuring module to ensure integrity. Medical imaging is a significant aspect of image research. So, we picked a medical image dataset for our research work. Breast cancer is the most striking cancer in women and the possibility of getting breast cancer is 1 in 8. Sometimes breast cancer can be predictable based on blood vessels. More research is required in that area. Moreover, forged images are a troublesome issue. To check the accuracy of our work, we initially processed natural image-based forgeries and finally checked mammograms. We developed a fused approach: advanced local binary pattern and gray level (ALBPVG) is the combination of local binary pattern (LBP) variants and a second-order statistical feature extraction algorithm that exposes any doctored image (e.g., images of lung and other types of cancer, brain-based images, natural images, dental images) and also outperforms the accuracy rates of other experiments.

1.4   PROPOSED METHODOLOGY

The mammogram image can be processed based on a second-order statistical feature extraction algorithm and LBP variants. In LBPVG, different machine learning methods are processed. Also, feature scaling results are used to remove noise

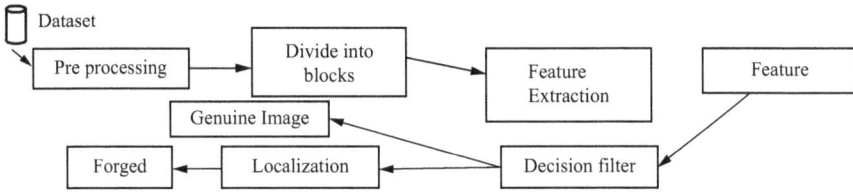

FIGURE 1.3   General flow of prediction.

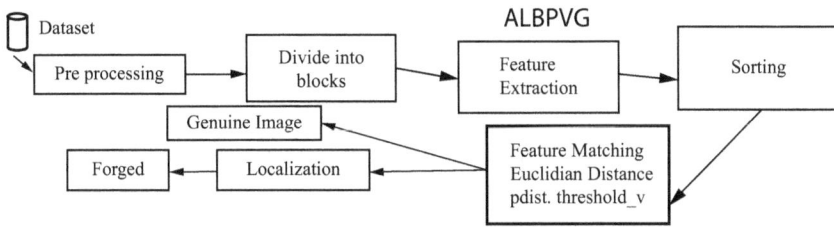

FIGURE 1.4   Proposed flow of prediction.

and redundant features. The supervised learning algorithms processed are the extreme learning machine (ELM), CatBoost, Naïve Bayes, decision trees, XGBoost, AdaBoost, bagging classifier, extra tree classifier, Bernoulli Naïve Bayes, passive aggressive classifier, support vector machine (SVM), k-neighbors classifier, logistic regression, random forest classifier, gradient boosting classifier, and linear discriminant analysis (Figures 1.3 and 1.4).

In future ALBPVG methods, it will be helpful to remove overfitting issues, with the help of bioinspired optimization techniques before moving to classifiers.

A *hybrid feature extraction approach* is the combination of LBP variants and second-order statistical feature extraction methods.

1.4.1   WORKING WITH ALBPVG TO DETECT IMAGE FORGERIES

- In *preprocessing*, as usual, a color image is converted to a grayscale image to reveal good and important features. In eye images, the process starts based on green layer extraction. As we take images from different datasets, our assumption is based on "no need for an image noise removal process".
- The dataset images used were from the Mammographic Image Analysis Society (MIAS) [1].
- Image manipulation paint was used for forgery image bulk creation. This product consists of different options. Images are taken based on the following way.
- Considered both single and multiple forgeries done based on our "image manipulation paint" product.
- Different image operations were done mainly based on copy–move, copy–rotation–paste, resizing, and adjusting brightness.

- In *feature extraction*, extraction was based on LBP variants and GLCM algorithms.

$$\alpha 1 = LBP_{N1,R1}(x1, y1) = \sum_{p1=0}^{N1-1} s(g_{p1} - g_{c1})2^{p1} \tag{1.1}$$

In Table 1.3 are the different types of LBP variants.

- In *feature matching*, 16 different feature matching methods are mentioned.
- Second-order statistical feature extraction and feature vector collection stages are explained next:

$$Feature\_Vector(FV)_{ALPvG1} = \{LBP_{N1,R1}(x,y), ILBP_{N1,R1}(x,y), MBP_{N1,R1}(x,y),$$

$$LTP_{N1,R1}(x,y), ILTP_{N1,R1}(x,y), RLBP_{N1,R1}(x,y,t_1), SLBP_{N1,R1}(x,y,k),$$

$$C_{i1,j1}, E_{i1,j1}, CO_{i1,j1}, H_{i1,j1}, AngularSecondMoment_{feature_{ALPvG}}, ContrastFeature_{ALPvG},$$

$$EntropyFeature_{ALPvG}, VarianceFeature_{ALPvG}, CorrelationFeature_{ALPvG},$$

$$InverseDifferenceMomentFeature_{ALPvG}, SumAverageFeature_{ALPvG},$$

$$SumVarianceFeature_{ALPvG}, SumVarianceFeature_{ALPvG},$$

$$SumEntropyAverage_{ALPvG}, InformationMeasuresCorrFeature1, 2_{ALPvG}\}$$

$$= 31 features$$

(1.2)

$$Feature\_Vector(FV)_{ALPvG2} = \{LBP_{N1,R1}(x,y), ILBP_{N1,R1}(x,y), MBP_{N1,R1}(x,y),$$

$$LTP_{N1,R1}(x,y), ILTP_{N1,R1}(x,y), RLBP_{N1,R1}(x,y,t_1), SLBP_{N1,R1}(x,y,k), SRE_{GLRLM}$$

$$LRE_{GLRLM}, GLN_{GLRLM}, RP_{GLRLM}, RLN_{GLRLM}, LGRE_{GLRLM}, HGRE_{GLRLM}\} = 14 features$$

(1.3)

$$Feature\_Vector(FV)_{ALPvG3} = \{LBP_{N1,R1}(x,y), ILBP_{N1,R1}(x,y), MBP_{N1,R1}(x,y),$$

$$LTP_{N1,R1}(x,y), ILTP_{N1,R1}(x,y), RLBP_{N1,R1}(x,y,t_1), SLBP_{N1,R1}(x,y,k), Contrast_{GLDM},$$

$$Angular\ second\ moment\ Entropy_{GLDM}, Mean_{GLDM}, Inverse\ difference\ moments_{GLDM}$$

$$= 11 features$$

(1.4)

- Features generated based on second-order statistical feature extraction algorithm are given next:

TABLE 1.3

LBP variants and second-order statistical feature extraction algorithms

$$\left(x_{p1}, y_{p1}\right) = \left(x_{c1} + R\cos(2\pi p / N), y_{c1} - R\sin(2\pi p1 / N)\right)$$

$$LBP_{N1,R1}\left(x, y\right) = \sum_{p1=0}^{N1-1} s(g_{p1} - g_{c1})2^{p1}$$

$$s(x) = \begin{cases} 1, x \geq 0 \\ 0, otherwise \end{cases}$$

$$ILBP_{N1,R1}\left(x, y\right) = \sum_{p1=0}^{N1-1} s(g_{p1} - g_{mean})2^{p1} + s\left(g_{c1} - g_{mean}\right)2^{N1}$$

$$g_{mean} = \frac{1}{N1+1}\left(\sum_{p1=0}^{N1-1} g_{p1} + g_{c1}\right) \quad [17, 19]$$

$$MBP_{N1,R1}\left(x, y\right) = \sum_{p1=0}^{N1-1} s(g_{p1} - g_{med})2^{p1} + s\left(g_{c1} - g_{med}\right)2^{N1}$$

$$g_{med} = median\left(\{g_0, g_1, \ldots, g_{N1-1}, g_{c1}\}\right) \quad [35\text{--}36]$$

$$LTP_{N1,R1}\left(x, y\right) = \sum_{p1=0}^{N1-1} s_3(g_{p1}, g_{c1}, t_1)2^{p1} \quad [18, 36, 16, 40]$$

$$s_3\left(g_{p1}, g_{c1}, t_1\right) = \begin{cases} 1, g_{p1} \geq g_{c1} + t_1 \\ 0, g_{c1} - t_1 \leq g_{p1} < g_{c1} + t_1 \\ -1, otherwise \end{cases}$$

$$ILTP_{N1,R1}\left(x, y\right) = \sum_{p1=0}^{N1-1} s_3\left(g_{p1} - g_{mean}\right)2^{p1} + s_3(g_{c1} - g_{mean})2^{N1} \quad [33]$$

$$RLBP_{N1,R1}\left(x, y, t_1\right) = \sum_{p1=0}^{N1-1} s(g_{p1} - g_{c1} - t_1)2^{p1}$$

$$SLBP_{N1,R1}\left(x, y, k\right) = \sum_{p1=0}^{N1-1} s(g_{p1} - g_{c1} - k)2^{p1} \quad [17, 19]$$

$$GLCM_{i1,j1} = \{C_{i1,j1}, E_{i1,j1}, CO_{i1,j1}, H_{i1,j1}\} \quad [15, 44, 43]$$

E1 is the feature for finding an image's uniformity of LBPVG and it is mathematically defined as the following equation [29]:

$$E1 = \sqrt{\sum_{i1=0}^{N1-1}\sum_{j1=0}^{N1-1} M1^2\left(i1, j1\right)}$$

C1 is the feature of LBPVG and it is mathematically defined as

$$C1 = \sum_{i1, j1=0}^{N1-1} M_{i1j1}(i1 - j1)^2 \quad (12)$$

[24] states variance and inertia details.

[32] states the calculation of intensity of an image and its neighborhood regions.

(Continued)

TABLE 1.3 CONTINUED

LBP variants and second-order statistical feature extraction algorithms

C1 is the feature of LBPVG and it is mathematically defined as

$$C1 = \sqrt{\sum_{i1=0}^{N1-1}(\sum_{j1=0}^{N1-1}[\{(i1\,j1)\,M\,(i1,j1)-u_{x1},u_{y1}\}/\{s\_x1,s\_y1\}])}$$

[41] states correlations for the feature calculator of GLCM algorithms methods which is the proportion of gray level linear dependence between the image element or its picture element.

H1 is the feature of LBPVG and it is mathematically defined as

$$H1 = \sqrt{\sum_{i1=0}^{N1-1}\sum_{j1=0}^{N1-1}M\,(i1,j1)/(1+(i1-j1)^2}$$

[18] states homogeneity usage and it acts like a feature calculator for the measuring of closeness in the GLCM against the diagonal regions or values of the matrix.

EVEN/ODD/FIRST/LAST$_{(\text{RANDOM FEATURES})}$ (FV)

- The procedure process is as follows:
- We collected 569 images from the MIAS Database [1].
- The features were processed by different ML methods: extreme learning machine, CatBoost, Naïve Bayes, decision trees, XGBoost, AdaBoost, bagging classifier, extra tree classifier, Bernoulli Naïve Bayes, passive aggressive classifier, support vector machine, k-neighbors classifier, logistic regression, random forest classifier, gradient boosting classifier, and linear discriminant analysis.
- Measures including precision, recall, F1 score, and classification accuracy will decide the authenticity proving (model stacking) stage.
- Forgery detection and recognition are shown in Figures 1.5 and 1.6.

1.4.2 EXTREME LEARNING MACHINE

The ELM algorithm (Figures 1.7 and 1.8) [36] and its hidden neuron limit were set (50–150). It's clear that it's not fixed and the optimal number of hidden neuron nodes is unknown. The number of nodes is chosen by trial and error [37].

1.5 EXPERIMENTATION AND RESULTS

The proposed ALBPGL Duplicate move fraud acknowledgment delivered high exactness by various artificial intelligence (AI)-based classifiers and convolutional neural networks (CNNs).

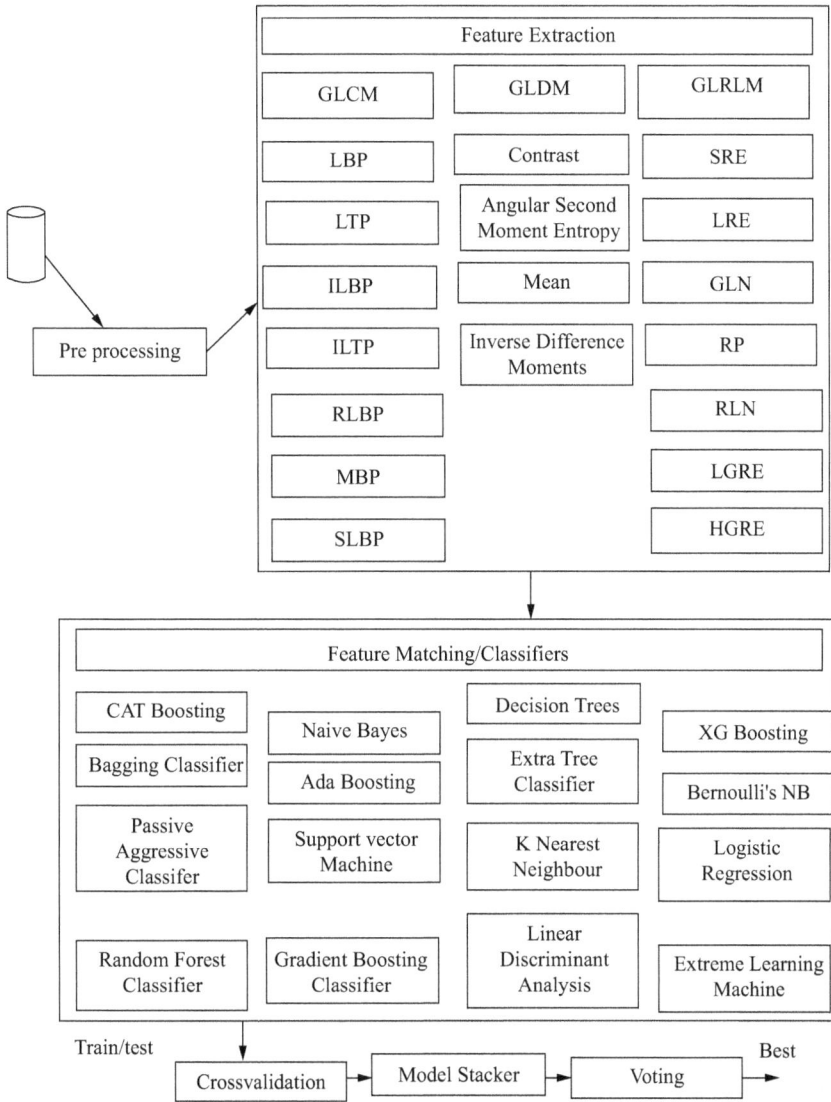

FIGURE 1.5 Proposed flow of advanced LBPVG for image forgery detection using ML.

The mammogram datasets were downloaded from Suckling's Mammogram Picture Examination Society [1], which contains the first 322 pictures at the 50-micron goal in the portable gray map (PGM) design and related information.

We used a proposed MIAS information base [1] for mammograms research for the "Picture filename", that is the prefix mdb, followed by a three-digit number; l or r for the left and right breast; and s, m, l, and x to demonstrate the image aspects. The model is "mdb001lm" (MIAS Reference Number).

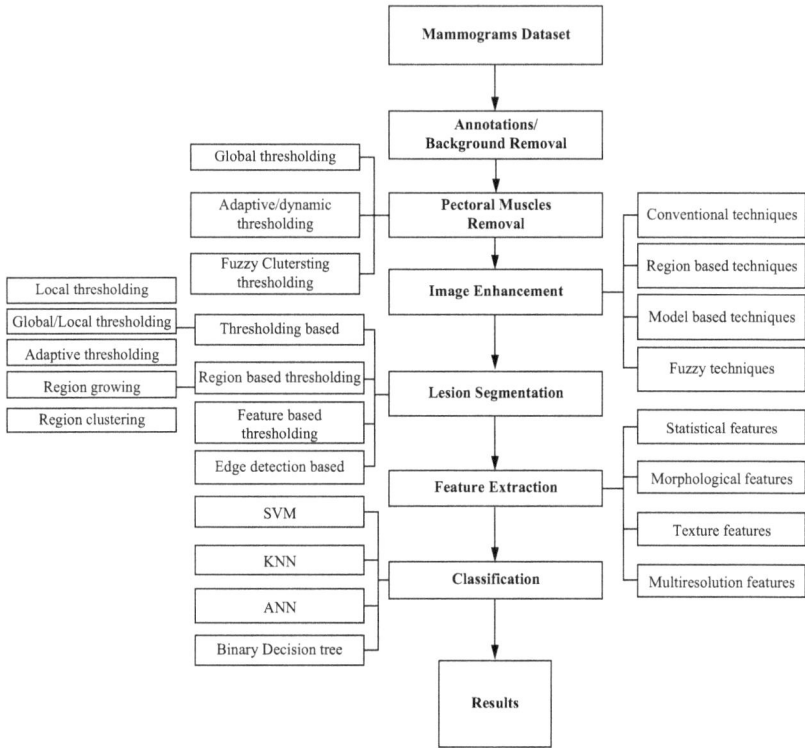

FIGURE 1.6   Mammogram processing.

We took 569 pictures for the research. We included extraction handled in light of LBP variations and second request statistical feature extraction algorithms, and GLCM, GLDM [12], and GLRLM [13–14] calculation. The values are the elements delivered by mixture LBPVG calculation.

mdb003ll was taken from Suckling's dataset [1]. mdb003ll_F("_F" signifies picture fashioned) we forged it for research purposes. Furthermore, the forged images were used only inside our lab; not moved or transferred to anybody else.

One picture element's equivalent closeness won't influence the whole list of capabilities. Extraction of elements won't reveal picture realness. Legitimacy should be demonstrated by "AI or a component matching method" not by "the extraction of feature(s)" alone.

1.6   PERFORMANCE EVALUATION OF LBPVG WITH ELM

- The presentation of the proposed LBPVG-based duplicate move falsification identification is assessed by specific execution measures. LBPVG is the cross-breed blend of LBP and a second-order statistical feature extraction algorithm (GLCM). Furthermore, the execution was done given an ELM AI approach. The LBP variations produced 7 elements; GLCM creates 24 different component pixel values.

Data: Dataset of Test and train Images
Result: Final Prediction either Genuine or Forged

$//Prediction Model Details//$
$Conv2D\_2\ 128,128,32$
$MaxPooling2D\ 42,42,32$
$Conv2D\_3\ 42,42,16$
$MaxPooling2D\_3\ 21,21,16$
$Flatten\_1\ 7056$
$dense\_2\ 8$
$dense\_3\ 3$
$For\ epochs = 1 \rightarrow 50$
Forged_Image = Image_manipulation_paint(Data)
Absolute_Diff = Data − Forged_Image
Resize = 64,64,3 of Data_images
Accuracy = Predictor,Optimizer
$EndFor$

$//Forgery\ region\ Localization//$
Data: Test Images
Result: Detection & Recognition of Genuine or Forged

$Forgery\ Image\ Creation$
$Absolute\ Difference\ Findings$
$Resize\ of\ Original\ Image$
$Model\ based\ Prediction$

$//Forgery\ Region\ Recognition//$
Dataset
Pre-processing using Wiener Filter
overlapping and non-overlapping block division
Feature Extraction
Feature Vector Calculation
Lexicographic Sorting
Euclidian Distance & Threshold Calculation
Feature Matching
Forged region localization
Algorithm 2: ALBPVG-A NOVEL APPROACH FOR MEDICAL
FORGERY DETECTION IN IMAGE TRANSMISSION using CNN

FIGURE 1.7 The optimization techniques.

Data: N-dimensional Feature Vector of ALBPVG
Result: Final Prediction either Genuine or Forged
Initialize $i \leftarrow 1, 2, \ldots, N$ training samples
$\beta \leftarrow [\beta_1, \beta_2, \ldots, \beta_L]^T$ output of matrix between hidden and output
neurons
$h(x) = [a_1, a_2, \ldots, a_n]$ hidden neuron outputs
x_i Randomized hidden feature
$h_i(x)$ i^{th} hidden neuron
$h_i(x) = G(a_i, b_i, x), a_i \in R^d, b_i \in R \ G(a_i, b_i, x)$ using hidden neuron
parameters (a, b), is a non − linear piecewise continuous function
Log Sigmoid $\leftarrow G(a, b, x) \leftarrow \frac{1}{1+\exp(-ax+b)}$
$\|H\beta − T\|$ where, Hiddenlayer(H), T, β is the procedure step of ELM
and 'H' is the randomized hidden layer output then it is notated below
$[g(x_1), g(x_2), \ldots, g(x_n)]$
$[t_1^1, t_2^2, \ldots, t_n^T]$
$\beta^* = H^+ T$
where, $H^+ T$ is Moore Penrose generalized inverse function +
ALBPVG based on ELM Algorithm

FIGURE 1.8 The ELM algorithm.

- GLCM + LBP variants = 31 features
- GLDM + LBP variants = 11 features
- GLRLM + LBP variants = 14 features
- AI approaches were utilized in light of neural networks, Naïve Bayes, SVM, and ELM for LBPVG copy–move forgery detection. ELM was highly effectively contrasted with the other three calculations. ELM is the best one for our examination work in view of execution assessment. Our calculation will work with all datasets that have a unique and manufactured pair.
- The boundaries precision (p), recall (r), F1 score, and exactness percentage are used. The precision and recall are assessed and tried with different clinical pictures. Execution estimates utilized here are depicted in the equations.

Tp1 is valid positive, TN1 is valid negative, Fp1 is misleading positive, and FN1 is bogus negative.

Precision (p): It connotes the right and exact discovery of a falsified picture. It connotes the accuracy of the strategy.

$$Calculated \_ \Pr ecision, Cp = \frac{T_{p1}}{T_{p1} + F_{p1}} = \frac{Fdetected_{Image} \cap Manipulated_{Image}}{FDetected_{Image}} \quad (1.5)$$

Recall (r): It is a negligible portion of the pertinent phony picture that is recuperated. It demonstrates the fortitude of the procedure.

$$Calculated \_ \mathrm{Re}\,call, Cr = \frac{T_{p1}}{T_{p1} + F_{N1}} = \frac{FDetected_{Image} \cap Manipulated_{Image}}{Manipulated_{Image}} \quad (1.6)$$

F1 score: The F1 score or F-measure is the proportion of test exactness. The exactness percentage is the extent of the classifier to make an exact forged picture grouping. For example, if the exactness yield is 96%, the significance is 96 authentic pictures and 4 forged pictures out of 100 pictures.

$$Calculated\_F1-score = \frac{2*pl*r}{Calculated\_Precision + Calculated\_R} \quad (1.7)$$

In Table 1.4, a CNN with an ADAM optimizer with a learning rate of .0005 with entropy loss was used. StandardScaler was used for the feature scaling process. For the cross-validation step, a 25% testing set was taken. Also, the MinMaxScaler with 50 epochs achieved 94.37% and 96.48% accuracy, and the StandardScaler with 40 epochs achieved 96.24% accuracy. Because of the most noted feature extraction utilizing scaling processes, the measure's higher value for the proposed approach is attained in some situations noted in Table 1.4.

The following are the main parameters used here: input LBPVs parameters, number of hidden neurons 30 (random value), output either genuine or forgery noted by binary values. The accuracy is calculated based on features extracted from the image(s) and the colors denoted by different machine learning approaches (in the plot itself).

Figure 1.9 depicts the primer evaluation based on the machine learning classifiers random forest, CatBoost, Gaussian Naïve Bayes, and decision tree. Table 1.4 shows XGBoost and AdaBoost classification accuracy. Figure 1.10 introduces the confusion matrix and different evaluation measure values. Figure 1.11 depicts LR, KNN (k-nearest neighbor), and AdaBoost confusion matrices. Figures 1.12, 1.13and 1.14 show the logistic regression precision recall evaluation curve and AdaBoost performance evaluation plot. Table 1.5 is the image forgery detection and recognition based on ALBPVG with the Euclidian distance method. The images considered are based on the image manipulation paint tool. The image manipulation paint tool is used to create forged images. The tool was developed for different types of forgery attack-based dataset creation. Although Photoshop and GIMP are already available, this tool is especially for researchers who are working in this field. It may help them to easily create datasets with lots of images instead of depending on Photoshop and other image tools. Photoshop and GIMP require lots of studies and editing skills, so it may negatively impact researchers to create dataset images.

Figure 1.15 depicts some sample images we used to process medical image forgery detection work. The height- and width-based image views can also be found in the figure. Figure 1.16 depicts the genuine images for the same experimental evaluation work.

1.7   CONCLUSION

Authenticating a picture has ended up being fundamental as a result of the abuse of images in various media to change their genuine portrayal. Trial results have shown

TABLE 1.4
Performance evaluation of CNN with epochs

Test data	Number of images	Number of features	Feature scaling process	Methods	Epochs	Loss	Accuracy	Val_loss	Val_accuracy
MIAS dataset breast cancer images, original and forged pair mixed	569	31	StandardScaler	CNN with ADAM optimizer with binary cross entropy loss	10	0.2248	0.9272	0.4102	0.8951
					20	0.1547	0.9460	0.2324	0.9301
					30	0.1209	0.9577	0.1656	0.9371
					40	0.1123	0.9624	0.1679	0.9510
					50	0.1202	0.9577 or 0.9648	0.1662	0.9580
			MinMaxScaler		10	0.2693	0.8967	0.5704	0.6713
					20	0.1765	0.9319	0.3832	0.8811
					30	0.1777	0.9272	0.2273	0.9371
					40	0.1608	0.9413	0.1562	0.9510
					50	0.1608	0.9437	0.1474	0.9510

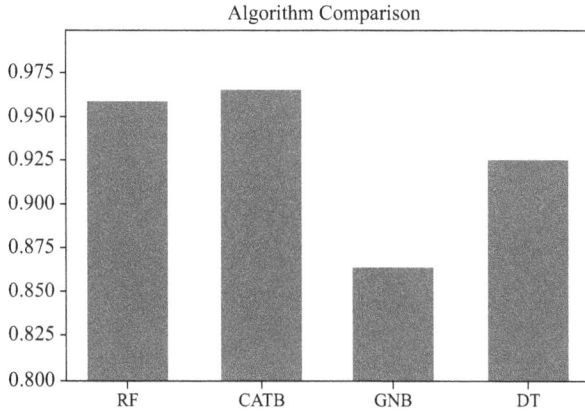

FIGURE 1.9 Proposed flow of prediction.

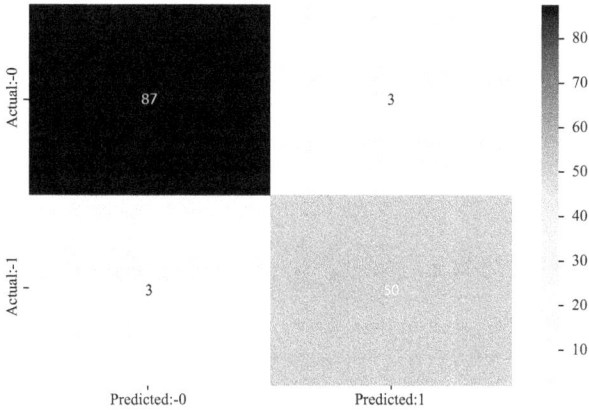

FIGURE 1.10A Confusion matrix based on Figure 1.9.

```
The acuuracy of the model = TP+TN/(TP+TN+FP+FN) =  0.958041958041958
 The Missclassification = 1-Accuracy =  0.04195804195804198
 Sensitivity or True Positive Rate = TP/(TP+FN) =  0.9433962264150944
 Specificity or True Negative Rate = TN/(TN+FP) =  0.9666666666666667
 Positive Predictive value = TP/(TP+FP) =  0.9433962264150944
 Negative predictive Value = TN/(TN+FN) =  0.9666666666666667
 Positive Likelihood Ratio = Sensitivity/(1-Specificity) =  28.301886792452837
 Negative likelihood Ratio = (1-Sensitivity)/Specificity =  0.05855562784645412
```

FIGURE 1.10B The different evaluation parameters identified and used for this work.

LR

87	3
3	50
0	1

KNN

86	4
4	49
0	1

ADA Boosting

87	3
4	50
0	1

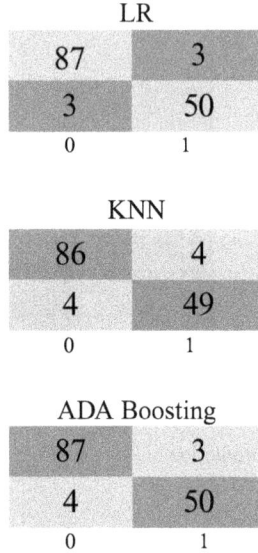

FIGURE 1.11   Collection of confusion matrices based on LR, KNN, and AdaBoost.

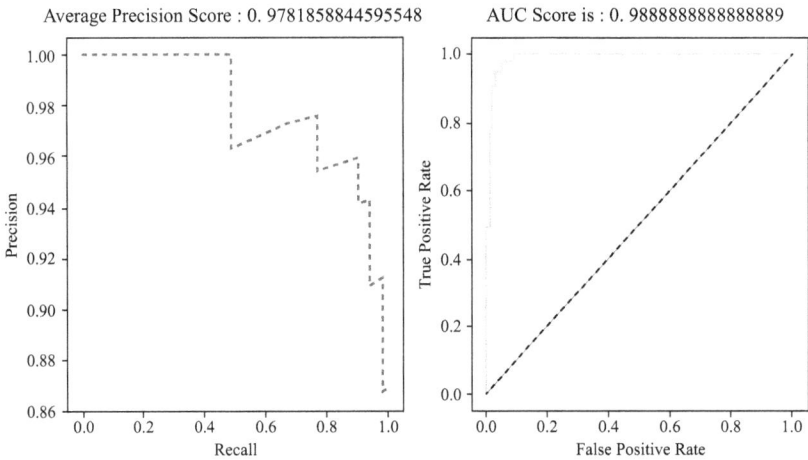

Average Precision Score : 0. 9781858844595548   AUC Score is : 0. 9888888888888889

FIGURE 1.12   Precision and recall curve based on logistic regression.

that this technique gives nearly great accuracy. The proposed approach demonstrates authenticity given various forgery changes. Among the supervised machine learning classifiers, ELM with various activation functions was productive with a high accuracy rate. The feature extracting algorithms are based on second-order statistical texture and LBP variants-based features. The performance was evaluated based on single as well as multiple merging of features using machine learning classification

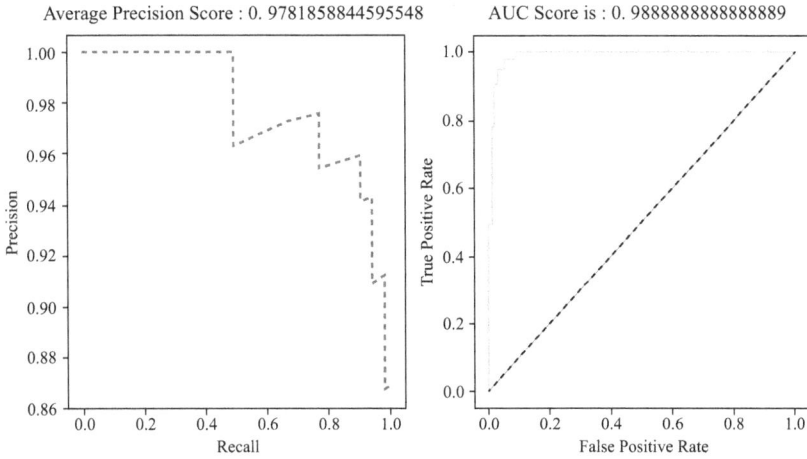

FIGURE 1.13   Precision and recall curve based on AdaBoost.

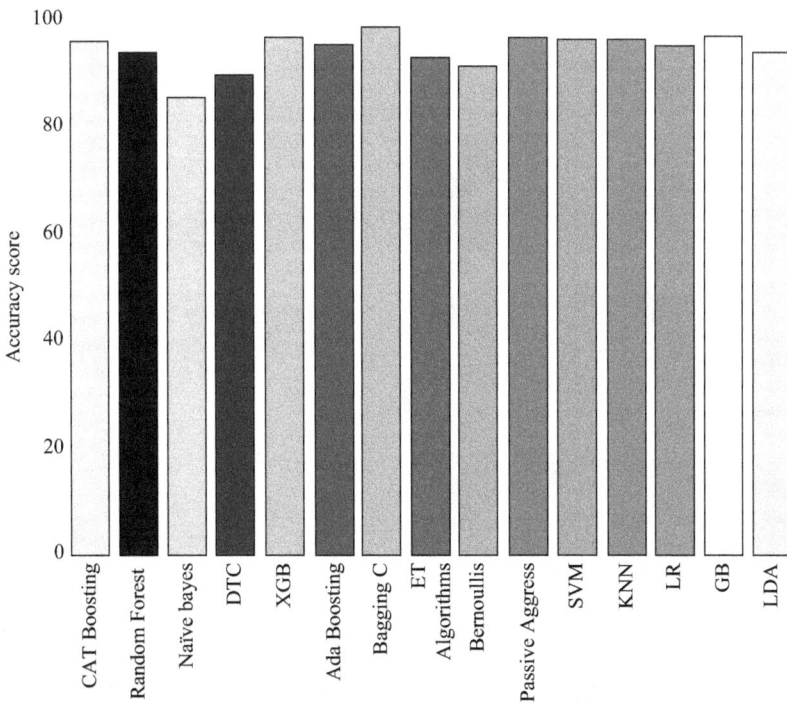

FIGURE 1.14   Accuracy statistics for 15 supervised classifiers considered for our work. The bagging classifier achieved the highest accuracy.

TABLE 1.5
Model stacking results

Model	Accuracy
CatBoost	96.50
Random forest	94.41
Naïve Bayes	86.01
DTC	90.21
XGBoost	97.20
AdaBoost	95.80
Bagging C	99.06
ET	93.01
Bernoulli	90.02
Passive aggressive	97.18
SVM	96.71
KNN	96.48
LR	95.77
GB	97.20
LDA	94.41
ELM	96.50

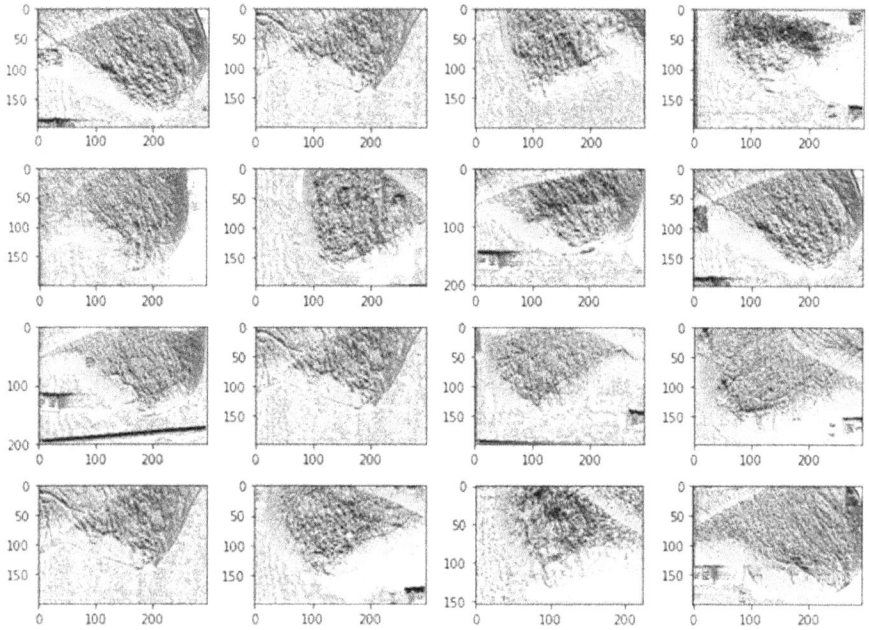

FIGURE 1.15   Breast cancer forged images.

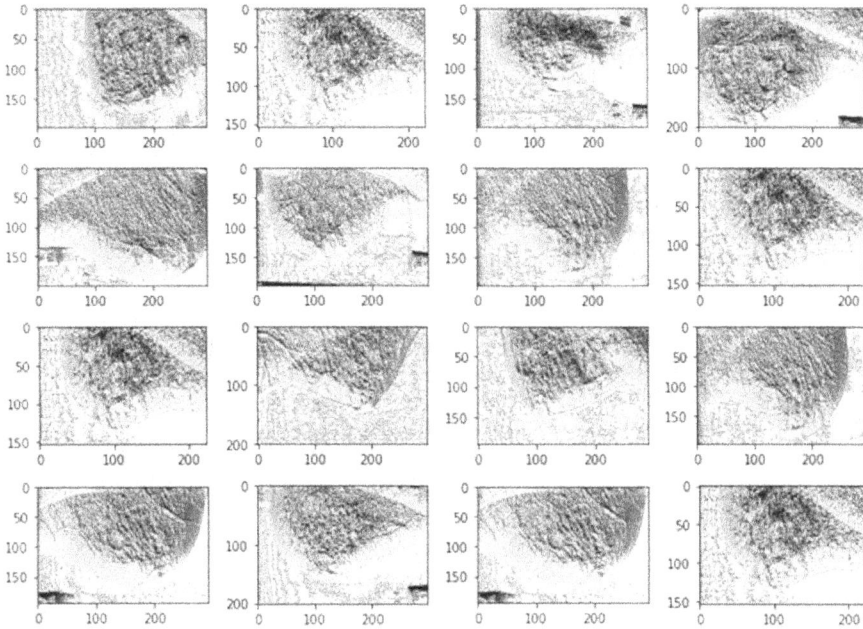

FIGURE 1.16   Breast cancer genuine images.

TABLE 1.6
Accuracy for different methods

Method	Accuracy %
FCID-HIST and FE [28]	76.33%–79.22%
Proposed (LBPVG + ELM)	96.05%
CNN based on medical images	83%
BusterNet [25]	78.0%

techniques. The cross-validation (stratified and repeated stratified k-fold) was performed, and performance was evaluated in terms of receiver operating characteristic (ROC) curve, precision, recall, and F-measure. Based on single-feature extracting strategies, the highest classification accuracy achieved was between 93% and 96%. Merging different local binary pattern variants feature extracting methods performed at an accuracy of 97%–99.06%. In the future, we may consider different bioinspired algorithms and pretrained models of CNN for the performance evaluation process based on the jackknife cross-validation k-fold method.

REFERENCES

1. Suckling, J., Parker, J., Dance, D., Astley, S., Hutt, I., Boggis, C., Ricketts, I., Stamatakis, E., Cerneaz, N., Kok, S-L., Taylor, P., Betal, D., Savage, J., *Mammographic Image Analysis Society Digital Mammogram Database*. Elsevier, 375–378, 1994.
2. Farid, H., "Image Forgery Detection." *IEEE Signal Processing Magazine* 26(2): 16–25, March 2009. DOI: 10.1109/MSP.2008.931079.
3. Chen, Jie, Kellokumpu, Vili, Zhao, Guoying, Pietikainen, Matti, *RLBP: Robust Local Binary Pattern*, 122.1–122.11, 2013. DOI: 10.5244/C.27.122.
4. Baek, Jeonghyun, Kim, Jisu, Kim, Euntai, *Part-Based Face Detection Using SLBP*, 1501–1503, 2014. DOI: 10.1109/ICCAS.2014.6987799.
5. Yang, Meng, Zhang, Lei, Zhang, Lin, Zhang, David, "Monogenic Binary Pattern (MBP): A Novel Feature Extraction and Representation Model for Face Recognition." *Proceedings – International Conference on Pattern Recognition*, 2680–2683, 2010. DOI: 10.1109/ICPR.2010.657.
6. Raths, Thomas, Otten, Jens, Kreitz, Christoph, "The ILTP Problem Library for Intuitionistic Logic: Release v1.1." *Journal of Automated Reasoning* 38: 261–271, 2007. DOI: 10.1007/s10817-006-9060-z.
7. Zhang, Tong, Su, Tonghua, Liu, Mingyi, Tu, Zhiying, Wang, Zhongjie, *LTP: A New Active Learning Strategy for CRF-Based Named Entity Recognition*, 2020.
8. Tian, Guangjian, Fu, Hong, Feng, David Dagan, Feng, *Automatic Medical Image Categorization and Annotation Using LBP and MPEG-7 Edge Histograms*, 51–53, 2008. DOI: 10.1109/ITAB.2008.4570523.
9. Malegori, Cristina, Franzetti, Laura, Guidetti, Riccardo, Casiraghi, Ernestina, "GLCM, an Image Analysis Technique for Early Detection of Biofilm." *Journal of Food Engineering* 185, 2016. DOI: 10.1016/j.jfoodeng.2016.04.001.
10. Yu, Wei, Gan, Lin, Yang, Sha, Ding, Yonggang, Jiang, Pan, Wang, Jun, Li, Shijun, "An Improved LBP Algorithm for Texture and Face Classification." *Signal, Image and Video Processing* 8, 155–161, 2014. DOI: 10.1007/s11760-014-0652-5.
11. Nasiri, Morteza, Behrad, Alireza, "Using Expectation-Maximization for Exposing Image Forgeries by Revealing Inconsistencies in Shadow Geometry." *The Journal of Visual Communication and Image Representation* 58, 323–333, 2019.
12. Ahmadi, Neda, Akbarizadeh, Gholamreza, "Iris Tissue Recognition Based on GLDM Feature Extraction and Hybrid MLPNN-ICA Classifier." *Neural Computing and Applications*, 2018. DOI: 10.1007/s00521-018-3754-0.
13. Sohail, Abu Sayeed Md., Bhattacharya, Prabir, Mudur, Sudhir P., Krishnamurthy, Srinivasan, "Local Relative GLRLM-Based Texture Feature Extraction for Classifying Ultrasound Medical Images." *IEEE CCECE, 2011–001092*.
14. Mishra, Sonali, Majhi, Banshidhar, Sa, Pankaj Kumar, "GLRLM-Based Feature Extraction for Acute Lymphoblastic Leukemia (ALL) Detection." Springer Nature Singapore Pte Ltd., Recent Findings in Intelligent Computing Techniques. *Advances in Intelligent Systems and Computing* 708. DOI: 10.1007/978-981-10-8636-6_41.
15. Abd, Nor Bakiah, Warif, Mohd, Idris, Yamani Idna, Wahab, Ainuddin Wahid Abdul, Salleh, Rosli, Ismail, Ahsiah, "CMF-iteMS: An Automatic Threshold Selection for Detection of Copy-Move Forgery." *FSI*, 2018. DOI: 10.1016/j.forsciint.2018.12.004.
16. Tralic, Dijana, Grgic, Sonja, Zovko-Cihlar, Branka, "Video Frame Copy-Move Forgery Detection Based on Cellular Automata and Local Binary Patterns." *International Symposium on Telecommunications (BIHTEL), Sarajevo, Bosnia and Herzegovina*, IEEE, 978-1-4799-4136-0/14, 27–29, October 2014.
17. Kylberg, Gustaf, Sintorn, Ida-Maria, "Evaluation of Noise Robustness for Local Binary Pattern Descriptors in Texture Classification." *EURASIP Journal on Image and Video Processing*, Springer, 2013.

18. Tan, X., Triggs, B., "Enhanced Local Texture Feature Sets for Face Recognition Under Difficult Lighting Conditions." *IEEE Transactions on Image Processing* 19(6), 635–650, 2007.
19. Kylberg, Gustaf, Sintorn, Ida-Maria, "On the Influence of Interpolation Method on Rotation Invariance in Texture Recognition." *EURASIP Journal on Image and Video Processing*, Springer, 2016.
20. Ravichandran, Dhivya, Praveenkumar, Padmapriya, Bosco Balaguru Rayappan, John, Amirtharajan, Rengarajan, "DNA Chaos Blend to Secure Medical Privacy." *IEEE Transactions on Nanobioscience* 16, 850–859, December 2017.
21. Mehrish, Ambuj, Subramanyam, A. V., Emmanuel, Sabu, "Joint Spatial and Discrete Cosine Transform Domain-Based Counter Forensics for Adaptive Contrast Enhancement." IEEE Access 7, 27183–27195, 13 March 2019.
22. Yan, Yanyang, Ren, Wenqi, Cao, Xiaochun, "Recolored Image Detection Via a Deep Discriminative Model." *IEEE Transactions on Information Forensics and Security* 14(1), 5–17, 2019.
23. Calberson, Filip L. G., Hommez, Geert M., De Moor, Roeland J., "Fraudulent Use of Digital Radiography: Methods to Detect and Protect Digital Radiographs." *American Association of Endodontists, JOE* 34(5), May 2008. DOI: 10.1016/j. joen.2008.01.019.
24. Ghoneim, Ahmed, Muhammad, Ghulam, Umar Amin, Syed, Gupta, Brij, "Medical Image Forgery Detection for Smart Healthcare: Advances in Next Generation Networking Technologies for Smart Healthcare." *IEEE Communications Magazine*, April 2018. DOI: 10.1109/MCOM.2018.1700817.
25. Wu, Yue, Abd-Almageed, Wael, Natarajan, Prem, "BusterNet: Detecting Copy-Move Image Forgery with Source/Target Localization." *Lecture Notes in Computer Science Book Series (LNCS, Volume 11210), Computer Vision – ECCV 2018*, pp. 170–186
26. Li, Wei, Yuan, Wei-qi, "Multiple Palm Features Extraction Method Based on Vein and Palmprint." *Journal of Ambient Intelligence and Humanized Computing*, February 2018. DOI: 10.1007/s12652-018-0699-1.
27. Tuncer, Turker, Dogan, Sengul, "Pyramid and Multi Kernel Based Local Binary Pattern for Texture Recognition." *Journal of Ambient Intelligence and Humanized Computing*, May 2019. DOI: 10.1007/s12652-019-01306-1.
28. Guo, Yuanfang, Cao, Xiaochun, Zhang, Wei, Wang, Rui, "Fake Colorized Image Detection." *IEEE Transactions on Information Forensics and Security* 13(8), 2018.
29. Heikkilä, M., Pietikäinen, M., "A Texture-Based Method for Modeling the Background and Detecting Moving Objects." *IEEE Transactions on Pattern Analysis and Machine Intelligence* 28(4), April 2006.
30. Albregsten, F., "Statistical Texture Measures Computed From Gray Level Co-Occurrence Matrices." Technical Note. Department of Informatics, University of Oslo, Norway, 1995.
31. Hadjer, Benchikh, Sara, Razi, Halima, Korichi, Oussama, Aiadi, "Content-Based Image Retrieval." University Kasdi Merbah Ouargla, 2016/17.
32. Raju, Priya Mariam, Nair, Madhu S., "Copy-Move Forgery Detection Using Binary Discriminant Features." *Journal of King Saud University – Computer and Information Sciences.* Elsevier, 2018. DOI: 10.1016/j.jksuci.2018.11.004.
33. Nanni, L., Brahnam, S., Lumini, A., "A Local Approach Based on a Local Binary Patterns Variant Texture Descriptor for Classifying Pain States." *Expert System Applications* 37(12), 7888–7894, 2010.
34. Azemin, Mohd Zulfaezal Che, Tamrin, Mohd Izzuddin Mohd, Hilmi, Mohd Radzi, Kamal, Khairidzan Mohd, "GLCM Texture Analysis on Different Color Space for Pterygium Grading." *ARPN Journal of Engineering and Applied Sciences* 10(15), August 2015.

35. Girisha, A. B., Chandrashekhar, M. C., Kurian, M. Z., "Texture Feature Extraction of Video Frames Using GLCM." *International Journal of Engineering Trends and Technology (IJETT)* 4(6), June 2013.

36. Yaseen, Zaher Mundher, Deo, Ravinesh C., Hilal, Ameer, Abd, Abbas M., Cornejo Bueno, Laura, Salcedo-Sanz, Sancho, Nehdi, Moncef L., "Predicting Compressive Strength of Lightweight Foamed Concrete Using Extreme Learning Machine Model." *Advances in Engineering Software*, 20 April 2017. DOI: 10.1016/j.advengsoft.2017.09.004.

37. Feng, Guorui, Huang, Guang-Bin, Lin, Qingping, Gay, Robert, "Error Minimized Extreme Learning Machine With Growth of Hidden Nodes and Incremental Learning." *IEEE Transactions on Neural Networks* 20(8), August 2009.

38. Yang, Fan, Li, Jingwei, Lu, Wei, Weng, Jian, "Copy-Move Forgery Detection Based on Hybrid Features." *Engineering Applications of Artificial Intelligence* 59, 73–83, 2017. DOI: 10.1016/j.engappai.2016.12.022.

39. Wang, Yuan, Tian, Lihua, Li, Chen, "LBP-SVD Based Copy Move Forgery Detection Algorithm." *IEEE International Symposium on Multimedia*, 2017. DOI: 10.1109/ISM.2017.108.

40. Tralic, Dijana, Rosin, Paul L., Sun, Xianfang, Grgic, Sonja, "Copy-Move Forgery Detection Using Cellular Automata." In P. Rosin (Ed.), *Cellular Automata in Image Processing and Geometry, 105 Emergence, Complexity and Computation 10*. Springer International Publishing, Switzerland, 10125, 2014. DOI: 10.1007/978-3-319-06431-4_6.

41. Díaz-Flores-García, V., Labajo-Gonzalez, E., Santiago-Saez, A., Perea-Perez, B., "Detecting the Manipulation of Digital Clinical Records in Dental Practice." In *The College of Radiographers*. Elsevier, 2017. DOI: 10.1016/j.radi.2017.05.003.

42. Roy, Aniket, Konda, Akhil, Chakraborty, Rajat Subhra, "Copy Move Forgery Detection With Similar But Genuine Objects." *ICIP, IEEE*, 2017. DOI: 10.1109/ICIP.2017.8297050.

43. Chakraborty, C., Othman, S. B., Almalki, F. A., Sakli, H., "FC-SEEDA: Fog Computing-Based Secure and Energy Efficient Data Aggregation Scheme for Internet of Healthcare Things." Neural Computing and Applications, 2023. DOI: 10.1007/s00521-023-08270-0.

44. Ben Othman, Soufiene, Bahattab, Abdullah Ali, Trad, Abdelbasset, Youssef, Habib, "PEERP: A Priority-Based Energy-Efficient Routing Protocol for Reliable Data Transmission in Healthcare using the IoT." *The 15th International Conference on Future Networks and Communications (FNC)*, Leuven, Belgium, 9–12 August 2020.

45. Ben Othman, Soufiene, Almalki, Faris A., Chakraborty, Chinmay, Sakli, Hedi, "Privacy-Preserving Aware Data Aggregation for IoT-Based Healthcare With Green Computing Technologies." *Computers and Electrical Engineering* 101, 108025, 2022. DOI: 10.1016/j.compeleceng.2022.108025.

46. Lee, Jen-Chun, Chang, Chien-Ping, Chen, Wei-Kuei, *Detection of Copy–Move Image Forgery Using Histogram of Orientated Gradients*. Elsevier, 2015. DOI: 10.1016/j.ins.2015.03.009.

47. Soni, Badal, Das, Pradip K., Thounaojam, Dalton Meitei, "Copy-Move Tampering Detection Based on Local Binary Pattern Histogram Fourier Feature." *ICCCT*, Allahabad, India, 24–26 November 2017. DOI: 10.1145/3154979.3155001.

48. Mondal, Satyajit, Mukherjee, Joydeep, "Image Similarity Measurement Using Region Props, Color and Texture: An Approach." *International Journal of Computer Applications* 121(22), July 2015.

49. Zhuo, Long, Tan, Shunquan, Zeng, Jishen, Li, Bin, "Fake Colorized Image Detection with Channel-wise Convolution Based Deep-learning Framework." *2018 Asia-Pacific Signal and Information Processing Association Annual Summit and Conference (APSIPA ASC)*, 12–15 November 2018. DOI: 10.23919/APSIPA.2018.8659761.

2 Multiple Lung Disease Prediction Using X-Ray Images Based on Deep Convolutional Neural Networks

Nagarjuna Telagam, Nehru Kandasamy,
Kumar Raja, Tharuni Gelli, and D Ajitha

2.1 INTRODUCTION

Machine learning models play a significant role in the medical industry and have significant applications. The main objective of this chapter is to predict the types of lung diseases, such as asthma, allergies, lung cancer, pulmonary diseases, and bronchitis. The authors proposed the work with various classifications with 323 instances with 19 attributes. The attributes were classified into two types – positive and negative – then the training of the system was analyzed. The accuracy of the various models is calculated with multiple machine learning models, out of which the logistic model tree achieved the highest accuracy (89.23%) [1]. The k-nearest neighbor (KNN) and Gaussian Bayes are used mainly as text and audio data classifiers, especially in diseases. Based on the doctor's advice, the patient information is recorded from different lung sounds from other subjects. The machine learning algorithms run on various datasets to classify patients into multiple types [2]. This chapter discusses the potential for medical diagnosis using neural networks. The neural network method is developed based on multilayer perceptron (MLP) with a backpropagation technique [3]. The various MLP functions are used to compare with the conventional methods. The MLP algorithm provides 96.3% accuracy in heart disease prediction [4]. The ANN-based histogram with genomic gradient characteristics is used to predict who developed lung cancer [5]. The MLP and radial base function are combined to predict lung disease, and the same dataset is used to analyze the accuracy, with 93.22% achieved. Neurologists examined the algorithms used for the medical diagnosis of patients [6]. The researchers used the diagnosis method for heart disease prediction with numerical analysis. The support vector machine (SVM) and MLP neural network are classifiers for heart

DOI: 10.1201/9781003366249-2

disease prediction with database prediction [7]. This chapter proposes a convolutional neural network (CNN) method for classifying lung disease images, and the accuracy is compared with a conventional neural classifier [8]. The researchers developed the early stage of cancer detection using particle swarm optimization with neural networks [9]. The researchers use the genetic k-means nearest neighbor algorithm for early-stage detection of lung cancer. The value of k is chosen as 50 or 100 for every iteration with various performance tests in the range of 90% [10]. The authors use KNN to distinguish cancer diseases with different image classifications [11]. The SVM is used as a classifier for lung cancer diagnosis. The CLAHE (contrast-limited adaptive histogram equalization) technique uses computed tomography (CT) scan graphic methods with random walk for segmentation [12].

The median filter is the filtering technique used for noise removal from images and signals. The features of the images are extracted using the particle swarm optimization algorithm method [13]. The genetic algorithm is used for heart disease prediction, with the KNN classifier used for predicting heart disease for different k values [14]. The features are derived from gray level co-occurrence matrix (GLCM) methods with a backpropagation algorithm for various classifications of images. These classifiers generated 95% precision in the evaluation levels [15]. The neural network is used to diagnose the different patterns of rubella and chickenpox based on skin symptoms. The artificial neural network can predict better than human doctors [16]. Two methods are integrated for the classification of diseases: predictive t-test and absolute ranking. Classification methods such as linear, proximal, and Newton support vector machines are explored [17]. The fractal image compression methods describe the image processing techniques for detecting diseases [18].

This book chapter discusses the machine learning methods, various architectures, and the researchers' hyperparameters used in neural networks. This chapter primarily focuses on different CNN methods with chest X-ray images and calculates the performance metrics. This chapter concludes with calculated metrics in multiple lung disease prediction.

Section 2.2 briefly introduces lung diseases in machine learning methods and different drawbacks from other research papers. Section 2.3 discusses the classified items, number of features, classification methods, and performance metrics used by the researchers in the last 5 years. Section 2.4 discusses the proposed system model. Section 2.5 discusses the impact of machine learning methods and their performance metrics on multiple lung disease predictions. Section 2.6 concludes the chapter with future scope.

2.2   LITERATURE SURVEY

The public suffers from dangers such as carbon dioxide levels, cigarette smoking, and respiratory health. The global temperature is increasing by 2 degrees every decade, significantly impacting human life [32]. People with some diseases, such as asthma and lung cancer, will be significantly impacted by these climate changes. Chronic obstructive pulmonary disease caused about 3.23 million deaths worldwide in 2019 [48].

Pulmonary disease increased in 2016, of which 3 million to 4 million people died [49, 50]. According to the World Health Organization, people in lower- and middle-income countries face air pollution and have more lung diseases like asthma and pneumonia. COVID-19 can cause severe lung damage, breathing problems, and other bacterial infections [51]. New advanced techniques such as deep neural networks and machine learning play a significant role in detecting lung disease. Many researchers have published numerous papers that help doctors and other researchers worldwide. The datasets play a substantial role in the accuracy of detecting diseases [52]. Coronavirus detection is possible only with the help of kits. Another alternative way to detect the disease is via a chest scan of the patient. The X-ray is a frequently used method, with machine learning and deep learning algorithms playing a significant role in identifying diseases. Jain et al. present a study with 1,832 images using data augmentation techniques and avoiding overfitting techniques. The deep neural network is implemented in two stages to differentiate COVID-19–based pneumonia from other cases using chest X-ray images. The authors achieved 97% accuracy [53]. The CT imaging system is valuable for detecting COVID-19. A light CNN algorithm is used to detect the disease based on CT images. The authors named it the light CNN method because they used a medium-end laptop without GPU acceleration for accuracy calculation [54]. The authors proposed a new deep neural network called CoroNet based on Xception architecture using a COVID-19 chest X-ray images dataset. The authors achieved 89.6% accuracy for the prepared dataset and promising results with substantial improvement with the current radiology-based tool in the COVID-19 cases [55].

The deep learning model with artificial intelligence is used for coronavirus detection. The fuzzy color technique is used as the preprocessing step. The stacked dataset was used to train the deep learning models in the next step. Finally, the efficient features are classified using a support vector machine [8]. The conventional method for treating COVID-19 patients is a transcription-polymerase chain reaction, which is quite expensive and time-consuming. Heidari et al. used a hybrid combination of deep neural networks and convolutional neural networks for disease diagnosis. The authors achieved 83.84% accuracy in detecting infected regions [56]. The tests to detect the virus in humans take a few hours to generate a result. The main aim of adopting deep learning for disease detection is threefold: The first part is to detect pneumonia in the chest X-ray. The second part is to discern between COVID-19 and pneumonia, and the third part is to localize the gaps in the X-ray. The proposed architecture was conducted based on 6,523 images within 2.5 seconds and achieved an accuracy of 97% [57]. The computer-aided diagnosis scheme of chest X-ray images to detect COVID-19–infected pneumonia was implemented. The CNN model divides the disease into three sets and achieves 94.5% accuracy in classifying the three sets. The study plays a significant role in developing a new deep learning computer-aided diagnosis model for chest X-ray images by adding two images in the preprocessing stage and generating a pseudocolor image to detect COVID-19 disease [58]. Many researchers have proposed a lung disease detection model based on machine learning. Different conventional algorithms have already been applied for lung disease prediction, and some methods have poor performance for rotated, tilted, and abnormal image orientation. A new method, called VGG data STN with CNN, exhibited an accuracy of 73% [59]. Table 2.1 shows survey on multiple lung diseases with features and accuracy.

2.3   DATASETS AND THE ROLE OF X-RAY IN DETECTING DISEASE

Figure 2.1 shows the X-ray image datasets for the detection of COVID-19.

2.3.1   ROLE OF CHEST X-RAY IN CONFIRMING CORONA DISEASES

The density of the lungs is the increase in COVID-19 pneumonia. Based on the severity levels, the radiography can observe the whiteness in the lungs. Due to the whiteness, lung markings are lost, indicating the consolidation stage, usually seen in severe diseases. Typical pneumonia has various appearances in the radiograph, such as ground glass opacity and linear opacities (see Figure 2.2).

2.3.2   ROLE OF CHEST X-RAY IN CONFIRMING PNEUMONIA DISEASES

Pneumonia infection causes lung inflammation because of viruses, bacteria, and fungi. The doctor will conduct a physical exam with chest X-ray, CT, and ultrasound to diagnose the lung disease condition. Also, the doctor can hear abnormal sounds like crackling and rumbling during the physical exam. In the chest X-ray, white spots on the lungs are observed. This test will determine the complications related to pneumonia, such as abscesses. The CT scan of the lungs will identify the more refined details within the lungs, and the scan shows the airway to detect the disease. Ultrasound technology is used to check the fluid surrounding the lungs. The doctor understands the causes of fluid and its determination. The MRI scan is used to evaluate pneumonia in the chest wall structure. The doctor can determine whether there is a tumor or infection. The doctor can request a biopsy to determine the cause of pneumonia. The MRI can detect biopsies of the lung, and details of the image are shown in Figure 2.3.

2.3.3   ROLE OF CHEST X-RAY IN CONFIRMING TUBERCULOSIS DISEASES

Persons with tuberculosis (TB) disease have symptoms such as coughing for 3 weeks, hemoptysis, fever, chest pain, weight loss, and fatigue. A TB X-ray is shown in Figure 2.3. Persons with symptoms may test negative for TB, or persons with no symptoms may test positive. The patient's diagnosis can be made by considering the risk factors. The person's medical history and chest X-ray data are other tests required for treatment. Drugs in high doses are used to treat the disease. The physical exam provides valuable information about the patient's condition, such as HIV infection. The tuberculin skin test or TB blood test is also used to identify TB disease. The detection can be revealed by radiography of the chest. The abnormalities in the chest of various sizes, shapes, and densities are observed in radiographs. The main problem with radiographs is that they will not rule out the possibility of

TABLE 2.1
Survey on multiple lung diseases with features and accuracy

Reference	Classified items	Number of features	Classification method	Accuracy
Kahya et al. [19]	COPD, lung disease	14	KNN	69.59%
Heckerling et al. [20]	Pneumonia	35	MLP	82.8%
Barua et al. [21]	Pulmonary	12	MLP	61.53%
Barua et al. [22]	Asthma	12	MLP	95.01%
Er et al. [23]	TB	38	MLNN, GRNN	95.08%
Er et al. [24]	COPD	38	MLNN	96.08%
Er et al. [25]	Pneumonia COPD	38	PNN, MLNN, AIS	94%
Temurtas et al. [26]	Thyroid disease	5	LVQ, MLNN, PNN	94.81%
Er et al. [27]	TB, lung cancer, asthma, COPD	38	RBF, GRNN, LVQ, MLNN	90%, 93.75%, 90.91%, 88%
Yamashita et al. [28]	Emphysema	—	HMM	88.7%
Amaral et al. [29]	COPD	7	KNN, SVM	95%
Rao et al. [30]	Lung disease	11	GMM, SVM, KNN	91.7%
Jayalakshmy et al. [31]	COPD	Automatic	CNN	83.78%
Goel et al. [33]	COVID-19	Automatic	CNN, grey wolf optimization	97.78%
Jain et al. [34]	COVID-19, pneumonia	Automatic	Inception V3, ResNeXt	97.97%
Apostolopoulos et al. [35]	COVID-19	Automatic	VGG19, MobileNet	96.78%
Alom et al. [36]	COVID-19	Automatic	NABLA-N network	98.78%
Minaee et al. [37]	COVID-19	Automatic	ResNet 18, ResNet 50	98%
Oh et al. [38]	COVID-19	Automatic	Patch-based CNN	88.9%
Kumar et al. [39]	COVID-19	Automatic	XGBoost	97.7%
Turkoglu et al. [40]	COVID-19	Automatic	SVM	99.18%
Wang et al. [41]	COVID-19	Automatic	3D ResNet	93.3%
Han et al. [42]	COVID-19	Automatic	3D multiple instance learning	97.9%
Ouyang et al. [43]	COVID-19	Automatic	3D CNN	87.5%
Kang et al. [44]	COVID-19	Automatic	SVM, latent representation learning, decision tree	95.5%
Chandra et al. [45]	COVID-19	Automatic	KNN	93.41%
Pham et al. [46]	COVID-19	Automatic	DenseNet-201	84.7%
Pham et al. [47]	COVID-19	Automatic	AlexNet	96%

Negative   Positive

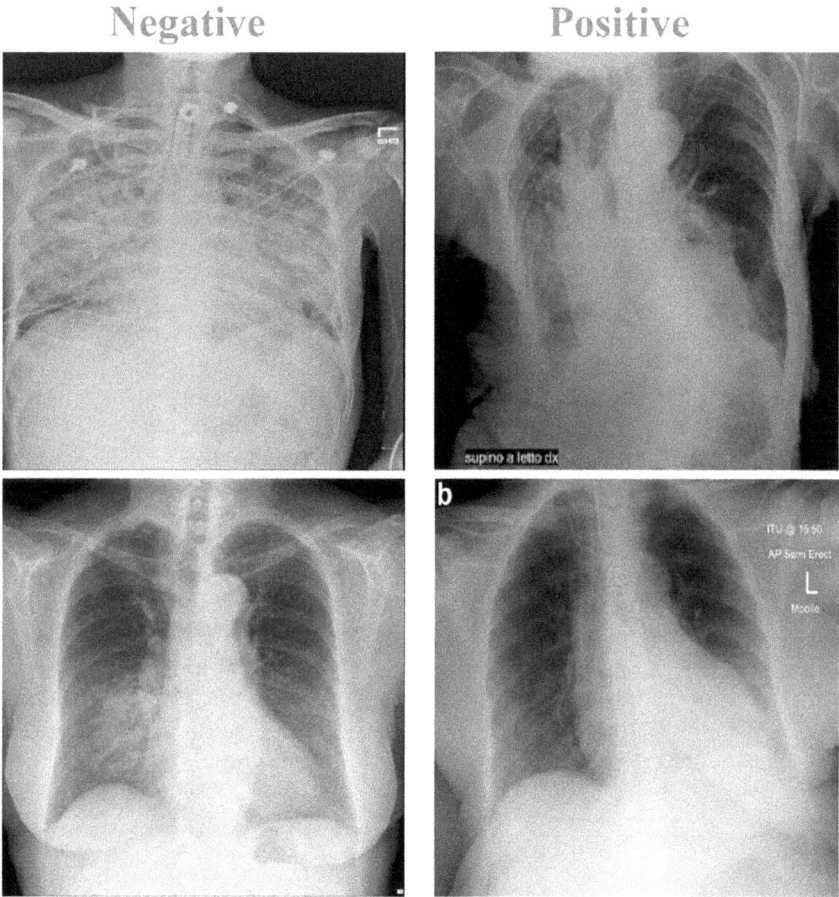

FIGURE 2.1   COVID-19 X-ray images [60].

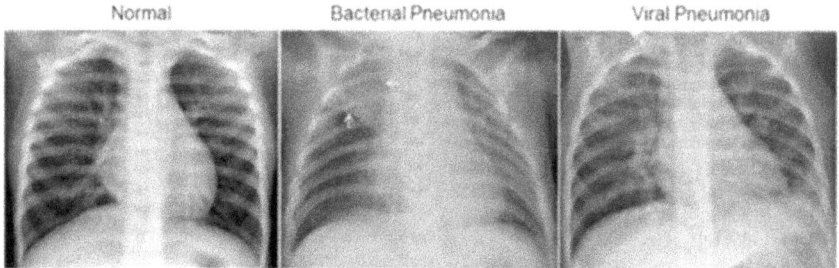

FIGURE 2.2   Pneumonia X-ray images [61].

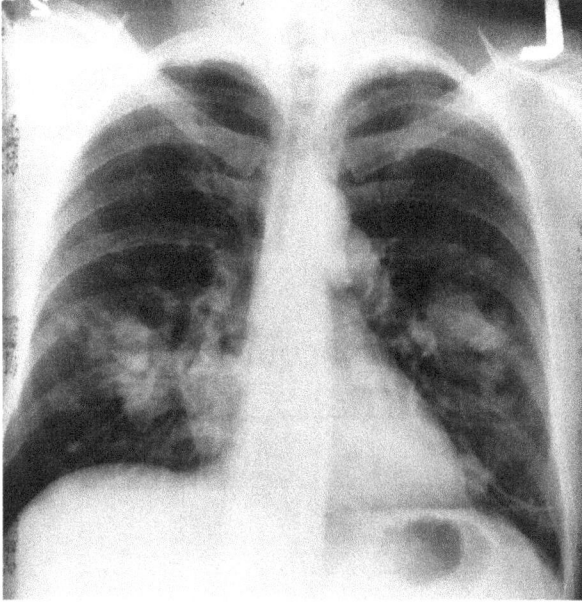

FIGURE 2.3 Tuberculosis X-ray image.

pulmonary TB even if the patient has had a positive reaction. The diagnosis of TB is not confirmed with an acid-fast bacilli on sputum smear. The drug resistance of the patient needs to be tested, and the opposition is a crucial part of ensuring effective treatment. The susceptibility result of the drug resistance should be noted.

2.4 PROPOSED SYSTEM MODEL

For any machine learning algorithm, the first step is gathering an image dataset, which can be of any data, such as time series and voice data. Significant data is required to detect lung diseases, including chest X-rays, CT scans, and histopathology images. The output of the first step is to check the images by training the model. The second step in machine learning is to preprocess the image datasets, and the images can be modified or enhanced to increase the quality [62, 63, 65, 64].

The image contrast can also be increased with histogram equalization. Various preprocessing algorithms can perform the region of interest or the modification. The data augmentation can also be applied to images to check the alternate data representation. The feature extraction can be applied to the image dataset to identify certain objects and classes. The image outputs are enhanced in the training data. The third step in machine learning is to train the data. Various deep learning algorithms are available, such as deep belief networks and recurrent neural networks. The different data types work well with certain algorithms, especially CNN works well with images. The ensemble method uses one more model with classification, mostly to reduce the training time, improve the classification, and reduce the overfitting. The output of this step is a model generated from the data learned. The final step is classification. The trained model will predict which class the image belongs to. In this case, the CNN model will differentiate healthy and infected lung X-ray images. The CNN model will also give a probability score for the images. The sequence of steps is shown in Figure 2.4.

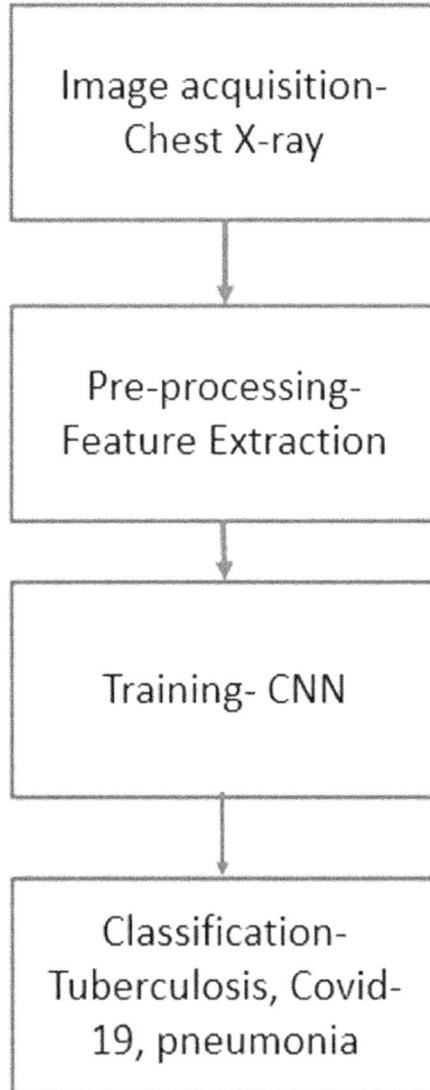

FIGURE 2.4   CNN model for three different datasets.

In computer vision, the features in the images are extracted to solve the problem. The features are mainly in the form of points, edges, and objects. The feature transformation process creates new features with the original features and has discriminatory power in spaces. The primary purpose of transforming the features with machine learning methods is to identify the object identification. Mainly, binary patterns, descriptors, color layout, and edge histograms are analyzed by using machine learning methods. The CNN method is adaptive learning with feature identification. This method is used to find the patterns in images. The neural networks in CNNs have neurons with variable weights with several inputs. The weighted sums are passed to the activation function and generate the output. The CNN consists of multiple layers, such as pooling, convolutional, and fully connected. With the convolution operator, the convolution method of linear operation is performed on the weights with inputs. The set of weights is called the kernel. The pooling layer reduces the spatial size of the network's parameters and computations. The rectified linear unit is added to the CNN to apply an activation function sigmoid to the previous layer. The CNN has two components: extraction and classification, primarily used for image classification and recognition. Figure 2.5 shows the proposed model for predicting multiple lung diseases.

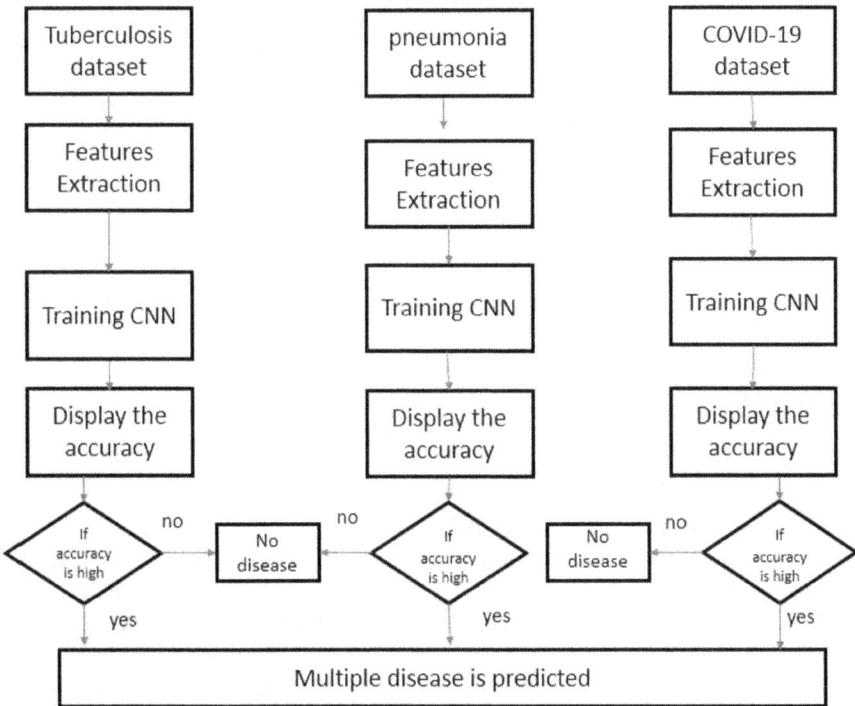

FIGURE 2.5　Proposed CNN model for three different datasets to predict multiple diseases.

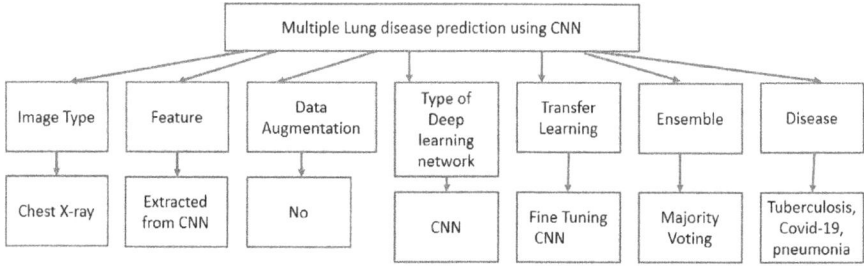

FIGURE 2.6 Taxonomy of the proposed model.

The taxonomy of the literature survey with the deep learning method is shown in Figure 2.6. The taxonomy shows a clear picture of the concepts with different attributes explained. The image datasets, feature extraction, and data augmentation are used to classify lung diseases. The world's researchers can use the taxonomy to improve efficiency and increase the applications in healthcare.

2.5   RESULTS AND DISCUSSION

The training accuracy versus epoch plots is shown in Figure 2.7. Epochs tell us the number of times we pass the entire dataset through the neural network. Epochs can have multiple intervals of 100 or even 1,000. If we keep increasing the epochs, more data is present on the dataset. After training the dataset multiple times, the system no longer provides improved accuracy. In our model, we have a limited number of epochs for the system at 10.

Precision and recall are significant performance metrics that are calculated based on the values in the confusion matrix. Precision is the ratio of correctly predicted measurements to the total number of measurements, and recall is the ratio of correctly predicted positive measurements to all measurements in the total class. The F1 score is another performance metric. It is the weighted average of both precision and recall measurements.

The testing accuracy versus epochs plot is shown in Figure 2.8.

Table 2.2 shows the performance metric comparison of machine learning methods.

2.6   CONCLUSIONS

Lung disease detection with deep learning plays a significant role in classifying different diseases using X-ray images. An extensive research survey is done in this chapter, especially concerning COVID-19 detection, pneumonia, and tuberculosis research. Existing works are analyzed in this chapter with different parameters. The taxonomy of the deep learning methods is presented in this chapter. The importance and applications of convolutional neural networks are deeply understood and implemented for various datasets. The performance of a model is highly dependent on the quality of preprocessing. The results of this study demonstrate that medical image

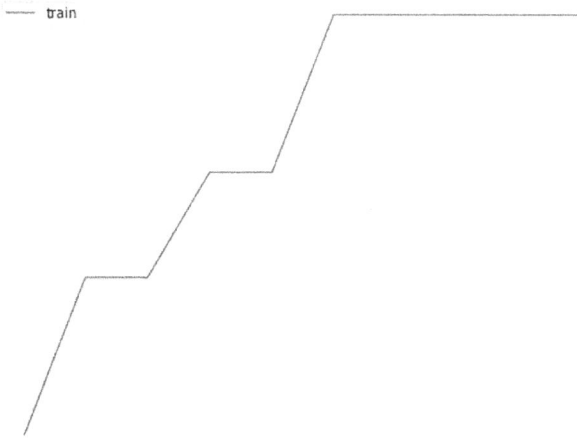

FIGURE 2.7   Training accuracy for the CNN model.

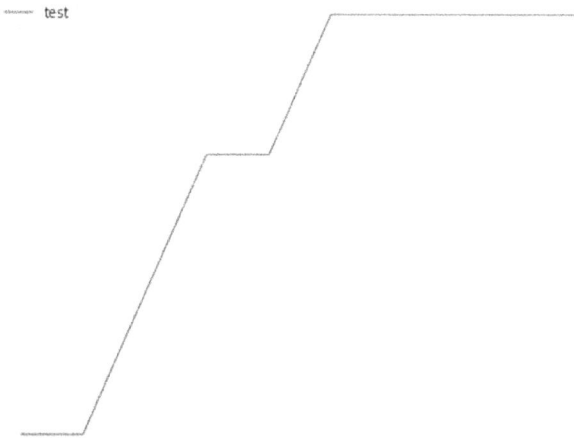

FIGURE 2.8   Testing accuracy for the CNN model

TABLE 2.2
Performance metrics comparison of machine learning methods

Attribute	COVID-19	Pneumonia	Tuberculosis
Recall	0.85	0.88	0.89
Precision	0.813	0.841	0.835
Accuracy	81.92%	83.2%	85%
F1 score	0.8315	0.8605	0.8625

processing helps us predict and cure diseases. To conclude, deep learning methods play a major role in disease classification. Future directions suggest that efficiency can be improved by increasing the number of deep learning methods.

REFERENCES

1. Sen, I., Hossain, M. I., Shakib, M. F. H., Imran, M. A., Al Faisal, F. Depth analysis of lung disease prediction using machine learning algorithms. In Bhattacharjee, A., Borgohain, S., Soni, B., Verma, G., Gao, X. Z. (Eds.), *Machine Learning, Image Processing, Network Security and Data Sciences. MIND 2020. Communications in Computer and Information Science*, Vol. 1241. Springer, Singapore, 2020.
2. Aykanat, M., Kılıç, Ö., Kurt, B., Saryal, S. B. Lung Disease Classification Using Machine Learning Algorithms. *International Journal of Applied Mathematics Electronics and Computers*, 8(4), 125–132, 2020. DOI: 10.18100/ijamec.799363.
3. Mantzaris, D. H., Anastassopoulos, G. C., Lymberopoulos, D. K. Medical Disease Prediction Using Artificial Neural Networks. *8th IEEE International Conference on BioInformatics and BioEngineering*, October 2008.
4. Durairaj, M., Revathi, V. Prediction of Heart Disease Using Back Propagation MLP Algorithm. *International Journal of Scientific Technology Research*, 4(8), August 2015.
5. Adetiba, Emmanuel, Olugbara, Oludayo O. Lung Cancer Prediction Using Neural Network Ensemble With Histogram of Oriented Gradient Genomic Features. *The Scientific World Journal*, 2015, Article ID 786013. DOI: 10.1155/2015/786013.
6. Gharehchopogh, Farhad Soleimanian, Mohammadi, Peryman. A Case Study of Parkinson's Disease Diagnosis Using Artificial Neural Networks. *International Journal of Computer Applications*, 73(19), July 2013.
7. Hasan, Tabreer T., Jasim, Manal H., Hashim, Ivan A. Heart Disease Diagnosis System Based on Multi-Layer Perceptron Neural Network and Support Vector Machine. *International Journal of Current Engineering and Technology*, 7, 2017.
8. Sasikala, S., Bharathi, M., Sowmiya, B. R. Lung Cancer Detection and Classification Using Deep CNN. *International Journal of Innovative Technology and Exploring Engineering (IJITEE)*, 8(2S), December 2018.
9. Senthil, S., Ayshwarya, B. Lung Cancer Prediction Using Feed Forward Back Propagation Neural Networks With Optimal Features. *International Journal of Applied Engineering Research*, 13(1), 318–325, 2018.
10. Bhuvaneswari, P., Brintha Therese, A. Detection of Cancer in Lung With K-NN Classification Using Genetic Algorithm. *2nd International Conference on Nanomaterials and Technologies*, 2014.
11. Thamilselvan, P., Sathiaseelan, J. G. R. An Enhanced k Nearest Neighbor Method to Detecting and Classifying MRI Lung Cancer Images for Large Amount Data. *International Journal of Applied Engineering Research*, 11(6), 4223–4229, 2016.
12. Sathishkumar, R., Kalaiarasan, K., Prabakaran, A., Aravind, M. Detection of Lung Cancer Using SVM Classifier and KNN Algorithm. *International Journal of Scientific Research and Review*, 8(3), 2019.
13. Kaur, Tejinder, Gupta, Neelakshi. A New Algorithm for Classification of Lung Diseases. *International Journal of Advances in Electronics and Computer Science*, 2(9), 2015.
14. Akhil Jabbar, M., Chandra, B. L. Deekshatulua Priti. Classification of Heart Disease Using k-Nearest Neighbor and Genetic Algorithm. *International Conference on Computational Intelligence: Modeling Techniques and Applications (CIMTA)*, 2013.

15. Adi, Kusworo, Widodo, Catur Edi, Widodo, Aris Puji, Gernowo, Rahmat, Pamungkas, Adi, Syifa, Rizky Ayomi. Detection Lung Cancer Using Gray Level Co-Occurrence Matrix (GLCM) and Backpropagation Neural Network Classification. *Journal of Engineering Science and Technology Review*, March 2018.

16. Monisha, M., Suresh, A., Rashmi, M. R. Artificial Intelligence Based Skin Classification Using GMM. *Journal of Medical Systems*, 43(1), 3, 2018.

17. Arunkumar Chinnaswamy, Ramakrishnan S. Two Step Feature Extraction Method for Microarray Cancer Data Using Support Vector Machines. *International Journal of Computer Applications*, 85(8), 34–42, 2014.

18. Loganathan, D., Amudha, J., Mehata, K. M. Classification and Feature Vector Techniques to Improve Fractal Image Coding. *IEEE Region 10 Annual International Conference, Proceedings/TENCON*, Vol. 4, Bangalore, pp. 1503–1507, 2003.

19. Kahya, Y. P., Guler, E. C., Sahin, S. Respiratory Disease Diagnosis Using Lung Sounds. In *Proceedings of the 19th Annual International Conference of the IEEE Engineering in Medicine and Biology Society. Magnificent Milestones and Emerging Opportunities in Medical Engineering (Cat. No. 97CH36136)* (Vol. 5, pp. 2051–2053). IEEE, October 1997.

20. Heckerling, P. S., Gerbera, B. S., Tapec, T. G., Wigton, R. S. Use of Genetic Algorithms for Neural Networks to Predict Community-Acquired Pneumonia. *Artificial Intelligence in Medicine*, 30, 71–84, 2004.

21. Barua, M., Nazeran, H., Nava, P., Granda, V., Diong, B. Classification of Pulmonary Diseases Based on Impulse Oscillometric Measurements of Lung Function Using Neural Networks. In *The 26th Annual International Conference of the IEEE Engineering in Medicine and Biology Society*, San Francisco, CA, USA (Vol. 2, pp. 3848–3851), September 2004.

22. Barua, M., Nazeran, H., Nava, P., Diong, B., Goldman, M. Classification of Impulse Oscillometric Patterns of Lung Function in Asthmatic Children Using Artificial Neural Networks. In *2005 IEEE Engineering in Medicine and Biology 27th Annual Conference*, Shanghai, China, pp. 327–331, January 2006.

23. Er, O., Temurtas, F., Tanrıkulu, A. Ç. Tuberculosis Disease Diagnosis Using Artificial Neural Networks. *Journal of Medical Systems*, 34(3), 299–302, 2008. DOI: 10.1007/s10916-008-9241-x.

24. Er, O., Temurtas, F. A Study on Chronic Obstructive Pulmonary Disease Diagnosis Using Multilayer Neural Networks. *Journal of Medical Systems*, 32(5), 429–432, 2008.

25. Er, O., Sertkaya, C., Temurtas, F., Tanrikulu, A. C. A Comparative Study on Chronic Obstructive Pulmonary and Pneumonia Diseases Diagnosis Using Neural Networks and Artificial Immune System. *Journal of Medical Systems*, 33(6), 485–492, 2009.

26. Temurtas, F. A Comparative Study on Thyroid Disease Diagnosis Using Neural Networks. *Expert Systems With Applications*, 36, 944–949, 2009.

27. Er, O., Yumusak, N., Temurtas, F. Chest Diseases Diagnosis Using Artificial Neural Networks. *Expert Systems With Applications*, 37(12), 7648–7655, 2010.

28. Yamashita, M., Matsunaga, S., Miyahara, S. Discrimination Between Healthy Subjects and Patients With Pulmonary Emphysema by Detection of Abnormal Respiration. *2011 IEEE International Conference on Acoustics, Speech and Signal Processing (ICASSP), Prague, Czech Republic*, pp. 693–696, May 2011.

29. Amaral, J. L. M., Lopes, A. J., Jansen, J. M., Faria, A. C. D., Melo, P. L. Machine Learning Algorithms and Forced Oscillation Measurements Applied to the Automatic Identification of Chronic Obstructive Pulmonary Disease. *Computer Methods and Programs in Biomedicine*, 105, 183–193, 2012.

30. Rao, A., Chu, S., Batlivala, N., Zetumer, S., Roy, S. Improved Detection of Lung Fluid With Standardised Acoustic Stimulation of the Chest. *IEEE Journal of Translational Engineering in Health and Medicine*, 6, 1–7, 2018.

31. Jayalakshmy, S., Sudha, G. F. Scalogram Based Prediction Model for Respiratory Disorders Using Optimised Convolutional Neural Networks. *Artificial Intelligence in Medicine*, 103, 101809, 2020.

32. Liu, Y., Wu, Y. H., Ban, Y., Wang, H., Cheng, M. M. Rethinking Computer-Aided Tuberculosis Diagnosis. In *Proceedings of the IEEE/CVF Conference on Computer Vision and Pattern Recognition* (pp. 2646–2655), 2020.

33. Goel, T., Murugan, R., Mirjalili, S., Chakrabartty, D. K. OptConet: An Optimised Convolutional Neural Network for an Automatic Diagnosis of COVID-19. *Applied Intelligence*, 51(3), 1351–1366, 2021.

34. Jain, R., Gupta, M., Taneja, S., Hemanth, D. J. Deep Learning Based Detection and Analysis of COVID-19 on Chest X-Ray Images. *Applied Intelligence*, 51(3), 1690–1700, 2021.

35. Apostolopoulos, I. D., Mpesiana, T. A. Covid-19: Automatic Detection From x-Ray Images Utilising Transfer Learning With Convolutional Neural Networks. *Physical and Engineering Sciences in Medicine*, 43(2), 635–640, 2020.

36. Alom, M. Z., Rahman, M. M., Nasrin, M. S., Taha, T. M., Asari, V. K. COVID MTNet: COVID-19 Detection With Multi-Task Deep Learning Approaches. *arXiv preprint arXiv:2004.03747,* 2020.

37. Minaee, S., Kafieh, R., Sonka, M., Yazdani, S., Soufi, G. J. Deep-Covid: Predicting Covid-19 From Chest X-Ray Images Using Deep Transfer Learning. *Medical Image Analysis*, 65, 101794, 2020.

38. Oh, Y., Park, S., Ye, J. C. Deep Learning Covid-19 Features on CXR Using Limited Training Data Sets. *IEEE Transactions on Medical Imaging*, 39(8), 2688–2700, 2020.

39. Kumar, R., Arora, R., Bansal, V., Sahayasheela, V. J., Buckchash, H., Imran, J., … Raman, B. Accurate Prediction of COVID-19 Using Chest X-Ray Images Through Deep Feature Learning Model With SMOTE and Machine Learning Classifiers. *MedRxiv*, 2020.

40. Turkoglu, M. COVIDetectioNet: COVID-19 Diagnosis System Based on X-Ray Images Using Features Selected From Prelearned Deep Features Ensemble. *Applied Intelligence*, 51(3), 1213–1226, 2021.

41. Wang, J., Bao, Y., Wen, Y., Lu, H., Luo, H., Xiang, Y., … Qian, D. Prior-Attention Residual Learning for More Discriminative COVID-19 Screening in CT Images. *IEEE Transactions on Medical Imaging*, 39(8), 2572–2583, 2020.

42. Han, Z., Wei, B., Hong, Y., Li, T., Cong, J., Zhu, X., … Zhang, W. Accurate Screening of COVID-19 Using Attention-Based Deep 3D Multiple Instance Learning. *IEEE Transactions on Medical Imaging*, 39(8), 2584–2594, 2020.

43. Ouyang, X., Huo, J., Xia, L., Shan, F., Liu, J., Mo, Z., .. & Shen, D. Dual-Sampling Attention Network for Diagnosis of COVID-19 From Community Acquired Pneumonia. *IEEE Transactions on Medical Imaging*, 39(8), 2595–2605, 2020.

44. Kang, H., Xia, L., Yan, F., Wan, Z., Shi, F., Yuan, H., … Shen, D. Diagnosis of Coronavirus Disease 2019 (COVID-19) With Structured Latent Multi-View Representation Learning. *IEEE Transactions on Medical Imaging*, 39(8), 2606–2614, 2020.

45. Chandra, T. B., Verma, K., Singh, B. K., Jain, D., Netam, S. S. Coronavirus Disease (COVID-19) Detection in Chest X-Ray Images Using Majority Voting-Based Classifier Ensemble. *Expert Systems With Applications*, 165, 113909, 2021.

46. Pham, T. D. A Comprehensive Study on Classification of COVID-19 on Computed Tomography With Pretrained Convolutional Neural Networks. *Scientific Reports*, 10(1), 1–8, 2020.

47. Pham, T. D. Classification of COVID-19 Chest X-Rays With Deep Learning: New Models or Fine Tuning? *Health Information Science and Systems*, 9(1), 1–11, 2021.

48. CDC - Data and Statistics—Chronic Obstructive Pulmonary Disease (COPD). (2021, June 14). Retrieved January 16, 2022, from https://www.cdc.gov/copd/data.html.

49. Bharati, S., Podder, P., Mondal, R., Mahmood, A., Raihan-Al-Masud, M. Comparative Performance Analysis of Different Classification Algorithm for the Purpose of Prediction of Lung Cancer. *Advances in Intelligent Systems and Computing*, 941, 447–457, 2020. DOI: 10.1007/978-3-030-16660-1_44.

50. Coudray, N., Ocampo, P. S., Sakellaropoulos, T., Narula, N., Snuderl,M., Fenyö, D., Moreira, A. L., Razavian, N., Tsirigos, A. Classification and Mutation Prediction From Non-Small Cell Lung Cancer Histopathology Images Using Deep Learning. *Nature Medicine*, 24, 1559–1567, 2018. DOI: 10.1038/s41591-018-0177-5.

51. Mondal, M. R. H., Bharati, S., Podder, P. Data Analytics for Novel Coronavirus Disease. *Informatics in Medicine Unlocked*, 20, 100374, 2020. DOI: 10.1016/j.imu.2020.100374.

52. Kuan, K., Ravaut, M., Manek, G., Chen, H., Lin, J., Nazir, B., Chen, C., Howe, T. C., Zeng, Z., Chandrasekhar, V. Deep Learning for Lung Cancer Detection: Tackling the Kaggle Data Science Bowl 2017 Challenge, 2017. https://arxiv.org/abs/1705.09435.

53. Jain, Govardhan, Mittal, Deepti, Thakur, Daksh, Mittal, Madhup K. A Deep Learning Approach to Detect Covid-19 Coronavirus With X-Ray Images. *Biocybernetics and Biomedical Engineering*, 40(4), 1391–1405, 2020.

54. Polsinelli, Matteo, Cinque, Luigi, Placidi, Giuseppe. A Light CNN for Detecting COVID-19 From CT Scans of the Chest. *Pattern Recognition Letters*, 140, 95–100, 2020.

55. Khan, A. I., Shah, J. L., Bhat, M. M. CoroNet: A Deep Neural Network for Detection and Diagnosis of COVID-19 From Chest X-Ray Images. *Computer Methods and Programs in Biomedicine*, 196, 105581, 2020.

56. Heidari, Morteza, Mirniaharikandehei, Seyedehnafiseh, Khuzani, Abolfazl Zargari, Danala, Gopichandh, Qiu, Yuchen, Zheng, Bin. Improving the Performance of CNN to Predict the Likelihood of COVID-19 Using Chest X-Ray Images With Preprocessing Algorithms. *International Journal of Medical Informatics*, 144, 104284, 2020.

57. https://www.kaggle.com/c/stat946winter2021/overview.

58. https://www.kaggle.com/datasets/paultimothymooney/chest-xray-pneumonia.

59. https://www.kaggle.com/datasets/tawsifurrahman/tuberculosis-tb-chest-xray-dataset.

60. Telagam, Nagarjuna, Venkata Kranti, B., Devarasetti, Nikhil Chandra. Cardiovascular Disease Prediction Using Deep Neural Network for Older People. In *Deep Learning for Targeted Treatments: Transformation in Healthcare*, 369–406, 2022.

61. Telagam, N., Kandasamy, N. Review of the Medical Internet of Things-Based RFID Security Protocols. In *Nanoelectronic Devices for Hardware and Software Security* (pp. 163–178). CRC Press, 2021.

62. Telagam, N., Ajitha, D., Kandasamy, N. Review on Hardware Attacks and Security Challenges in IoT Edge Nodes. In *Security of Internet of Things Nodes: Challenges, Attacks, and Countermeasures*, 211, 2021.

63. Chakraborty, C., Othman, S. B., Almalki, F. A., Sakli, H. FC-SEEDA: Fog Computing-Based Secure and Energy Efficient Data Aggregation Scheme for Internet of Healthcare Things. *Neural Computing & Applications*, 2023. DOI: 10.1007/s00521-023-08270-0.

64. Ben Othman, Soufiene, Bahattab, Abdullah Ali, Trad, Abdelbasset, Youssef, Habib. PEERP: A Priority-Based Energy-Efficient Routing Protocol for Reliable Data Transmission in Healthcare Using the IoT. *The 15th International Conference on Future Networks and Communications (FNC)*, Leuven, Belgium, 9–12 August 2020.

65. Ben Othman, Soufiene, Almalki, Faris A., Chakraborty, Chinmay, Sakli, Hedi. Privacy-Preserving Aware Data Aggregation for IoT-Based Healthcare With Green Computing Technologies. *Computers and Electrical Engineering*, 101, 108025, 2022. DOI: 10.1016/j.compeleceng.2022.108025.

3 Analysis of Machine Learning and Deep Learning in Health Informatics, and Their Application

*Tharuni Gelli, Challa Sri Gouri, D Ajitha,
Nagarjuna Telegam, and Ben Othman Soufiene*

3.1 INTRODUCTION

Machine learning and deep learning artificial intelligence (AI) models are playing a beneficial role in health informatics. But the use cases are not limited to medical research; they can also be integrated with clinical decision-making support and risk assessment by following patient insights with high predictive analysis. Since the beginning, AI has made a huge impact in many fields including business, gaming, manufacturing, automobiles, and education. But it is evident that in the near future, AI can be completely incorporated into healthcare services. Neural networks in medical diagnosis can perform classification, detection, segmentation, and registration for complete diagnosis with precision medication. AI can also be used in data mining, data acquisition, follow-up planning, and aided reporting. In earlier iterations, rule-based algorithms were popularly used for medical diagnoses, but there are various drawbacks to those algorithms such as accuracy interpretation, high cost, and continuous changes in the system. However, in recent years modern AI-based prediction systems have brought a revolutionary change in the medical field with their versatility in using various techniques of data extraction in any complex environment. To bring together all the aforementioned details, AI specialists must put focus on the structure of AI models and consider AI strengths and weaknesses to improve performance in health informatics.

3.2 BASICS OF AI AND ANN

The artificial neural network (ANN) is considered a subclass of AI. It mimics the human neuron system in predicting the output from the given input. In 1957, the first

DOI: 10.1201/9781003366249-3

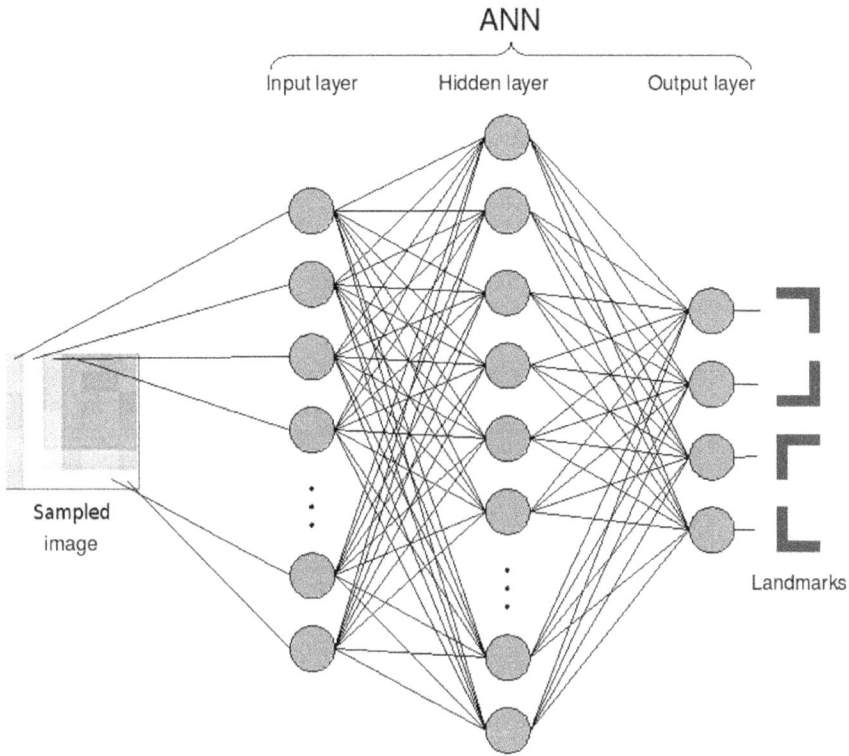

FIGURE 3.1 Architecture of ANN.

neural network prototype, called perceptron, was created by Frank Rosenblatt [1]. The main aim of ANN is to take low-level input data and predict high-level output. It consists of a huge number of interconnected nodes that carry information. The ANN with many layers (depth) is the best-known sophisticated implementation of AI that can process data and recognize patterns using a set of algorithms. As shown in Figure 3.1, the layers in the network are the input layer, hidden layer, and output layer. The function of the input layer is to take information from the surrounding environment, which helps the model derive conclusions and give output. The hidden layer consists of a set of neurons that performs computations on the derived data; generally, any number of hidden layers can be present in the algorithm. The output layer, which comprises one or more nodes, its function is to make conclusions from the computed data. So, the three layers of the ANN follow the forward propagation mechanism by following the whole process.

3.2.1 SUPERVISED LEARNING

Supervised learning is one of the approaches for creating artificial intelligence, where an algorithm is fed with labeled training data so that system can predict particular output. The underlying patterns can be detected by the system until it finds the relationships among the given input to give accurate output. There are two phases: training and testing. During system training, the labeled datasets instruct the model to relate output to a particular input value. In the testing phase, the system is fed with test data, but labels are not revealed to the model. The system on its own will perform algorithms on the unlabeled data and predict the output. Comparing the performance with humans, medical image processing using supervised learning has shown exceptional results [2, 3]. To use supervised learning in neural network algorithms, the model should be trained to reach target accuracy.

The following determines the level of accuracy in supervised learning:

1) Large datasets for training the model for yielding higher accuracy, because samples determine how well the algorithm performs while testing new cases.
2) The data used for training must be cleaned and balanced. Any duplicates in the data can skew the model's understanding.
3) One major issue is sometimes the model can suffer from overfitting, i.e., high accuracy obtained by overtuning to a particular dataset is paradoxically not a good indication. These systems are unreliable in real time as they can't be interfaced with generalized applications.

Results obtained by supervised learning are of two kinds: classification and regression.

3.2.1.1 Classification Algorithms

The algorithm aims to sort the given inputs into classes or categories based on the labels specified in the data. However, classification can be implemented in many ways, such as binary, multiclass, and multilabel algorithms. For example, classification in the medical field can be used for diabetes disease using a support vector machine (SVM) along with a radial basis function which improves performance parameters. It can be used to detect heart disease with data mining techniques and tuberculosis using the decision tree algorithm. The most popular algorithms of classification used in health informatics are CART, C4.5, C5.0, ID3, and SVM. C4.5 gives higher accuracy in the prediction of breast cancer and prognosis among all the available classification algorithms [4].

3.2.1.2 Regression Algorithms

The main aim of the model is to find the mathematical relation between the given input and output data. Based on the given predictor variables, the model finds the correlation among variables and predicts the output variables. Regression algorithms are used along with classification in medical analysis. For example, in an analysis of elderly people to determine the length of hospital stay, first, the stay was measured in days using regression and then grouped by weeks using classification analysis for prediction. Usage of these tools and techniques in the orthopedic department will be a scorecard for doctors by reducing overall resources, time, and cost utilized [5].

In conclusion, when choosing a supervised learning algorithm, things to consider are bias, variance, and complexity of the model. Also, ensure enough flexibility of the model and the learning capability of the system. For implementing the model in sensitive areas such as health care, accuracy, redundancy, and heterogeneity of data should be analyzed before an algorithm is chosen.

3.2.2 Unsupervised Learning

Unsupervised learning uses machine learning algorithms for uncovering hidden patterns for data grouping, considering the similarities and differences in data provided without human intervention. This clustering process enables the model to be implemented in image recognition, data analysis, and customer segmentation.

The following tasks can be achieved using unsupervised learning:

1) Clustering can be done by grouping unlabeled data considering their features. These algorithms are used for processing unclassified or raw data objects into clusters by patterns in the given information. The different types of clustering algorithms include hierarchical, probabilistic, exclusive, and overlapping clustering.

a) *Hierarchical clustering*: Hierarchical cluster analysis (HCA) is an unsupervised hierarchical clustering that can be classified as agglomerative or divisive clustering, but their processes work in opposite ways. Agglomerative clustering follows a bottom-up approach, by which the isolation of data points is done by grouping at initial stages and then merging repeatedly until a single cluster is formed based on their similarities. In the case of divisive clustering, it follows a top-down approach. Here the data points are separated at each iteration by breaking down a single cluster based on its differences. This algorithm is not as popular as agglomerative.

b) *Exclusive and overlapping clustering*: Exclusive clustering is a mode of clustering where a particular data point belongs to only a single cluster, which constituently results in hard clustering. K-means clustering is an example of exclusive clustering, whereas overlapping clustering allows data points to appear in multiple clusters, which have separate degrees of membership. Soft k-means is an example of overlapping clustering.

c) *Probabilistic clustering*: In this clustering mode the data, points are clustered according to their likelihood to which particular distribution they belong. It helps in solving soft clustering and density estimation problems. The Gaussian mixture model (GMM) is popularly used in probabilistic clustering.

2) The association rule is based on rules to determine the relationships among variables in the data provided. A priori algorithm is the most widely used association rule. This algorithm uses the hash tree with a breadth-first operation that counts items and navigates through the dataset. For example, different kinds of recommendation engines use this algorithm in implementation.

3) Dimensionality reduction is used when large datasets are fed into machine learning models in order to produce high accuracy, which in turn impacts the model with overfitting. It reduces the dataset to a manageable size without affecting the characteristics of the dataset. Principal component analysis, singular value decomposition, and autoencoders are some examples of dimensionality reduction methods [6].

In conclusion, unsupervised learning plays a vital role in medical imaging by integrating all the aforementioned algorithms in radiology and pathology diagnosis by image classification, detection, and segmentation to ensure the correctness of patient health reports.

3.2.3 SEMI-SUPERVISED LEARNING

Semi-supervised learning is a middle ground between supervised and unsupervised learning, which combines labeled and a huge amount of unlabeled data. The main aim of this learning is to overcome the drawbacks occurred due to supervised and unsupervised learning. In supervised learning, the data should be labeled, which is expensive as hand-labeling must be done by data scientists or machine learning specialists. Whereas unsupervised learning has limited application, introducing semi-supervised learning can be an exceptional replacement in these cases by using clustering for similar data along with the unsupervised learning model. This helps in labeling the unlabeled data. The process flow of semi-supervised learning is as follows: it uses pseudo-labeling for training the model with fewer labeled data. At first, the model is trained similarly to supervised learning with less training data until higher accuracy is obtained. Then unlabeled data with pseudo labels are fed into the model, but the results may not be accurate. Now pseudo labels and labels with training data are linked together and similarly, the labeled dataset and unlabeled dataset as well. Again, the model is trained from step 1 in order to reduce errors and improve the model's overall accuracy. Existing models of semi-supervised learning are random forest methods, which are replaced by graph-based entropy to overcome the challenges in medical imaging [7].

Application of semi-supervised learning in the medical sector is imminent; protein sequence classification requires highly active human intervention and now that can be completely replaced with semi-supervised learning.

3.2.4 REINFORCEMENT LEARNING

Reinforcement learning is a specialized category of machine learning and deep learning combined. This learning algorithm is applied in potentially complex or uncertain environments where the agent is trained until it achieves the goal by employing a trial-and-error method; it gets either rewards or penalties based on its performance. But the ultimate goal of the system is to maximize its rewards. It almost resembles superhuman skills at the end of training, because its task is to maximize its leverage power. These features made reinforcement learning one of the most powerful algorithms in AI. Human involvement is minimal in training the model; most of it is focused on preventing exploitation of the system.

Challenges in reinforcement learning include the following:

1) The simulation environment is one of the main challenges that define the complexity of training the model. It depends on the application where the model is going to be applied; in some applications, building a realistic simulating environment is very difficult. This makes the algorithms unreliable to implement in real time.
2) The only way to train the model is through rewards and penalties, which make the model forget the old knowledge gained by acquiring new knowledge. This phenomenon is known as catastrophic forgetting [8].
3) Another challenge of reinforcement learning is local optimum. In this case, the model acquires high rewards but not in an optimal way. By not performing the task specified, sometimes the model gets maximum rewards by optimizing the prize.

One of the promising applications of reinforcement learning in medical research is the precise musculoskeletal model. This model was designed by the Stanford neuromuscular biomechanics laboratory to model the human walk more easily and efficiently by automatically recognizing human body locomotion.

3.2.5 EVOLUTIONARY LEARNING

Evolutionary learning is also known as evolutionary computation for classification because classification algorithm uses many evolutionary machine learning techniques. It consists of evolutionary algorithms, which are highly heuristic and inspired by natural evolution.

There are two key factors in this learning:

1. *Variational reproduction*: This factor is used to randomly generate a population from the search space, and an objective function value is computed for each sample. The selection operator is used to select specific values of the computed objective function and select those samples for the next step. The variation operator is used to make additional samples from the selected samples from the search space.
2. *Superior selection*: This factor selects the best solution by eliminating relatively poor solutions from the population produced.

Reproduction and removal of solutions are repeated until the stop criterion is met.

3.2.5.1 Evolutionary Cycle

Whenever an evolutionary algorithm enters into the first step of the cycle, the reproduction of new solutions takes place using mutation and recombination. This process of using mutation and recombination is called crossover. Mutation works like a random function, which generates new functions from old ones. The recombination function combines formed solutions to make new ones. The accuracy of newly generated solutions is measured using the fitness function, by which the model ends the cycle when the criterion is met, such as no improvement in solution using predefined iterations, resources running out of budget, or the predefined quality of the solution being met.

In conclusion, evolutionary learning is applied in machine learning algorithms to solve optimization problems in complicated environments, for example, in artificial neural networks, optimizing architectures and learning rules. In biomedical applications, evolutionary machine learning techniques are developed for gene mapping, analysis of DNA, structure prediction, gene sequence analysis, and biomarker identification. Many evolutionary machine learning methods are also used in the prediction of the 3D structure of protein, materials design, and drug discovery [9].

3.2.6 Deep Learning

Deep learning is a neural network that is a subset of machine learning that tries to simulate the human brain. Using multiple nonlinear transformations of multiprocessing layers, this method does the data processing function [10]. It can learn from large amounts of data, which includes hidden layers for optimizing the accuracy of predicted output.

3.2.6.1 Working of Deep Learning

In fields such as bioinformatics, computer vision, natural language processing, and speech and audio recognition, deep learning has had a remarkable influence in recent years [11]. Three main factors for deep learning are inputs, weights, and bias, which work together for the recognition, classification, and prediction of outputs.

1. At the interconnection of multiple layers, the output of one layer is fed as input to another. The model refines and optimizes the prediction through each layer. The visible layers of the deep learning network are the input and output layers. Input is fed through the input layer and prediction is taken at the output layer. This progression is known as forward propagation.
2. There is one more method known as backward propagation; an algorithm used in this is gradient descent. It calculates the errors in outputs and uses the bias function for adjusting the error by moving backward. Overall, the algorithms become more accurate by minimizing errors.

There are two types of neural networks:

1) *Convolutional neural networks*: Widely used for image classification or recognition, or object or pattern detection in computer vision.
2) *Recurrent neural networks*: Used in speech recognition and natural language processing.

The usage of efficient algorithms for replacing manual acquisition techniques used in semi-supervised and unsupervised feature extraction is the main advantage of deep learning [12]. Deep learning techniques can be implemented in the medical sector for digitalization. For radiology, medical imaging with neural networks can be used.

3.3   ROLE OF MACHINE LEARNING IN MEDICAL IMAGING

Machine learning is widely used in medical imaging. With the help of medical imaging, one can analyze medical images by recognizing the various patterns applied to them. Most of the time, people fail in understanding its perfect application which results in its wrong usage. There is a stepwise procedure in the application of machine learning for medical imaging. In the first step, we usually start the process of computing the various features of an image, which are used for the predictions of the diagnosis methods. The type of learning that is often used in robot control or game playing is reinforcement learning [13]. Every machine learning algorithm has advantages and disadvantages. The analysis must be given high priority.

A new medical image segmentation architecture, U-Net, was proposed in the year 2015 [14]. With the improved technology and the results obtained from various analyses of medical imaging using machine learning, one can find the assurance to improve the health of the patients by constant monitoring and perfect diagnosis. Even though we are getting highly improved results through these methods, there are certain challenges with the data and the methods that are developed for assessing. In every step of this process, we encounter many potential biases and problems. In this section, we will explore a few algorithms used for medical imaging and some of the problems raised during their application.

Precision medicine prediction is one of the most popular techniques used. It is an initiative in which analysis of an individual's genes, environment, and lifestyle is done. This can be considered as a special help to doctors to predict which kind of treatment helps which kind of people. This makes their process of treatment much easier. Using this process, one can develop methods of treatment and prevention strategies for a person. This term seems new to most of us, but this concept started early in the history of medicine.

The most widely used model of machine learning for medical imaging is supervised learning in which we train the model with the help of various datasets. With the help of the data collected, machine learning algorithms will help us in finding multidimensional solutions. Machine learning not only helps in solution finding, but it also proves to be very efficient in collecting and organizing data. The various applications in the medical field that are designed with the help of medical imaging can be stated as follows:

1. Predicting the outbreak of various kinds of viruses
2. Maintaining health records
3. Improving clinical trials
4. Developing various drugs
5. Radiotherapy

In classification, the most used classifier for machine learning is SVM. Using the SVM algorithm, one can create the best line or the decision boundary that is used to segregate the available n-dimensional space into classes. The extreme cases used are known as support vectors. This method is used mainly for the process of image classification. The two types of SVM are:

1. Linear SVM
2. Nonlinear SVM

The kernel trick gives us a brief idea of kernel principal component analysis and kernel ridge regression. Kernels are defined as similarity measures on the space x of inputs. Kernel methods are used for the pattern analysis. This approach can be used for any domain. It offers a kind of flexible approach to the design of learning systems.

To improve the accuracy of breast cancer detection algorithms, a challenge named Dream using digital mammography was organized in 2017 [15]. To conclude, machine learning in medical diagnosis can help in decreasing the risk of incorrect examination. It improves the patient's confidence. One can easily predict the outcomes of various kinds of treatments and can decide which holds the most promise. With this, the patient can get a complete analysis report of their health, which helps them in determining their health condition in the best possible manner.

3.4   DEEP LEARNING IN MEDICAL IMAGING

Deep learning is a domain that has a wide range of applications in the medical field. Deep learning has various special features, including versatility, high generalization capacity, multidisciplinary uses, and high performance, which made the entire scientific community focus on the possibilities. The concept of deep learning starts with the simple aspects of artificial neural networks and then extends to attention models, convolutional structures, and recurrent structures. The important aspects of deep learning that are used especially in medical imaging are medical image classification and segmentation.

In today's world, deep learning has a great impact on the field of diagnosis. We can detect the abnormalities in X-ray images, and analyze and classify them into different types of diseases. With the help of deep learning, one can get accurate results in less assessment time. For the prediction of Alzheimer disease, a new model was developed using 18F-FDG PET using deep learning techniques [16]. Especially in radiology, these techniques play a key role. Let us discuss the steps used in deep learning in detail.

1. *Image classification*: The process of image classification starts with the identification of the type of malignancy. As we have images of various sizes and different patterns of diseases, it becomes complicated for the CNN model to be directly trained with these kinds of patterns. To provide deeper insights into data, conventional statistical analysis along with ANN can be

used [17]. The major challenge with deep learning is that it requires a large amount of data for the process of reducing overfitting and enhancing performance. It becomes hard to analyze a few medical images. We must opt for the best techniques to deal with small datasets. The combined features of the radiomic and the multilayer perceptron network classifier are perfectly applicable to magnetic resonance imaging (MRI) protocols for small datasets.

2. *Object identification*: The process of finding and categorizing the objects is termed object identification. In the process of detection of biomedical images, box coordinates are used to locate a patient's lesions. This technique is broadly categorized into two types. They are as follows:
   - Region proposal-based algorithm
   - Regression method as one-stage network

   In the region proposal-based algorithm, various patches are extracted with the help of a selective search algorithm from the input images. After the completion of this process, a decision will be made by the trained model about the existence of multiple images in each patch, and classification is done based on the region of interest. The advantage of this technique is it increases the speed of detection.

In the other technique, called the regression method as one-stage network, the box coordinates and class probabilities are directly found and detected from the image pixels in whole images. The region proposal approach is considered better in terms of its accuracy, whereas the regression method as one-stage network proved to be efficient in terms of speed and accuracy.

3. *Image segmentation and registration*: In segmentation and registration, these deep learning techniques are proved to be much more efficient. Methods such as dependent thresholding and close-contour methods are used to improve the performance of targeted segmentation. The excessive number of deaths is reduced with the help of breast cancer imaging, for early detection screening is considered as one of the best options to increase survival rates [18]. At the same time, registration is also applied to the segmentation. Many kinds of attempts are made for the process of segmentation of tumors and other structures in various parts. Deep learning networks are being continuously developed for the process of improving segmentation.

4. *Image generation*: Obtaining high-quality, balanced datasets with various kinds of labels is challenging. Generated images in the studies are used for the process of data augmentation. Anomaly detection in medical imaging is the most interesting application of generative adversarial networks (GANs). In synthetic images, the process of classification and segmentation accuracies is important.

5. *Image transformation*: Recent studies show that CNN is the most frequently used.

The deep learning development framework is a software development framework that is also booming. Deep learning is a technology that can operate on any kind of dataset that does not require human intervention. With the evolution of convolutional neural networks, there has been a tremendous change in the field of deep learning since 2012 [19]. After the enhancements that happened in the field of deep learning, it is being used to deal with a variety of image problems. With these advancements, many doctors are using medical image processing and recognition is being performed with the help of various machine learning techniques. In the current scenario, we are using deep learning technologies mainly for medical image classification and segmentation.

To conclude this section, we realize that deep learning has become one of the most important tools for the process of analyzing the image. This technology is being implemented successfully in detection, segmentation, registration, and classification. As we are aware, deep learning deals with a large number of ideas. With the various characteristics in the medical field, there is a high scope of big data, which makes it even more suitable for these applications. Deep learning is being used for various applications in the medical field such as ophthalmology, neuroimaging, and ultrasound. An obvious solution to overcome small datasets and grow large ones quickly is to share data across medical centers. Sharing data through medical centers enables us to initiate the rapid growth of large datasets, but with the existing data privacy policies, this seems to be a little difficult [20]. Deep learning is mostly inseparable from the various kinds of medical practices that are performed by a doctor. Now we have a large number of algorithms that have diverse uses that work efficiently in completing the task we planned for. There are certain diseases that we cannot analyze using these techniques. This can be considered as one of the challenges that can be used as a step for building potential solutions. Deep learning proves to be efficient not only in the detection of common diseases but also can help us in finding rare diseases. Now with the advancements, we are more focused on a software framework that makes our tasks even simpler.

3.5   APPROACH WITH NEURAL NETWORKS

3.5.1   Classification

Classification for medical imaging has two methods: one that follows traditional models and another that uses deep learning models. Out of all the deep learning methods for image classification, the convolutional neural network is a widely used structure. The AlexNet-based CNN model, proposed by Krizhevsky et al. in 2012, had remarkable results in image classification. From then, deep learning in image classification applications began to rise. The major challenge of CNN is overfitting, which was overcome by using global average pooling in the year 2013 by Lin et al. GoogLeNet and VGGNet models have improved the overall accuracy of the ImageNet dataset in the year 2014. In later years, a few more versions of GoogLeNet were introduced to improve the models' performance further [21]. One more challenge in CNN is the fixed input size. To overcome this challenge, the spatial pyramid pooling technique was introduced. Advancement in deep learning techniques is continued by introducing residual networks, which overcome the model degradation problem.

The AlexNet algorithm uses an eight-layer network structure: five layers of convolution and three layers that are connected. Convolution is performed in convolutional layers to maximize the pooling performed and to reduce the size of the data. After the completion of convolution in the five layers, the output in the form of a feature matrix is sent to the fully connected layers. In the first fully connected layer, a network dropout operation is performed with 4,096 kernels. The last two layers produce the prediction results with float-type data output.

The steps of classification involve segregation or prediction of whether something belongs to a particular class or not. As discussed earlier, there are many types of classifications; predicting something to know which of two categories it falls into is known as binary classification. Multiclass classification has more than two categories of classes. Multilabel classification has more than one label for one category. Similar patterns that are in the training data are analyzed with the help of data correlation, analysis, and clustering algorithms [22].

Steps involved in classification:

1) Import the necessary libraries.
2) Create the dataset.
3) Based on the dataset chosen, define labels. Example: Binary classification (1 or 0).
4) Now visualization of data should be done so that we can know what kind of predicting model we have to build.
5) While building the neural network, make sure that both the input feature and output feature size are the same.
6) Model the neural networks by creating, compiling, and fitting a model.
7) After completing the preceding steps, the model accuracy should be checked. If its performance is poor, visualized the data again and modify the number of layers or the optimizer function until you obtain the best performance.

In conclusion, in the case of binary classification of nonlinear datasets for better accuracy and optimization, one should use nonlinear activation functions.

3.5.1.1 Image Classification

Image classification classifies and assigns labels by grouping the images or vectors within the image. There are two types: single label and multilabel. In single label, each image is assigned to only one label, whereas multiple labels can be given to a single image in the case of multilabel classification.

Working of image classification:

1) *Preprocessing*: This involves the preparation of data through various steps. Here removal of duplicates, cutting of irrelevant data, filtering of unwanted outliers, detecting missing data, and fixing structural errors will be done on the data to make it ready for processing in the AI model so that no

inaccuracies can occur. This whole process is referred to as the cleaning or cleansing of data. To set up the best AI model for classification, well-organized datasets play a major role.

2) *Object detection*: This helps in locating objects within the image. This does segmentation on the picture to determine the location of objects in it.

3) *Object recognition and training*: In this stage, the model is given labels as well as training data so that it recognizes the patterns within the data and learns from them for classifying the test data.

4) *Object classification*: Here it classifies the images into predefined classes by comparing patterns within the image.

Finally, the model can be integrated with AI workflow. Example models for image classification are SVM, bag-of-words, k-nearest neighbor, logistic regression, and face landmark estimation. To obtain better classification and generalization results, fuzzy system-based approaches are applied in ANNs [23].

3.5.1.2   Video Classification

Video classification differs from image classification such that the video is a set of frames in which the CNN model is applied to all frames of the video. As each frame passes through the model, they are individually classified, and based on probability one label is chosen and that will be given to frame output. Model prediction using multiple video frames is used for the calculation of accuracy [24]. Applying CNN of image classification to video classification can lead to prediction flickering. This can be prevented by using K predictions while predicting each frame. The average of those K predictions can be done, and then a label assigned to the frame.

3.5.2   DETECTION

During classification, one image can fit into more than one class. But with object detection, we have to find all the objects in a given image and recognize them. In this stage a new term is introduced, region of interest, in which we need to make boundary boxes for the detected objects in the image. The image is considered in a hierarchal graph using the selective search algorithm, by which five similarity criteria images are iteratively segmented; a superpixel algorithm is used for this process [25]. U-Net is considered one of the best latent representations, which is used by autoencoder architecture in the medical imaging domain [26]. Object detection is a combination of both image classification and object localization. After classification, the image undergoes object localization which locates the position of the object in the image. There may be multistage detection or single-stage detection in object detection.

- *Multistage detection*: Here there will be two stages for detection purposes. In the first stage, extraction of a region of the image is done, and then classification for obtaining the final result.
- *Single-stage detection*: Here the feature extraction and classification are done at the same time.

3.5.3 SEGMENTATION

Image segmentation is one of the most important applications of deep learning. In segmentation, image parts are clustered as per the segment they belong. The image is divided into certain regions considering properties such as texture and brightness [27, 28]. Segmentation involves pixel-level classification, where images are partitioned into segments based on their pixel values. The combination of mutually related elements is called texture [29]. The spatial relation between pixels is structure and pixel intensity properties are used to measure tone [30, 31].

The approach may be semantic or instance segmentation. If it is classified based on semantic labels, then it's known as semantic segmentation. Otherwise, the partitioning of objects is done, which is referred to as instance segmentation. The region of interest is used to represent the detected region of a medical image effectively with the help of feature extraction [32]. Traditional methods for image segmentation comprise k-means, histogram based, region growing, and thresholding. The most popular and advanced algorithms of segmentation are sparsity based, Markov random, active contours, and graph cut methods.

In medical imaging, segmentation can be applied for measuring tissue volumes and boundary extraction of tumors. It can also be used for detection of fast-spreading diseases such as coronavirus.

3.5.4 REGISTRATION

Image analysis involves registration as a base concept because registration calculates the transform function value in which the coordinate system moves from one image to another. Computation results are made efficient and semantic image meanings are dealt with effectively [33]. In medical diagnosis, various image modality properties are analyzed and their complementary information is brought together.

Based on the nature of registration, the methods are categorized into intrinsic and extrinsic [34]. There are various frameworks for the registration process, but the base framework is the same.

1) Creation of synthetic data from existing datasets.
2) Generation of truthful data that can be used for training and testing purposes.
3) CNN and deep learning methods can be used for the extraction of multimodal images as registers.
4) Automatic image registration through classification of image modalities.

The presence of transformation parameters, which are easily computed, helps these methods to work without complex optimization algorithms [35]. Image registration can be applied in medical diagnosis for treatment planning and predictive guided surgery. For example, consider CT, PET, or MRI scans of a patient during different times by showing the results of surgery by considering the pre- and postoperative analysis of the scan.

3.6 AI APPLICATIONS IN MEDICAL IMAGING

Artificial intelligence is the kind of technology where computerized algorithms are used to evaluate complex and complicated data. AI finds a huge number of applications in medical imaging. For tasks based on regression, when the output variable is continuous, and for classification-based tasks, when the output variable is categorical supervised, machine learning is used [36]. Among the various applications offered by AI in medical, imaging diagnostic imaging and mounting attention are the most important. Studies have shown that these computerized algorithms have high accuracy, sensitivity, and good specificity to detect radiographic abnormalities. Radiomic feature extraction and selection are considered AI approaches for detecting lung cancer [37].

The application of AI in medical imaging is still being studied extensively. Since it has shown good sensitivity and high accuracy, it is expected that it can be suitable for even tissue-based detection and characterization. However, people, especially radiologists, fear that they might be replaced by AI. Natural selection and natural genetics are imitated with the development of an algorithm known as stochastic search [38]. The following sections explore various areas where AI is being used extensively, its importance in the medical field, and user satisfaction.

3.6.1 AI AND DESIGN THINKING

As AI has become a part of our lives, there are other ways in which we can benefit through AI. Many researchers are in the process of experimenting with AI with the application they want but are not realizing its potential in adding business value. AI is a powerful technological tool. Design thinking is a creative process of crafting business solutions in a stepwise process. When we combine AI with design thinking, then the result is creativity driven by powerful technology to provide optimum results and create business value. Incidental radiographic findings that reflect malignancy are termed adrenal nodules [39]. In this aspect, we particularly focus on how design thinking can be applied to projects that deal with AI technology.

In this methodology, everyone is encouraged to observe problems around them and then apply the approach of AI combined with that of design thinking to create a solution that creates and captures value. When compared with the human reader, the process of analyzing brain MRI with the machine learning application is more efficient [40]. In an AI ecosystem along with the technology, there are certain stakeholders including users, consumers or customers, organizations, and businesses. This approach helps everyone to understand the various functionalities exhibited by AI.

To start any project, choosing the best and appropriate methodology is considered to be crucial. It has great potential in helping us to find the problems faced by the target groups. AI-based solutions have become very common in every field. In AI design thinking, our primary focus will be on the process of designing AI systems that have the capability of working in an unpredictable environment with very few resources. There is no universal approach to design thinking in AI. Accountability is considered to be very important for AI-based products. Deep learning processes will not follow logic and explanations all the time. Radiologists must understand that application of AI will make them even more productive [41, 42]. So, we must make sure that there is logic behind how AI works in certain situations.

The various stages of design thinking in AI are as follows:

1. Empathize
2. Define
3. Ideate
4. Prototype
5. Test

To sum up this discussion, design thinking is the most powerful and efficient procedure to be used with products that are developed based on AI technology. To implement this, we need a team that is reliable and provides the best testing and development of a product to provide accurate results.

3.6.2 DATA USAGE AND DEVELOPMENT

The availability of a large amount of data helps in using the technologies to retrieve valuable information in medical images. Artificial intelligence is one such revolutionary technology in the field of medicine. The moment we develop robust algorithms, it is clear that we need data in the form of medical images. Before the application of the AI algorithms, we must get ready with the appropriate data.

Let us examine the various steps involved in the preparation of data.

1. Image acquisition
2. Image de-identification
3. Data curation
4. Image storage
5. Image annotation

In the first step, data is acquired. After image acquisition, it is important to take care that the user privacy is maintained and their data is removed; this stage is termed image de-identification. For this step, permissions must be received from the clinical sites' ethical committees. This is to ensure that local data protection regulations are followed. Data curation is performed to check that the linked or associated data such as headers are correct and there are no errors. For the perfect management and storage of data, a guiding principle called FAIR is used, which stands for findable, accessible, interoperable, and reusable. Image annotation is used to describe the boundaries considered significant for both the training and testing of the AI algorithms. These are the various steps that are involved in the preparation of data before the application of AI algorithms.

To perform each step, there are certain tools to make the process easier. The tools that are used for the process of deidentification are called patient privacy-preserving tools as they are meant to safeguard the user's information. Patient data is usually considered the most sensitive resource. This information is categorized as protected health information and personally identifiable information. In medical imaging, four kinds of file formatting are used, including DICOM (Digital Imaging and Communications in Medicine). For each stage, we have certain sets of tools that are used to ensure the perfect curation of data.

As per medical experts, AI is widely used for general as well as medical imaging. There are still certain issues that need to be addressed when we apply AI. Thus far, AI was successful in completely replacing humans in the process of image segmentation. It also plays a very crucial role when it comes to decision-making. Also without AI technology, it would be very difficult to collect and organize these huge amounts of data optimally. Even though we have many open-source tools for data preparation, certain challenges should be addressed. They are as follows:

1. Anonymization
2. Curation
3. Annotation
4. Storage

Along with the data preparation, certain aspects must be taken into consideration. They are data augmentation and synthesis, federated learning, ethical issues in AI, and uncertainty estimation. So, before starting the analysis of any AI model, data preparation plays a very crucial role and forms the basis of the entire process.

3.6.3 Implementation of Idea

3.6.3.1 Breast Cancer Prediction

In hematologic diseases, cancer diagnosis has become a challenging task for medical practitioners. Machine learning, with its highly predictive nature, can be implemented for detecting breast cancer in its early stages. Diagnosis and analysis using supervised machine learning can decrease the percentage of breast cancer patients and death rates.

Various methods of predicting breast cancer are the usage of biosensors such as tissue based, optical, sensors, and piezoelectric. These biosensors continuously monitor biomarkers, which are placed inside the body. They detect any tumors by finding abnormalities via biomolecular analytics. Screening techniques can also be used for prediction, but nanosized molecules can't be seen by the naked eye or detected in the early stages. Data analytics is also another approach to cancer prediction that uses big data or cross databases techniques. All the aforementioned methods have a few drawbacks such as sensitivity and cost.

3.6.3.2 Proposed Methodology

Many machine learning algorithms are being implemented for breast cancer prediction such as decision trees, logistic regression, SVM, and KNN classifiers.

Efficiencies with these algorithms are not accurate. The proposed model uses the XGBoost classifier of machine learning.

Figure 3.2 depicts the whole process flow for this prediction. In the first step, we need to import all the required libraries such as NumPy, Seaborn, pandas, and matplotlib. Then the breast dataset is loaded as a CSV file.

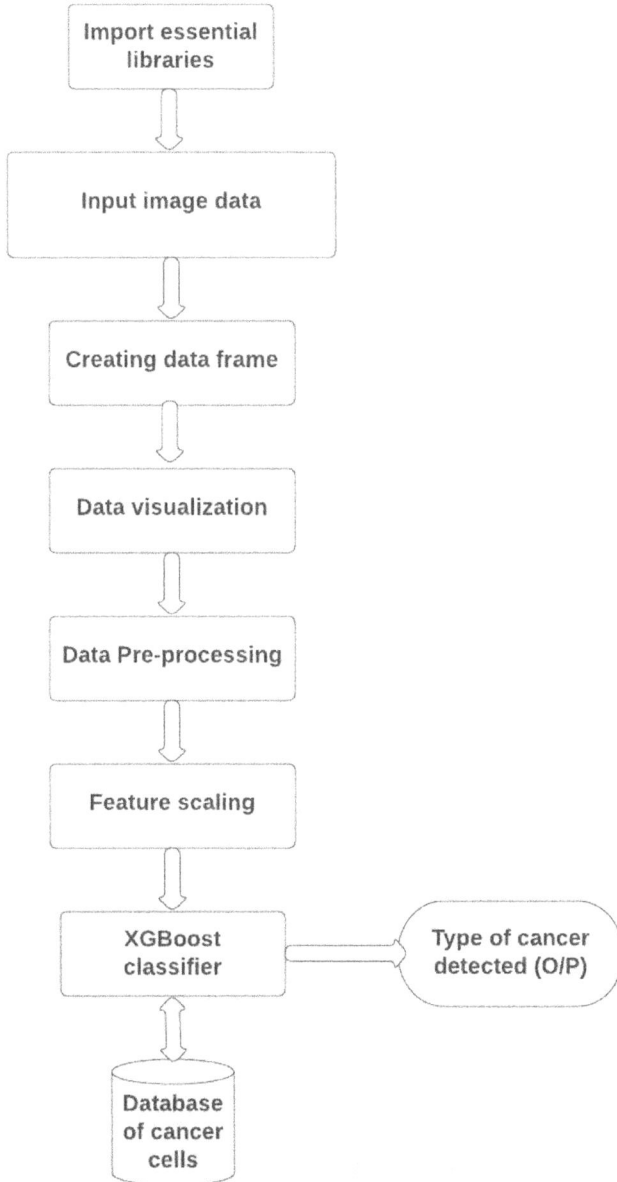

FIGURE 3.2 Process flowchart.

1) A data frame with feature names is created. Numeric values for extracted features are assigned, such as 0 for benign tumors and 1 for malignant tumors.
2) In the data visualization stage, a pair plot is drawn for breast cancer data and numeric distribution.
3) Splitting of training and testing data is done in the data preprocessing stage. Then all the units and magnitudes are converted into one unit.
4) Lat, the data is fed into the XGBoost classifier, and breast cancer is predicted, and whether it's benign or malignant is given as the output.

3.6.3.3 Results

From Figure 3.3 we can observe that the obtained accuracy using the XGBoost classifier is 98.34%, which shows that this classifier can perform accurate predictions and can be implemented in the detection of breast cancer.

3.6.4 REGULATION OF TECHNOLOGY

AI-based algorithms are used in improving the efficiency, accuracy, and safety of the diagnosis process. The proposed regulatory frameworks have proven to be effective, but there are still many issues that are not addressed by them. The Internet of Things (IoT) application of body sensors is considered to be one of the most advancing technologies [43]. There are many regulatory frameworks for the software to be used in medical applications, but there are gaps that must be filled.

To ensure that safety is maintained and effectiveness is not disturbed, special rules and frameworks have been developed by regulators. On the other hand, these regulations may lead to limited adoption of algorithms. To ensure safety, quality

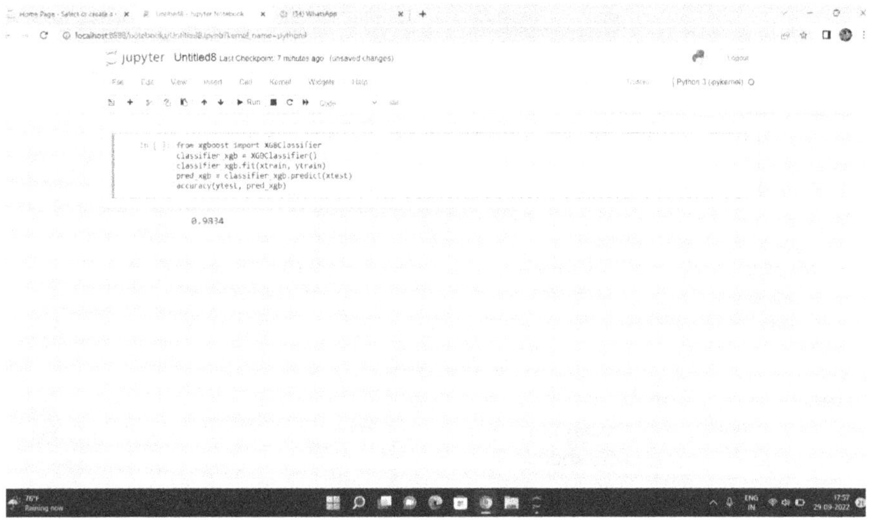

FIGURE 3.3 Observed result for accuracy.

management system principles for SaMD (software as a medical device) applications have been proposed by the International Medical Device Regulators Forum (IMDRF).

These regulatory frameworks address many issues, including the effectiveness of a system and safety. But some of the gaps are:

1. Insufficient characterization of safety and performance elements
2. Unable to assess performance at each installed site
3. Inherent conflicts of interest

To improve performance, fill these gaps, and overcome some of the issues, the following steps can be used.

1. Usually, the algorithm is considered as part and parcel of the diagnostic task. We must ensure that we separate the task of diagnosis from the algorithm.
2. When defining the elements, consider going beyond accuracy.
3. To make sure that the problems are rectified, try dividing or categorizing the evaluation process into discrete steps as follows:
   a. Diagnostic task definition
   b. Capability
   c. Effectiveness in terms of real-world performance
   d. Effectiveness in terms of local validity
4. Durability

To sum up, even though regulators have come up with a variety of frameworks that laid the foundation, there are still certain issues to consider in order to evaluate the model in any kind of unpredictable situation. The aforementioned suggestions can help in increasing performance in terms of efficiency, accuracy, safety, and reliability.

3.6.5 PATIENT EXPERIENCE

When people are suffering from diseases such as cancer and tuberculosis, early detection with accurate results helps. However, the increase in population, poor infrastructure and facilities, and limited caretakers are considered to be the major challenges in the health sector [44]. With improved technologies in the field of AI, we can enhance the user experience. When a patient comes for a consultation, they trust doctors to provide accurate results. The more satisfied the patient, the better the implementation of technology. With more focus on the patient experience, we move toward patient-centric care.

Certain important factors impact a patient's experience. They can be briefly stated as follows:

1. Time taken for getting the appointment
2. Waiting time

3. Comfort during check-ins
4. Navigation
5. Care taken
6. Dealing with priority cases first
7. Correct analysis of disease and proper treatment

For the success of any advancement in the medical field, patient experience is key. AI is bringing major changes to the health sector. This is considered to be an ideal tool. An increase in care time helps in getting the best feedback results. This also develops trust between a doctor and a patient. Larger datasets are required to improve the patient experience with more research and examples. The various technologies being used in the health sector are not completely reliable. Sometimes AI may also lead to incorrect data transmission; this can have an everlasting effect on patient experience [45]. An accurate diagnosis will encourage people to consider their health as a priority and take precautions according to the results. To conclude, the patient experience plays a vital role.

3.7   CONCLUSION

Various technologies are involved in the process of medical imaging, and every technology has its pros and cons. If we could overcome the limitations, we can improve the precision by which diseases are recognized and diagnosed. Considering this factor, we worked on breast cancer prediction using the XGBoost classifier algorithm and found that the proposed algorithm is more efficient than existing ones. With these algorithms, we can get accurate results. This chapter focused on the various ways in which new applications can be developed for existing artificial intelligence models.

3.8   FUTURE SCOPE

Research plays a very important role in the development of various applications in the medical field. With the help of a rich set of algorithms, we can come up with the best applications for efficient diagnosis. Even though much research has been done, we find very little scope in implementing the proposed algorithms. Apart from the computerized algorithms, it's equally important to focus on people's trust as it plays a vital role in acquiring efficient diagnosis. By using certain algorithms, we can increase the efficiency achieved. We are restricted to very narrow applications in this domain, but if we start analyzing and implementing various algorithms, we can explore a wide range of applications.

REFERENCES

1. Rosenblatt, F. (1958). The perceptron: A probabilistic model for information storage and organization in the brain. *Psychological Review, 65*(6), 386.
2. Ker, J., Wang, L., Rao, J., & Lim, T. (2017). Deep learning applications in medical image analysis. *IEEE Access, 6*, 9375–9389.

3. Li, Q., Cai, W., Wang, X., Zhou, Y., Feng, D. D., & Chen, M. (2014, December). Medical image classification with convolutional neural network. In *2014 13th International Conference on Control Automation Robotics & Vision (ICARCV)* (pp. 844–848). IEEE.

4. Venkatesan, E., & Velmurugan, T. (2015). Role of classification algorithms in medical domain: A survey. In *International Conference on Information, System and Convergence Applications*, June (pp. 24–27).

5. Ricciardi, C., Ponsiglione, A. M., Scala, A., Borrelli, A., Misasi, M., Romano, G., … & Improta, G. (2022). Machine learning and regression analysis to model the length of hospital stay in patients with femur fracture. *Bioengineering, 9*(4), 172.

6. Raza, K., & Singh, N. K. (2021). A tour of unsupervised deep learning for medical image analysis. *Current Medical Imaging, 17*(9), 1059–1077.

7. Gu, L., Zhang, X., You, S., Zhao, S., Liu, Z., & Harada, T. (2020). Semi-supervised learning in medical images through graph-embedded random forest. *Frontiers in Neuroinformatics, 14*, 601829.

8. Kaplanis, C., Shanahan, M., & Clopath, C. (2018, July). Continual reinforcement learning with complex synapses. In *International Conference on Machine Learning* (pp. 2497–2506). PMLR.

9. Li, N., Ma, L., Yu, G., Xue, B., Zhang, M., & Jin, Y. (2022). Survey on evolutionary deep learning: Principles, algorithms, applications and open issues. *arXiv Preprint arXiv:2208.10658.*

10. LeCun, Y., Bengio, Y., & Hinton, G. (2015). Deep learning. Nature, *521*(7553), 436–444.

11. Deng, L., & Yu, D. (2014). Deep learning: Methods and applications. *Foundations and Trends® in Signal Processing, 7*(3–4), 197–387.

12. Song, H. A., & Lee, S. Y. (2013, November). Hierarchical representation using NMF. In *International Conference on Neural Information Processing* (pp. 466–473). Springer, Berlin, Heidelberg.

13. Kaelbling, L. P., Littman, M. L., & Moore, A. W. (1996). Reinforcement learning: A survey. *Journal of Artificial Intelligence Research, 4*, 237–285.

14. Ronneberger, O., Fischer, P., & Brox, T. (2015, October). U-Net: Convolutional networks for biomedical image segmentation. In *International Conference on Medical Image Computing and Computer-Assisted Intervention* (pp. 234–241). Springer, Cham.

15. Schaffter, T., Buist, D. S., Lee, C. I., Nikulin, Y., Ribli, D., Guan, … & DM DREAM Consortium. (2020). Evaluation of combined artificial intelligence and radiologist assessment to interpret screening mammograms. *JAMA Network Open, 3*(3), e200265.

16. Ding, Y., Sohn, J. H., Kawczynski, M. G., Trivedi, H., Harnish, R., Jenkins, N. W., … & Franc, B. L. (2019). A deep learning model to predict a diagnosis of Alzheimer disease by using 18F-FDG PET of the brain. *Radiology, 290*(2), 456–464.

17. Balthazar, P., Harri, P., Prater, A., & Safdar, N. M. (2018). Protecting your patients' interests in the era of big data, artificial intelligence, and predictive analytics. *Journal of the American College of Radiology, 15*(3), 580–586.

18. Saadatmand, S., Bretveld, R., Siesling, S., & Tilanus-Linthorst, M. M. (2015). Influence of tumour stage at breast cancer detection on survival in modern times: Population based study in 173 797 patients. *BMJ, 351*, h4901.

19. Kirzhevsky, A., Sutskever, I., & Hinton, G. E. (2012). Imagenet classification with deep convolutional neural networks. *Advances in Neural Information Processing Systems, 25*, 1097–1105.

20. Rieke, N., Hancox, J., Li, W., Milletari, F., Roth, H. R., Albarqouni, S., … & Cardoso, M. J. (2020). The future of digital health with federated learning. *NPJ Digital Medicine, 3*(1), 1–7.

21. Cai, L., Gao, J., & Zhao, D. (2020). A review of the application of deep learning in medical image classification and segmentation. *Annals of Translational Medicine*, *8*(11), 713.
22. Miranda, E., Aryuni, M., & Irwansyah, E. (2016, November). A survey of medical image classification techniques. In 2016 *International Conference on Information Management and Technology (ICIMTech)* (pp. 56–61). IEEE.
23. Dhawan, A. P., & Dai, S. (2008). Clustering and pattern classification. In *Principles and advanced methods in medical imaging and image analysis* (pp. 229–265).
24. Madani, A., Arnaout, R., Mofrad, M., & Arnaout, R. (2018). Fast and accurate view classification of echocardiograms using deep learning. *NPJ Digital Medicine*, *1*(1), 1–8.
25. Felzenszwalb, P. F., Girshick, R. B., McAllester, D., & Ramanan, D. (2010). Object detection with discriminatively trained part-based models. *IEEE Transactions on Pattern Analysis and Machine Intelligence*, *32*(9), 1627–1645.
26. Ronneberger, O., Fischer, P., & Brox, T. (2015, October). U-Net: Convolutional networks for biomedical image segmentation. In *International conference on medical image computing and computer-assisted intervention* (pp. 234–241). Springer, Cham.
27. Gonzalez, R. C., Woods, R. E., & Eddins, S. L. (2004). *Digital image processing using MATLAB*. Pearson Education India.
28. Pal, N. R., & Pal, S. K. (1993). A review on image segmentation techniques. *Pattern Recognition*, *26*(9), 1277–1294.
29. Sonka, M., Hlavac, V., & Boyle, R. (2014). *Image processing, analysis, and machine vision*. Cengage Learning.
30. Haralick, R. M. (1979). Statistical and structural approaches to texture. *Proceedings of the IEEE*, *67*(5), 786–804.
31. Julesz, B. (1981). Textons, the elements of texture perception, and their interactions. *Nature*, *290*(5802), 91–97.
32. Nagarajan, G., Minu, R. I., Muthukumar, B., Vedanarayanan, V., & Sundarsingh, S. D. (2016). Hybrid genetic algorithm for medical image feature extraction and selection. *Procedia Computer Science*, *85*, 455–462.
33. Suzuki, K. (Ed.). (2012). *Machine learning in computer-aided diagnosis: Medical imaging intelligence and analysis*. IGI Global.
34. Hajnal, J. V., & Hill, D. L. (2001). *Medical image registration*. CRC Press.
35. Avanzo, M., Pirrone, G., Vinante, L., Caroli, A., Stancanello, J., Drigo, A., & Sartor, G. (2020). Electron density and biologically effective dose (BED) radiomics-based machine learning models to predict late radiation-induced subcutaneous fibrosis. *Frontiers in Oncology*, *10*, 490.
36. Amoroso, N., La Rocca, M., Bellantuono, L., Diacono, D., Fanizzi, A., Lella, E., & Bellotti, R. (2019). Deep learning and multiplex networks for accurate modeling of brain age. *Frontiers in Aging Neuroscience*, *11*, 115.
37. Lopez Torres, E., Fiorina, E., Pennazio, F., Peroni, C., Saletta, M., Camarlinghi, N., … & Cerello, P. (2015). Large scale validation of the M5L lung CAD on heterogeneous CT datasets. *Medical Physics*, *42*(4), 1477–1489.
38. Militello, C., Vitabile, S., Rundo, L., Russo, G., Midiri, M., & Gilardi, M. C. (2015). A fully automatic 2D segmentation method for uterine fibroid in MRgFUS treatment evaluation. *Computers in Biology and Medicine*, *62*, 277–292.
39. Oren, O., Blankstein, R., & Bhatt, D. L. (2020). Incidental imaging findings in clinical trials. *JAMA*, *323*(7), 603–604.
40. Lee, H., Lee, E. J., Ham, S., Lee, H. B., Lee, J. S., Kwon, S. U., … & Kang, D. W. (2020). Machine learning approach to identify stroke within 4.5 hours. *Stroke*, *51*(3), 860–866.

41. Oren, O., Kebebew, E., & Ioannidis, J. P. (2019). Curbing unnecessary and wasted diagnostic imaging. *JAMA*, *321*(3), 245–246.
42. Pesapane, F., Codari, M., & Sardanelli, F. (2018). Artificial intelligence in medical imaging: Threat or opportunity? Radiologists again at the forefront of innovation in medicine. *European Radiology Experimental*, *2*(1), 1–10.
43. Chakraborty, C., Othman, S. B., & Almalki, F. A. (2023). FC-SEEDA: Fog computing-based secure and energy efficient data aggregation scheme for internet of healthcare things. *Neural Computing & Applications*. Advance online publication. https://doi.org/10.1007/s00521-023-08270-0
44. Ben Othman, S., Bahattab, A. A., Trad, A., & Youssef, H. (2020). PEERP: A priority-based energy-efficient routing protocol for reliable data transmission in healthcare using the IoT. In *The 15th international conference on future networks and communications (FNC)*, Leuven, Belgium, 9–12 August 2020.
45. Ben Othman, S., Almalki, F. A., Chakraborty, C., & Sakli, H. (2022). Privacy-preserving aware data aggregation for IoT-based healthcare with green computing technologies. *Computers and Electrical Engineering*, *101*, 108025. https://doi.org/10.1016/j.compeleceng.2022.108025

4 Automated Acute Lymphoblastic Leukemia Detection Using Blood Smear Image Analysis

Chandan Kumar Jha, Arvind Choubey,
Maheshkumar H. Kolekar, and
Chinmay Chakraborty

4.1 INTRODUCTION

Red blood cells (RBCs), platelets, and white blood cells (WBCs) are three constituents of blood that are responsible for specific functions of the biological system of the human body [1]. RBCs transport oxygen from the heart to all tissues and remove carbon dioxide. In the overall volume of blood, up to 50% is comprised of RBCs. Platelets or thrombocytes are responsible for blood clotting to prevent bleeding. WBCs are important for the body's immune system, as they fight against different infectious diseases. There are two types of WBCs: granulocytes and agranulocytes. Granulocytes include basophils, eosinophils, and neutrophils, whereas agranulocytes include lymphocytes and monocytes. Blood cells are affected by various diseases such as malaria and leukemia [2].

In the bloodstream, when normal blood cell growth is hampered by the exponential growth of abnormal blood cells, it is known as blood cancer. There are three types of blood cancer: leukemia, myeloma, and lymphoma [3]. Leukemia is the leading cause of death in most countries, as it spread through the bloodstream to blood-forming organs [4]. Leukemia is a cancerous blood tumor that originates from the bone marrow and results in collateral damage to the human body. As per the report of the Leukemia & Lymphoma Society, New York [5], there were 61,780 cases of leukemia in the US in the year 2019. Cancer Research UK [6] reports 9,900 new cases of leukemia every year. In India, the Global Cancer Observatory [7] reported 42,055 cases of leukemia in 2018 [8].

Hematologists categorize leukemia based on the cell-line origin and progression of the disease. Based on cell-line origin, there are two types of leukemia: myeloid and lymphoid. Based on the rate of progression of the disease, there are also two types of leukemia: acute and chronic. Thus, leukemia is widely categorized into four

DOI: 10.1201/9781003366249-4

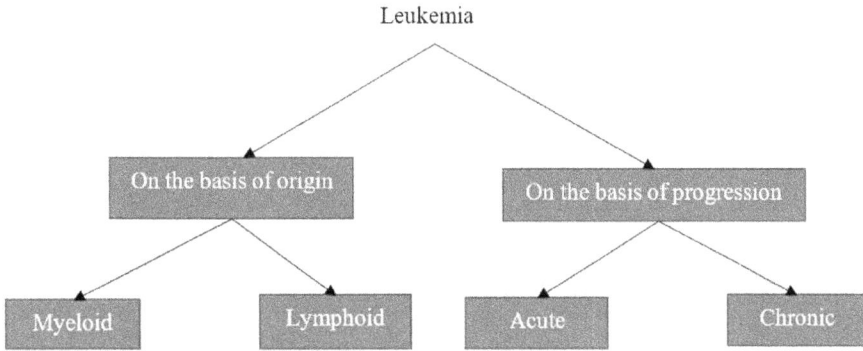

FIGURE 4.1 Types of leukemia.

types: acute myeloid leukemia (AML), acute lymphoblastic leukemia (ALL), chronic myeloid leukemia (CML), and chronic lymphocytic leukemia (CLL) [8, 2]. The classification of leukemia is shown in Figure 4.1. In the case of ALL and AML, the word "acute" indicates a fast-growing disease that may be fatal when it is not diagnosed at an early stage.

The abnormal proliferation of WBCs results in ALL, which produces a deficiency of normal blood cells. Primarily, ALL is diagnosed based on the symptoms of patients and a complete blood count (CBC) test using peripheral blood smear (PBS) image analysis. In the CBC test of ALL patients, it is observed that the number of WBCs is high, whereas RBCs and platelets are lower in number. Manual analysis of PBS images is difficult and prone to interobserver variations [9, 10]. Therefore, many automated PBS image analysis techniques have been developed in the past few decades. Computer-aided PBS image analysis is widely used for ALL detection. In the PBS images, the normal WBCs are known as lymphocytes and the abnormal WBCs are known as lymphoblasts. Figure 4.2 shows a few PBS images taken from the ALL-IDB. It shows PBS images with the lymphoblasts and healthy lymphocytes. Computer-aided automated ALL detection techniques facilitate quick and objective results. It can also handle a large amount of data efficiently. An automated ALL detection model is shown in Figure 4.3 that classifies a given input PBS image into a specific type.

4.2 RELATED WORKS

In automated ALL detection using blood smear image analysis, significant contributions have been made by researchers during the past few decades. In Table 4.1, details of some recently developed automated ALL detection techniques are summarized. Jha and Dutta [4] proposed a deep CNN-based acute lymphocytic leukemia detection technique that utilizes statistical and local directional pattern (LDP) features extracted from segmented images. In this method, a deep CNN classifier based on a chronological sine and cosine algorithm is used while image segmentation is performed using a mutual information-based hybrid model.

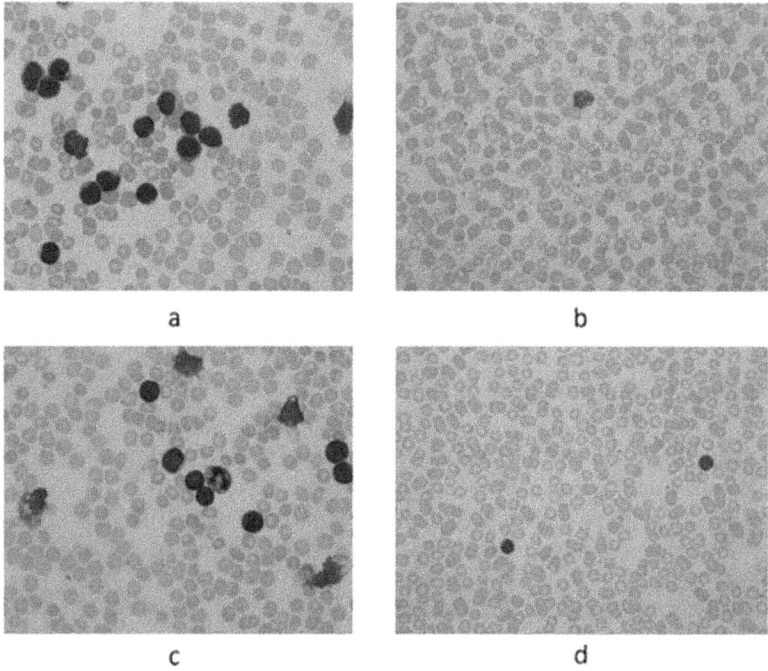

FIGURE 4.2   (a and c) Images with lymphoblasts. (b and d) Images with lymphocytes.

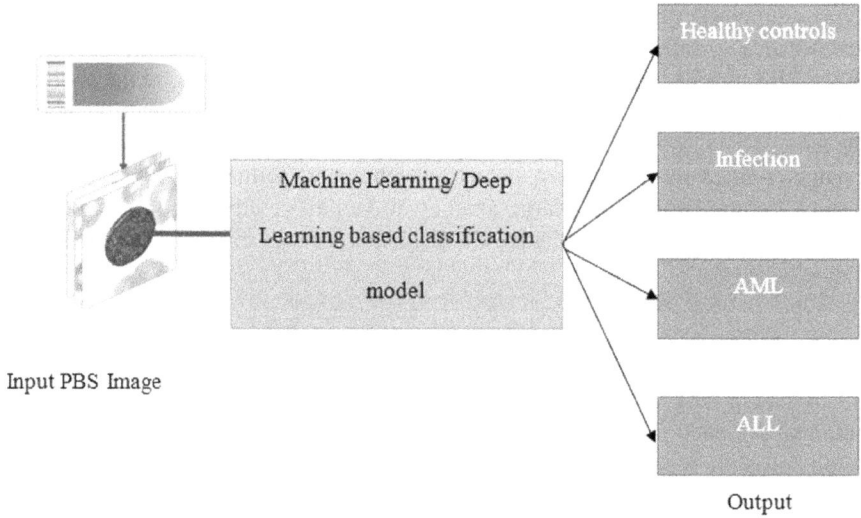

FIGURE 4.3   Automatic ALL detection system.

TABLE 4.1
ALL detection techniques

Reference	Database	Features	Classifier	Performance
[4]	ALL-IDB2	Statistical and LDP	Deep CNN	Accuracy: 98.70 %
[11]	Hospital Clinic of Barcelona	NA	Sequential CNN (VGG16 and VGG19)	Accuracy: 100%
[1]	ALL IDB + C-NMC datasets	Deep features	VGGNet + Swarm optimization	Accuracy: 96.11%
[3]	SN-AM Dataset	NA	Dense CNN	Accuracy: 97.20%
[8]	ASH Dataset	NA	Deep CNN	Accuracy: 94.12%
[12]	ALL-IDB1 + ALL-IDB2	NA	Hybrid deep CNN	Accuracy: 99.39% Accuracy: 97.18%
[13]	Cropped Images	Shape features: area, perimeter, circularity, convexity, solidity Color features Texture features	NN, autoencoders, CNN	Accuracy: 99.80% Accuracy: 99.00%
[14]	ALL-IDB and C-NMC-2019 dataset	NA	YOLOv4	MAP: 96.06% MAP: 98.74%
[15]	ALL-IDB1 dataset	DOST+LDA	AdaBoost algorithm + RF	Accuracy: 99.66 %

A deep learning model ALNet is proposed by Boldú et al. [11] that utilizes VGG16 and VGG18 as a sequential CNN classification system. In module 1 of the classification system, VGG16 is used, which classifies the input blood smear images as lymphocyte, monocyte, reactive lymphocyte, abnormal promyelocyte, and blast. Further, diagnostic orientation is determined based on this classification as healthy control, infection, promyelocytic leukemia, and acute leukemia. In the second module of the classification system, VGG19 is used that classifies the blast cell as a myeloid blast and B-lymphoblast. Further, diagnostic orientation is determined as myeloid leukemia and lymphoid leukemia from the classification results. This work produces 100% accuracy in leukemia detection.

A white blood cell leukemia detection technique has been proposed that uses VGGNet to obtain deep features that are further filtered using a statistically enhanced Salp Swarm Algorithm [1]. This algorithm selects 1,000 deep features out of the 25,000 that produce 96.11% classification accuracy. In this work, the classification model is trained and validated on the C-NMC dataset, whereas testing is performed using the ALL-IDB dataset. An ALL detection technique based on optimized dense

CNN has also been proposed that offers 97.2% classification accuracy. This work experimented on the blood smear images of the SN-AM dataset [3].

A deep CNN-based classification model, LeukNet, was developed by Anilkumar et al. [8] that uses the architectural characteristics of AlexNet. The developed classification model uses the American Society of Hematology (ASH) dataset for training, validation, and testing of the classification model. This technique classifies ALL B-cell and T-Cell with 94.12% accuracy.

Another ALL detection technique based on hybrid deep CNN has been proposed that uses MobileNetV2 architecture in the form of two blocks: mobleNetV2 block1 (MVB1) and mobileNetV2 bolck2 (MVB2) [12]. The proposed hybrid deep CNN model based on mobleNetV2 is trained and tested using the ALL-IDB1 and ALL-IDB2 datasets. The proposed classification model yields 99.39% and 97.18% accuracy with 70% training and 30% testing of the ALL-IDB1 and ALL-IDB2 datasets, respectively, while it achieves 97.92% accuracy with 50% training and 50% testing of the ALL-IDB1 and ALL-IDB2 datasets, respectively.

A comparative study of traditional image processing techniques and deep learning–based methods to classify white blood cells using PBS images was presented by Hedge et al. [13]. This study found that the neural network classifier yields an average accuracy of 99.8% with handcrafted features such as shape features, color features, and texture features, of PBS images. On the other hand, full training and transfer learning approaches of CNN results in 99% accuracy. In this study, it was concluded that the performance of traditional image processing techniques depends on different steps: image segmentation, feature extraction, and classification. The presence of a dark nucleus in a white blood cell makes the segmentation process easy using various image processing methods, but accurate border detection and overlapping of WBCs in a PBS image make the segmentation task difficult. Apart from this, the efficiency of features and different classification parameters also affect the performance of traditional PBS image analysis methods. The deep learning–based method does not require image segmentation and feature extraction steps, which makes this method advantageous.

A deep learning–based approach using the You Only Look Once (YOLO) algorithm is proposed by Khandekar et al. [14] for ALL detection. In this approach, version 4 of the YOLO algorithm is implemented, which is trained and tested using the PBS images of the ALL-IDB and C-NMC-2019 datasets. This technique achieves a mean average precision (MAP) of 95.57% for the ALL-IDB dataset and 98.7% for images of the C-NMC dataset.

An ALL detection technique that utilizes two-dimensional (2D) discrete orthonormal Stockwell transform (DOST)-based features of PBS images was tested by Mishra et al. [15]. Dimensions of the extracted features are reduced using principal component analysis (PCA) and logistic discriminant analysis (LDA). Further, dimensionally reduced features are used to classify PBS images using the AdaBoost algorithm with the random forest (RF) classifier. This technique achieves 99.6% classification accuracy to distinguish the ALL cell of a PBS image.

Although many automated ALL detection techniques have been developed, there is a need for an optimal solution to handle variations present in microscopic blood

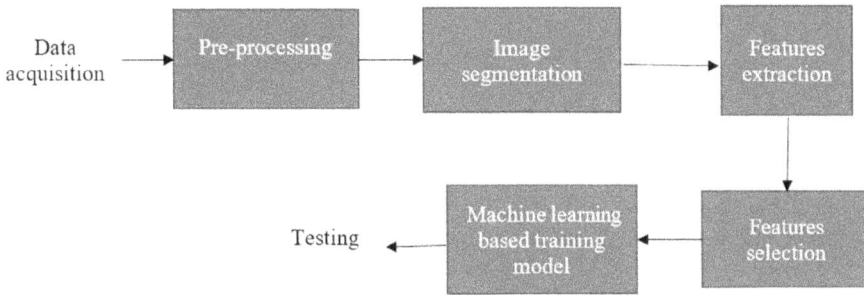

FIGURE 4.4 Different steps of machine learning–based ALL detection techniques.

smear images. Also, there is a requirement for a reliable automated system that can achieve high classification performance to classify WBCs into healthy control and lymphoblasts to reduce the workload of hematologists. Based on the studies of previous work, this chapter presents the methodological analysis of the few existing techniques. Based on methodological steps, automated ALL detection techniques are categorized into two types: machine learning–based methods and deep learning based–methods. Figure 4.4 depicts the different steps of the machine learning–based automated ALL detection technique using a block diagram.

4.3 MACHINE LEARNING–BASED ALL DETECTION TECHNIQUES

Machine learning–based ALL detection techniques are implemented using the following steps: data acquisition, image segmentation and augmentation, feature extraction, feature selection, and classification. In the automated ALL detection techniques, data acquisition is performed in the form of PBS images. The existing machine learning–based techniques widely used publicly open databases such as ALL-IDB, C-NMC, SN-AM, and ASH datasets to acquire PBS images. These images are processed further through different classification methods.

- *Preprocessing*: Blood smear images of different databases are acquired at a different magnification that introduces noise and unwanted background effects. It affects the classification performance. Hence, the preprocessing step includes noise removal techniques of PBS images. The image preprocessing step also includes image resizing that regulates the image segmentation smoothly.
- *Image segmentation*: In ALL detection, the presence of WBCs and platelets in PBS images is not desirable. Therefore, different image processing methods such as background subtraction and triangle method [16] for thresholding are used to extract WBCs. A PBS image may contain more than one WBC. For ALL detection, the region of interest must contain one WBC per image. Therefore, the marker-based watershed method [17] is used to segment grouped cells of a PBS image.

TABLE 4.2
Features used for classification of ALL

Type	Features
Shape	1. Area
	2. Perimeter
	3. Circularity
	4. Convexity and solidity
	5. NC ratio
Color	1. Mean and variance of R, G, B components of RGB image
	2. Mean and variance of H, S, V components
	3. Mean and variance of L, A, B components
Texture	1. Mean, variance, skewness, and kurtosis
	2. Spatial gray level dependence matrix (SGLDM)
	3. Laws' texture features from grayscale representation
	4. Laws' texture features from local binary pattern (LBP)

- *Feature extraction and selection*: After performing segmentation, features extracted from the region of interest play a major role in the machine learning–based classification of WBCs. In segmented WBCs, there are two parts: nuclei and cytoplasm. For a given WBC, shape features are extracted from nuclei, while color and texture features are extracted from both nuclei and cytoplasm. Table 4.2 lists the different shape, color, and texture features used for the classification of WBCs [13]. The shape features include area, perimeter, circularity, convexity, and solidity of nuclei of WBCs. It also includes the nucleus-to-cell (NC) ratio. All these features are extracted from the binary representation of nuclei of WBCs. In the PBS images of WBCs, the color of normal and abnormal nuclei varies significantly. Therefore, the color features in the form of mean and variance of R, G, B, components are extracted to detect abnormal WBC nuclei. In addition to this, H, S, V components of HSV images and L, A, B components of CIE Lab images of WBCs are also taken as features to classify ALL. Apart from this, transformation methods such as 2D-DOST [15] and wavelet transform [18] are also used to distinguish different classes of WBCs including ALL.

However, a large number of features increases the computational time of the classification model. Therefore, extracted features are dimensionally reduced using different methods such as PCA and LDA [15]. The reduced features are further used for the training and testing of machine learning–based classification models.

4.3.1 TRAINING AND TESTING FOR CLASSIFICATION

The reduced feature sets are used to train the classification model based on different machine learning methods. In machine learning–based ALL detection, the Naïve

Bayes classifier [19, 20], artificial neural network (ANN) [21, 22], support vector machine (SVM) [23–27], and k-nearest neighbor (KNN) [28–30] are widely used.

For ALL detection, the machine learning–based automated classification approach has been addressed in the last four decades. In these methods, a different classification model is used. A Naïve Bayes classifier for WBCs classification, proposed by Mathur et al. [20], reports an accuracy of around 92%.

Another Naïve Bayes classifier developed by Prinyakupt and Pluempitiwiriyawej [19] had a 98% WBCs classification accuracy. ANN-based WBC classification approaches developed by Nazlibilek et al. [21] evaluated the performance of ANN with PCA and without PCA. They found that ANN yields 65% classification accuracy without PCA, whereas it yields 95% classification accuracy with PCA. Many automated WBCs classification approaches [23–27] have also been developed based on SVM. Sinha and Ramakrishnan [23] compared the performance of WBC classification between ANN and SVM, which yielded an average classification accuracy of around 97% using ANN and 94% using SVM. Mohapatra et al. [18] proposed a method for the detection of ALL using PBS images. Several classifiers, namely, Naïve Bayes, KNN, multilayer perceptron (MLP), SVM, and ensemble of classifiers, were evaluated for detection of ALL. KNN [28–30] used for ALL detection achieves around 90% classification sensitivity. Since, machine learning–based methods include several steps such as preprocessing, image segmentation, feature extraction, and feature selection, it increases the computational load of the classification model. Presently, the deep learning–based classification model is widely used in automated ALL detection.

4.4 DEEP LEARNING–BASED ALL DETECTION TECHNIQUES

Deep learning–based ALL detection techniques directly learn features from raw pixels of PBS images. These techniques are robust to noise and illumination variations of PBS images, hence they are widely used in biomedical image analysis. A block diagram of deep learning–based ALL detection is shown in Figure 4.5. It does not require feature extraction and selection. Hence, it is computationally more efficient than machine learning–based methods. The deep learning–based ALL detection techniques widely use CNN [31–39] architecture for WBC classification, Other deep neural architectures, including VGGNet, ResNet, MobileNet, and YOLOv4, have been developed that are used for the classification of WBCs to detect ALL.

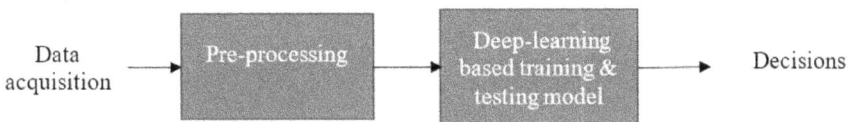

FIGURE 4.5   Deep learning–based ALL detection model.

4.5 PERFORMANCE ASSESSMENT

The classification performance of WBC classifiers is assessed using the following performance measures:

$$Accuracy = \frac{TP + TN}{P + N} \times 100\%$$

$$Sensitivity = \frac{TP}{TP + FN} \times 100\%$$

$$Specificity = \frac{TN}{TN + FP} \times 100\%$$

Here, P and N indicate total positive and total negative output, respectively, of the prediction model. True positive and true negative predictions are denoted by TP and TN, respectively. False positive and false negative predictions are denoted by FP and FN, respectively.

4.6 CONCLUSION

ALL is a type of blood cancer related to WBCs. It affects the blood cells of bone marrow and results in an increased number of immature lymphocytes, known as blast cells. The color and shape of lymphoblasts are different from normal lymphocytes. ALL is detected using peripheral blood smear image analysis. Manual analysis of peripheral blood smear images is time-consuming and prone to human error producing wrong diagnoses. Hence, automated ALL detection techniques based on machine learning and deep learning methods are widely used in this field. This chapter comprehensively studies automated ALL detection techniques based on machine learning and deep learning methods. This study found that machine learning–based methods require the feature extraction and selection steps separately, which are not required for deep learning–based methods. In the analysis, it is also observed that the performance of both machine learning–based and deep learning–based methods are good, but deep learning–based methods are advantageous over machine learning–based methods as they require less computational load.

REFERENCES

1. A. T. Sahlol, P. Kollmannsberger, and A. A. Ewees, "Efficient Classification of White Blood Cell Leukemia With Improved Swarm Optimization of Deep Features," *Sci Rep*, vol. 10, no. 1, Dec. 2020, doi: 10.1038/s41598-020-59215-9.
2. S. S. Al-jaboriy, N. N. A. Sjarif, S. Chuprat, and W. M. Abduallah, "Acute Lymphoblastic Leukemia Segmentation Using Local Pixel Information," *Pattern Recog Lett*, vol. 125, pp. 85–90, Jul. 2019, doi: 10.1016/j.patrec.2019.03.024.

3. D. Kumar, N. Jain, A. Khurana, S. Mittal, S. Chandra Satapathy, R. Senkerik, and J. D. Hemanth, "Automatic Detection of White Blood Cancer From Bone Marrow Microscopic Images Using Convolutional Neural Networks," *IEEE Access*, vol. 8, pp. 142521–142531, 2020, doi: 10.1109/ACCESS.2020.3012292.

4. K. K. Jha and H. S. Dutta, "Mutual Information Based Hybrid Model and Deep Learning for Acute Lymphocytic Leukemia Detection in Single Cell Blood Smear Images," *Comput Methods Programs Biomed*, vol. 179, Oct. 2019, doi: 10.1016/j.cmpb.2019.104987.

5. "The Leukemia & Lymphoma Society, New York, 2020."

6. "Cancer Research UK."

7. "The Global Cancer Observatory."

8. K. K. Anilkumar, V. J. Manoj, and T. M. Sagi, "Automated Detection of B Cell and T Cell Acute Lymphoblastic Leukaemia Using Deep Learning," *IRBM*, 2021, doi: 10.1016/j.irbm.2021.05.005.

9. F. Xing and L. Yang, "Robust Nucleus/Cell Detection and Segmentation in Digital Pathology and Microscopy Images: A Comprehensive Review," *IEEE Reviews in Biomedical Engineering*, vol. 9. Institute of Electrical and Electronics Engineers, pp. 234–263, 2016, doi: 10.1109/RBME.2016.2515127.

10. Z. Moshavash, H. Danyali, and M. S. Helfroush, "An Automatic and Robust Decision Support System for Accurate Acute Leukemia Diagnosis From Blood Microscopic Images," *J Digit Imaging*, vol. 31, no. 5, pp. 702–717, Oct. 2018, doi: 10.1007/s10278-018-0074-y.

11. L. Boldú, A. Merino, A. Acevedo, A. Molina, and J. Rodellar, "A Deep Learning Model (ALNet) for the Diagnosis of Acute Leukaemia Lineage Using Peripheral Blood Cell Images," *Comput Methods Programs Biomed*, vol. 202, Apr. 2021, doi: 10.1016/j.cmpb.2021.105999.

12. P. K. Das, and S. Meher, "An Efficient Deep Convolutional Neural Network Based Detection and Classification of Acute Lymphoblastic Leukemia," *Expert Syst Appl*, vol. 183, Nov. 2021, doi: 10.1016/j.eswa.2021.115311.

13. R. B. Hegde, K. Prasad, H. Hebbar, and B. M. K. Singh, "Comparison of Traditional Image Processing and Deep Learning Approaches for Classification of White Blood Cells in Peripheral Blood Smear Images," *Biocybern Biomed Eng*, vol. 39, no. 2, pp. 382–392, Apr. 2019, doi: 10.1016/j.bbe.2019.01.005.

14. R. Khandekar, P. Shastry, S. Jaishankar, O. Faust, and N. Sampathila, "Automated Blast Cell Detection for Acute Lymphoblastic Leukemia Diagnosis," *Biomed Signal Process Control*, vol. 68, Jul. 2021, doi: 10.1016/j.bspc.2021.102690.

15. S. Mishra, B. Majhi, and P. K. Sa, "Texture Feature Based Classification on Microscopic Blood Smear for Acute Lymphoblastic Leukemia Detection," *Biomed Signal Process Control*, vol. 47, pp. 303–311, Jan. 2019, doi: 10.1016/j.bspc.2018.08.012.

16. G. W. Zack, W. E. Rogers, and S. A. Latp, "Automatic Measurement of Sister Chromatid Exchange Frequency," 1977.

17. S. Mishra, B. Majhi, P. K. Sa, and L. Sharma, "Gray Level Co-Occurrence Matrix and Random Forest Based Acute Lymphoblastic Leukemia Detection," *Biomed Signal Process Control*, vol. 33, pp. 272–280, Mar. 2017, doi: 10.1016/j.bspc.2016.11.021.

18. S. Mohapatra, D. Patra, and S. Satpathy, "An Ensemble Classifier System for Early Diagnosis of Acute Lymphoblastic Leukemia in Blood Microscopic Images," *Neural Comput Appl*, vol. 24, nos. 7–8, pp. 1887–1904, 2014, doi: 10.1007/s00521-013-1438-3.

19. J. Prinyakupt and C. Pluempitiwiriyawej, "Segmentation of White Blood Cells and Comparison of Cell Morphology by Linear and Naive Bayes Classifiers," *Biomed Eng Online*, vol. 14, no. 1, pp. 1–19, 2015.

20. A. Mathur, A. S. Tripathi, and M. Kuse, "Scalable System for Classification of White Blood Cells From Leishman Stained Blood Stain Images," *J Pathol Inform*, vol. 4, no. 2 Supplement, p. 15, 2013.

21. S. Nazlibilek, D. Karacor, T. Ercan, M. H. Sazli, O. Kalender, and Y. Ege, "Automatic Segmentation, Counting, Size Determination and Classification of White Blood Cells," *Measurement*, vol. 55, pp. 58–65, 2014.

22. S. H. Rezatofighi, and H. Soltanian-Zadeh, "Automatic Recognition of Five Types of White Blood Cells in Peripheral Blood," *Comput Med Imaging Graphics*, vol. 35, no. 4, pp. 333–343, 2011.

23. N. Sinha, and A. G. Ramakrishnan, "Automation of Differential Blood Count," in *TENCON* 2003. *Conference on Convergent Technologies for Asia-Pacific Region*, 2003, vol. 2, pp. 547–551.

24. Q. Li, Y. Wang, H. Liu, X. He, D. Xu, J. Wang, and F. Guo, "Leukocyte Cells Identification and Quantitative Morphometry Based on Molecular Hyperspectral Imaging Technology," *Comput Med Imaging Graphics*, vol. 38, no. 3, pp. 171–178, 2014.

25. S. Osowski, R. Siroic, T. Markiewicz, and K. Siwek, "Application of Support Vector Machine and Genetic Algorithm for Improved Blood Cell Recognition," *IEEE Trans Instrum Meas*, vol. 58, no. 7, pp. 2159–2168, 2008.

26. M. M. Amin, S. Kermani, A. Talebi, and M. G. Oghli, "Recognition of Acute Lymphoblastic Leukemia Cells in Microscopic Images Using k-Means Clustering and Support Vector Machine Classifier," *J Med Signals Sens*, vol. 5, no. 1, p. 49, 2015.

27. J. Rawat, A. Singh, H. S. Bhadauria, J. Virmani, and J. S. Devgun, "Computer Assisted Classification Framework for Prediction of Acute Lymphoblastic and Acute Myeloblastic Leukemia," *Biocybern Biomed Eng*, vol. 37, no. 4, pp. 637–654, 2017.

28. P. Umarani, and P. Viswanathan, "Z-Score Normalized Features With Maximum Distance Measure Based k-NN Automated Blood Cancer Diagnosis System," *ECS Trans*, vol. 107, no. 1, p. 11945, 2022.

29. E. Purwanti and E. Calista, "Detection of Acute Lymphocyte Leukemia Using k-Nearest Neighbor Algorithm Based on Shape and Histogram Features," *J Phys Conf Ser*, 2017, vol. 853, no. 1, p. 12011.

30. N. Z. Supardi, M. Y. Mashor, N. H. Harun, F. A. Bakri, and R. Hassan, "Classification of Blasts in Acute Leukemia Blood Samples Using k-Nearest Neighbour," in *2012 IEEE 8th International Colloquium on Signal Processing and its Applications*, 2012, pp. 461–465.

31. Z. Gao, L. Wang, L. Zhou, and J. Zhang, "HEp-2 Cell Image Classification With Deep Convolutional Neural Networks," *IEEE J Biomed Health Inform*, vol. 21, no. 2, pp. 416–428, 2016.

32. S. Shafique and S. Tehsin, "Acute Lymphoblastic Leukemia Detection and Classification of Its Subtypes Using Pretrained Deep Convolutional Neural Networks," *Technol Cancer Res Treat*, vol. 17, p. 1533033818802789, 2018.

33. A. Rehman, N. Abbas, T. Saba, S. I. Ur Rahman, Z. Mehmood, and H. Kolivand, "Classification of Acute Lymphoblastic Leukemia Using Deep Learning," *Microsc Res Tech*, vol. 81, no. 11, pp. 1310–1317, 2018.

34. P. Tiwari, J. Qian, Q. Li, B. Wang, D. Gupta, A. Khanna, J. P. C. Rodrigues, and V. H. C. de Albuquerque, "Detection of Subtype Blood Cells Using Deep Learning," *Cogn Syst Res*, vol. 52, pp. 1036–1044, 2018.

35. J. W. Choi, Y. Ku, B. W. Yoo, J.-A. Kim, D. S. Lee, Y. J. Chai, H.-J. Kong, and H. C. Kim, "White Blood Cell Differential Count of Maturation Stages in Bone Marrow Smear Using Dual-Stage Convolutional Neural Networks," *PLoS One*, vol. 12, no. 12, p. e0189259, 2017.

36. F. Qin, N. Gao, Y. Peng, Z. Wu, S. Shen, and A. Grudtsin, "Fine-Grained Leukocyte Classification With Deep Residual Learning for Microscopic Images," *Comput Methods Programs Biomed*, vol. 162, pp. 243–252, 2018.

37. C. Chakraborty, S. B. Othman, F. A. Almalki, and H. Sakli, "FC-SEEDA: Fog Computing-Based Secure and Energy Efficient Data Aggregation Scheme for Internet of Healthcare Things," *Neural Comput Appl*, 2023, doi: 10.1007/s00521-023-08270-0.

38. S. Ben Othman, A. A. Bahattab, A. Trad, and H. Youssef, "PEERP: A Priority-Based Energy-Efficient Routing Protocol for Reliable Data Transmission in Healthcare Using the IoT," *The 15th International Conference on Future Networks and Communications (FNC)*, Leuven, Belgium, 9–12 August 2020.

39. S. Ben Othman, F. A. Almalki, C. Chakraborty, and H. Sakli, "Privacy-Preserving Aware Data Aggregation for IoT-Based Healthcare With Green Computing Technologies," *Comput Electr Eng*, vol. 101, p. 108025, 2022, doi: 10.1016/j.compeleceng.2022.108025.

5 Smart Digital Healthcare Solutions Using Medical Imaging and Advanced AI Techniques

P Divyashree and Priyanka Dwivedi

5.1 INTRODUCTION

Medical imaging has had a breakthrough with digital diagnosis innovation in recent times. The emergence of various medical image modalities has created a revolution in providing smart digital healthcare solutions with the amalgamation of advanced artificial intelligence (AI) technologies. Diagnosing, classifying, predicting, and prognosis (analyzing the progression) of a disease is possible through radiomics-based healthcare, as shown in Figure 5.1. Radiomic healthcare is the computational analysis of medical imaging (radiographs) to get meaningful interpretations of the health condition. Radiomics extract useful information from medical imaging data through AI techniques. The clinical decision support system was established for the diagnosis, prognosis, and prediction of health abnormalities [1]. AI applied to radiographs creates a new path for automated and digital approaches to disease diagnosis. An in-depth analysis of the region of interest in medical images is possible through advanced AI techniques. The broad exploration and advancement toward digitization, improved imaging modalities for healthcare applications, and AI boosted the evolution of smart healthcare solutions [2]. Radiology and AI created an unprecedented breakthrough in the field of digital healthcare solutions. The traditional way of humans capturing radiographs suffers from several technical concerns, including lack of standard expertise, the stress of individuals while scanning might produce inadequate images, and lack of technical expertise to analyze the radiographs. Radiologists and the naked eye cannot discern the finer details of medical images and could fail to properly diagnose the disease. Computer-aided diagnosis can be a robust solution for analyzing qualitative and quantitative medical images through AI [3]. AI acts as a guiding tool for physicians to determine a valid imaging-based diagnosis [4]. Though it has the potential to replace humans, AI possesses few setbacks, as it cannot perform with human-level cognition toward building a complete end-to-end radiograph-based diagnosis and treatment. However, in the future, AI

DOI: 10.1201/9781003366249-5

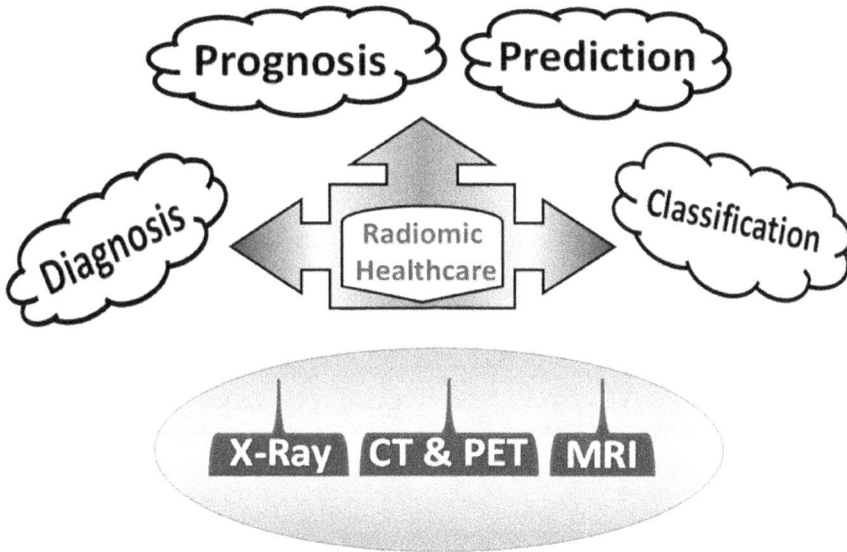

FIGURE 5.1 Medical imaging modalities for healthcare applications.

might possess the capability to replace traditional radiologists who do not use AI in their practice [5, 6, 7]. Explainable AI is the future technology that assists in building human trust toward technological decisions [8].

This chapter is organized to provide a bird's-eye view of the advanced technologies and AI for the realization of the smart health monitoring system through medical imaging. Section 5.2 comprises a discussion of the medical imaging modalities, their functioning, and the broad scope of applications in disease identification. Section 5.3 discusses the challenges of medical data acquisition for smart prediction of health status. Section 5.4 emphasizes the AI techniques for enhancing medical image quality for precise diagnosis. Section 5.5 presents novel healthcare solutions using AI algorithms from radiology scans. Section 5.6 provides the strategy of fusing various medical imaging modalities to diagnose disease with enhanced accuracy. Section 5.7 presents the idea of remote healthcare and various technologies that assist in achieving this goal. Section 5.8 is dedicated to providing the current limitations of AI utility in the healthcare domain. Then, Section 5.9 is the conclusion and the future perspective of digital diagnosis using AI and advanced technologies.

5.2 MEDICAL IMAGING MODALITIES

5.2.1 X-RAY

X-ray is one of the most commonly used radiology techniques for healthcare diagnosis. In this technique, X-rays are passed through the human body to capture internal details. Typically, humans are positioned in the middle of the X-ray source machine and photographic film. X-rays are passed through the body and based on the intensity of the body part these rays get adsorbed at different levels. Thus, the harder body parts, such as bone, are displayed in white since the rays are mostly adsorbed and do not reach the other side of the X-ray film. Similarly, when X-rays are passed through the air in the lungs almost all of the X-rays will reach the photographic film and appears dark. For fat and muscle tissue, an X-ray will appear in shades of gray. Through X-rays, diagnosis of bone degeneration, dislocations, fractures, tumors, infections, cancer, and pneumonia can be precisely performed. In special cases, contrast mediums like barium or iodine will be injected into the target region to extract greater details in the images. In the case of X-ray, if we want to extract the 3D image of the internal organ, then several X-ray photographs from different angles should be captured and analyzed by combining all of the acquired images [9]. In patient-centric radiography, deep learning techniques in radiology and image-guided therapeutics are possible through the analysis of X-ray imaging [5].

5.2.2   COMPUTED TOMOGRAPHY (CT) AND POSITRON EMISSION TOMOGRAPHY (PET)

Computed tomography (CT) provides high-quality and detailed images of the internal organs with 3D structure realization of the internal body through radiography. The 360° images of the spine vertebrae, bone, blood vessels, soft tissue, and organs can be captured. Typically, while performing CT scans, the patient lies on a sliding table that will pass through the tunnel of the CT scan machine. The CT scan machine rotates as simultaneously X-rays are passed and cross-section images of the body are generated. Through these radiographs, the doctor can diagnose health ailments such as cancer, appendicitis, heart disease, trauma, musculoskeletal disorders, infectious diseases, tumors in the lung, chest-related problems, and much more [10]. The advanced version of CT is positron emission tomography (PET) in which a tracer composed of glucose and radioactive material is sent into the patient's target region for radiography before undergoing the scanning. This tracer can be provided through injection, swallowing, or inhalation. The injected tracer will spread in the region of interest and collect in areas of higher levels of chemical activity. The tracer will show as white spots on the radiograph. Thus, a potential disease can be identified. Through PET scans, the diagnosis of brain diseases, cancer, and heart problems can be performed.

5.2.3   MAGNETIC RESONANCE IMAGING (MRI)

MRI is the radiography technique that uses strong magnets along with radio waves. Unlike X-rays and CT scanning, MRI is radiation-free and safer. Typically, an MRI scan captures a highly detailed cross-sectional image of the body through powerful magnets. Radio waves are used to obtain the radiographs, which are transferred to a remote computer for medical analysis. The person lying on the table is passed into a tunnel-shaped machine and then a magnetic field is applied. Humans are composed of 70% water molecules, which consist of hydrogen and oxygen. Each molecule has a proton that is sensitive to the magnetic field. MRI has two powerful magnets. One magnet aligns all the protons in water molecules to a specific direction (south or north), while the other magnet switches on and off in pulse format. This changes the alignment of the hydrogen atom when on and returns to relax state when off. The energy released by the proton to reach an equilibrium state depends on the chemical composition of the tissue. Thus, the internal composition can be captured. MRI is the preferred imaging technique for repeated diagnoses due to no harmful radiation. Through MRI, the human body can be analyzed in greater detail. Some of the applications of MRI include the detection of anomalies in the brain and spinal cord, identifying tumors and cysts, breast cancer screening, abnormalities in heart functioning, disease in the liver and abdominal organs, evaluation of pelvic cancer such as fibroids, uterine anomalies, and injuries of the joints, knees, and back. Functional MRI (fMRI) is the technique to measure cognitive operations. Standard MRI will signify the anomalies in the tissue structure, however, fMRI is useful to detect the anomaly in the activity. That is, fMRI captures the functioning of tissue rather than structural details [11, 12].

5.3 DATA CHALLENGES OF MEDICAL IMAGING AND AI AS A SOLUTION

Data acquisition for medical images takes a lot of time. The procedure to get medical data includes ethical committee permissions and consent from the patients as well as family members. Most important, the healthcare data is obtained in limited quantity due to challenges concerning patient confidentiality and convenience. It is also a major challenge to build an automated diagnosis model based on AI techniques. Though healthcare data is available, it suffers from several limitations. The medical data is usually of high dimensions, which makes the diagnostic models more complex. Moreover, due to high-dimensional data, there is a chance of noise and sparsity issues. To reduce the data dimensionality, feature extraction and selection of relevant features show a significant impact. Nonlinear dimensional reduction with deep learning and principal component analysis are a few techniques to get the required medical information from large datasets. Sometimes, due to improper data collection and lack of documentation, there is a chance of data loss with missing values and noise due to coding inaccuracies. Irregularity is one of the major issues in big data analytics for healthcare models. This issue could be resolved through the use of baseline features (data obtained on the first visit to the hospital) and relevant data transformation methods [13]. Thus, in the healthcare sector, diagnosis through advanced AI methods possesses numerous challenges concerning healthcare data availability, data integration, and analytics.

5.4 MEDICAL IMAGE ENHANCEMENT USING AI

Medical imaging is one of the unprecedented technologies that could benefit from digital techniques. Medical images acquired through various radiology equipment need to be further enhanced in terms of their resolution and feature appearance for the development of precise healthcare applications. Thus, one of the specific technologies in AI is generative adversarial networks (GANs), which possess tremendous scope for enhancement of the quality of medical images with super-resolution. E. C. de Farias et al. proposed GAN-based super-resolution on CT-scanned lesion (cancer)-focused medical radiomic images. The authors added spatial pyramid pooling with GANs, which are constrained by identical, residual, and cyclic ensemble techniques. This novel approach could achieve perpetual image quality with 2× super-resolution which is similar to state-of-the-art 4× super-resolution architectures [14]. Y. Xia et al. developed a super-resolution algorithm with GANs with the integration of optical flow components. The super-resolution of cardiac MRI could potentially synthesize 3D isotropic images from the learned visual properties and structures from the radiographs [15]. J. Zhu et al. proposed the Medical Image Arbitrary Scale Super-Resolution (MIASSR) model. MIASSR incorporates meta-learning with GANs that could super-resolve MRI radiographs with a magnification factor of 1 to 4. This model is flexible to scale to other medical modalities such as cardiac MRI, chest CT, and COVID-CT [16]. Thus, the super-resolution of the medical image is the prerequisite step in image-guided healthcare predictive models. Moreover, through medical image enhancement, the analysis for disease identification could be done more efficiently without an increase in the computation time. Therefore, advanced AI techniques such as GANs for super-resolution of medical images are an essential step toward image-guided diagnosis.

5.5 NOVEL HEALTHCARE SOLUTIONS FOR RADIOLOGY-BASED DIAGNOSIS USING AI

The previous sections covered various imaging techniques in the medical field and the techniques to enhance medical image quality with super-resolution. In this section, the emphasis will be on the use of quantitative analysis for medical images. The novel emerging field radiomics will be explored to attain the ultimate goal of precision healthcare. Radiomics is the statistical approach to analyzing various medical imaging modalities, including X-ray, CT, PET, and MRI. In the current state of the art, there is numerous research aiming for personalized healthcare solutions using radiomics. In medical scenarios, the knowledge of shape, intensity, and texture at the region of interest signifies important analytics for determining the disease as well as the health condition. Hence, this analysis through radiomics will be a breakthrough innovation toward noninvasive diagnosis for smart healthcare applications [17]. Noninvasive diagnosis is the booming innovation in recent times that transformed the traditional functioning of healthcare solutions in leaps and bounds. Radiology has become an emerging tool for capturing the finer details of health ailments through medical imaging protocols. In this section, insights into using the major radiography methodologies for diagnosing specific diseases will be discussed. The amalgamation of medical imaging along with AI technologies will impart a unique healthcare solution to diagnose, monitor, and set treatment standards. Thus, the noninvasive techniques of healthcare solutions are achieved through radiology.

Figure 5.2 illustrates the ideology of using AI in medical image modalities, such as X-ray, CT, PET, and MRI, to diagnose disease.

In the 21st century, the COVID-19 pandemic caused adverse effects on humans, society, and nations concerning the deaths of people, psychological trauma, and economic recession. T. Hu et al. proposed a deep learning architecture for the identification of COVID-19 through X-ray images. The proposed model comprises of a convolution neural network (CNN)-based feature extraction algorithm followed by extreme learning machines for the final detection of COVID-19. The authors examined and elucidated that the extreme learning machine could perform better generalization because of the small weight and minor training errors [18]. P. L. Bartlett, who studied the relationship between generalization and the size of neurons, supported this conclusion. The author contemplated that in the classification model if weights are small they correspond to a small, squared error. In such cases, generalization performance is the function of size and weight rather than the number of weights [19].

M. Chakraborty et al. developed a Corona–Nidaan algorithm for the diagnosis of COVID-19 infection. The COVID-19, pneumonia, and normal multiclass classification model was built using X-ray radiographs of the chest. A two-phase oversampling approach was used to solve the data balance issue with the minority class. Phase one includes the generation of sharp, blurred, red channel, green channel, and blue channel counterpart images. In phase two for each image generated in phase one, standard data augmentation techniques were applied. Therefore, minority class data balance is achieved with oversampling of COVID-19 images. The authors utilized a depth-wise separable convolution architecture that reduced multiplication complexity [20]. D. Ardila et al. developed a deep learning–based algorithm for the estimation of lung cancer from low-dose CT scan radiographs of the chest [21]. M. Kirienko et al. analyzed textural images from the radiomic signature obtained through PET/CT radiographs in non-small-cell lung cancer patients undergoing surgery [22]. S. A. Abdelaziz Ismael et al. developed a residual network to estimate brain tumors using MRI scan images [23]. M. Hu et al. proposed a 2D- and 3D-based CNN model for the determination of schizophrenia. The authors integrated a multimodal dataset with structural MRI images and diffusion MRI images to better classify the disease

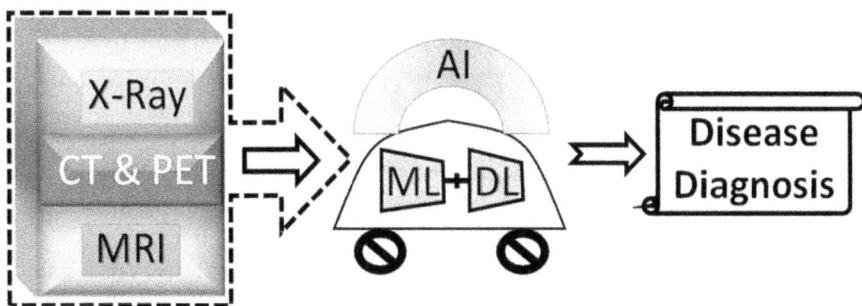

FIGURE 5.2   Graphical abstract for radiology-based disease diagnosis using AI.

[24]. E. E. Bron et al. developed a support vector machine (SVM) and CNN-based network to classify Alzheimer's disease (AD) in mild cognitive impairment (MCI) patients. To diagnose these cognitive disorders, minimally processed MRI radiographs were employed. The MRI images were transformed into modulated gray matter maps for building the classifier model [25]. E. Yee et al. proposed a lightweight 3D CNN model to classify stable dementia of the Alzheimer's type (sDAT) and common control. The authors transformed the MRI images into probabilistic dementia scores by extracting useful neurodegenerative patterns to develop a 3D CNN model. Additionally, the authors used dilated convolution that has holes inserted in the kernels. This process increases the reception field. The proposed compact model, in which sampling was done subject-wise, enables fast training with promising generalization. Through this novel approach, the authors provided a compact solution to solving the hardware limitations and memory constraints for real-world implementation [26].

5.6 FUSION OF MEDICAL IMAGE MODALITIES FOR ENHANCED DIAGNOSIS

In the previous section, the diagnosis of various diseases with specific medical imaging modalities was discussed. In this section, emphasis will be given to the fusion of different image modalities that will improve the disease classification performance. Alzheimer's is the most suffered form of dementia and, as reported by the United Nations, by 2050 1 in 85 people may have this disease [27]. D. Zhang et al. combined CSF (cerebrospinal fluid) biomarkers, FDG-PET (fluorodeoxyglucose-PET), and MRI to classify MCI and AD. The atlas warping algorithm was utilized to extract 93 features from 93 regions of interest in MRI and FDG-PET radiographs; for CSF, their raw values were used as features. Henceforth, multimodal classification with the fusion MRI, PET, and CSF biomarkers was proposed. The SVM kernel combination method was used to classify the MCI and AD, which showed better performance compared to individual modalities in the classification [28]. P. K. Choudhary et al. formulated the novel Fourier–Bessel series expansion-based decomposition (FBSED) method to diagnose pneumonia in COVID-19 patients. The fusion of chest CT and chest X-ray radiographs over the pretrained CNN architecture gave 100% accuracy in the classification of COVID-19 [29].

5.7 REMOTE HEALTHCARE USING AI

Remote healthcare using AI is a technological innovation that gained demand in recent times. Figure 5.3 graphically illustrates the AI-based analytics on the healthcare data acquired from people at their homes.

This AI-computed decision concerning diseases is communicated across healthcare professions in the smart hospital to further guide treatment procedures. Therefore, smart remote healthcare can be proposed with the integration of AI, the Health Internet of Things (H-IoT), and smart apps [30]. With the COVID-19

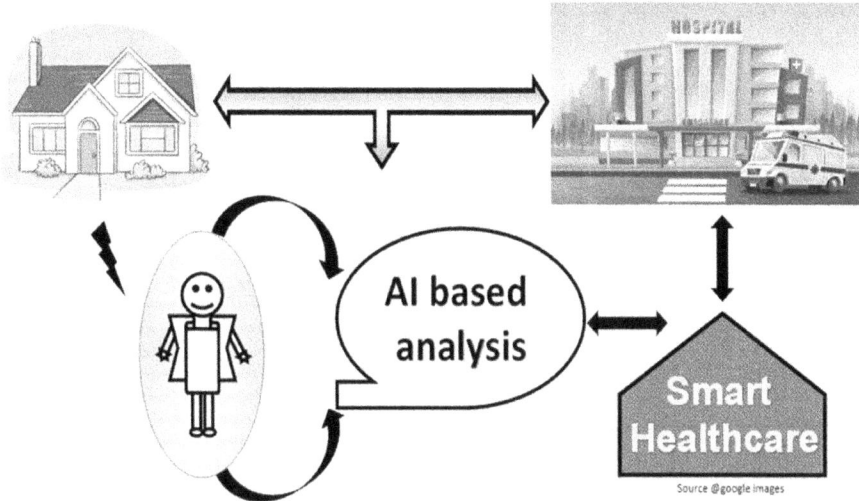

FIGURE 5.3 Representation of remote healthcare using AI.

pandemic, there was a need to develop continuous monitoring technology solutions remotely. H. Rohmetra et al. reviewed the novel methodology of remote monitoring of COVID-19 through vital signs. Vital signals, such as blood pressure, pulse rate, heart rate, oxygen saturation, and body temperature, are biomarkers for the detection of COVID-19 [31]. The emergence of numerous micro-/nanodevices, sensors, and wearable devices combined with AI and IoT can be a breakthrough for the sustainable healthcare infrastructure [32]. AI is the application of science and technology for developing intelligent machines. In the remote healthcare sector, AI provides an intelligent solution in two branches. In the virtual branch, AI analyzes patient electronic records to diagnose specific diseases and guide physicians with the treatment process. The physical branch comprises AI integrated with computer vision, robotics, nanobots, and intelligent algorithms for real-time healthcare solutions. The physical branch of AI represents smart healthcare solutions using automated drug delivery, remote operations, robotic helper, etc. [33]. The AI for remote healthcare with both virtual and physical treatment is depicted in Figure 5.4.

The continuous monitoring of health conditions, remotely predicting disease, proposing useful suggestions for treatment planning, and healthcare robots are the key aspects of remote healthcare using AI. Treatment with interventional radiology, such as laparoscopy, is a minimally invasive technique. A robot guided to move through the human body can perform the surgery process with reliable precision [34].

Digital pathology is a novel emerging technology in which the digital images of the pathology sample will be captured and transferred to the respective scientific laboratory for testing. The emergence of whole-slide imaging, cheaper storage solutions, and faster networks increase the pace of digital pathology. The incorporation of AI to perform computational analysis on the digitized pathology samples

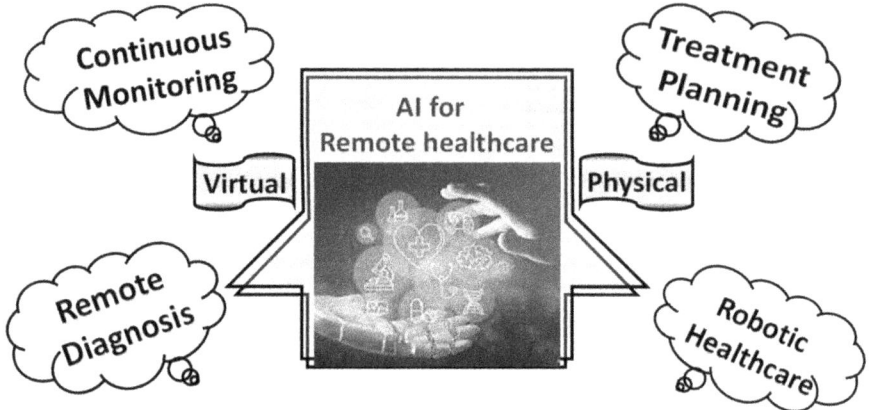

FIGURE 5.4   Graphical abstract to use AI branches for remote healthcare applications.

could be diagnosed at a greater efficiency than traditional techniques of humans diagnosing the pathology [35, 36]. Y. Hei et al. studied and concluded from their intensive research compilations that the combination of a graph convolution neural network with traditional deep learning models will enhance the performance of digital pathology [37]. Digital pathology is a revolution for remote diagnosis, as digital images can be shared instantaneously with far-away experts for treatment planning. So, during an emergency, the right guidance can be provided to save lives. Standard operating procedures through the digital workflow will keep up the turnaround time supporting remote healthcare [38]. Digital pathology aids remote diagnosis and treatment guidelines and is extensively used for research and development. In the education sector, through video conferencing introducing histopathological samples to students remotely, is possible. Henceforth, innovation in the treatment procedure can be developed by researchers studying digital pathology [39]. The perfect visualization of human organs is very crucial for the physician to take the proper decision. Thus, the human organ 3D view is regenerated by stacking several 2D sliced image sequences, known as 3D image reconstruction. M. I. A. Supriyanto et al. proposed an optical flow method for 3D image reconstruction after interpolation that enhanced reconstruction of the state-of-the-art algorithms [40]. In the healthcare sector, the cost of diagnosis and treatment needs to be minimized to be affordable and accessible to everyone. Medical imaging prospects have a key role even in the reduction of diagnosing costs. The 2D/3D registration and mapping of 3D atlases to 2D radiographs can help avoid undergoing costly CT scanning [41]. Thus, advancement in the processing of medical images is an opportunity for cost minimization for digital and remote diagnosis that in turn has the potential to save many lives. Moreover, computer-aided surgery, treatment planning, and continuous monitoring of health conditions are the tech innovations that are possible with the intelligent amalgamation of medical imaging and advanced AI techniques. Table 5.1 shows the various AI techniques used in medical imaging modalities for diagnosing different diseases.

TABLE 5.1
State of the art for radiology-based diagnosis

Model	Imaging	Disease	Accuracy (%)	Reference
CNN and ELM	X-ray	COVID-19	>99.11	[18]
CNN	X-ray	COVID-19, pneumonia, normal	95	[20]
Deep learning	CT	Lung cancer	—	[21]
Texture analysis	PET/CT	Lung cancer	—	[22]
Residual network	MRI	Brain cancer	99	[23]
2D and 3D CNN	MRI	Schizophrenia	79.27	[24]
SVM and CNN	MRI	AD and MCI	69.5	[25]
3D CNN	MRI	sDAT	88	[26]
SVM kernel combination	MRI, PET, and CSF	AD and MCI	91.8 and 75.6	[28]
CNN	X-ray and CT	COVID-19	100	[29]

5.8   LIMITATIONS OF USING AI FOR HEALTHCARE

AI has limitations for implementation in the healthcare domain. Hence, high precision, accuracy, fast computing, and communication of the right decision are very important, as it could be a matter of life and death. This section highlights a few of the drawbacks of AI being used for medical analysis. AI usually does not possess experience with real life. Therefore, the skill for generalization and abstraction is limited. Moreover, the possibility of misdiagnosing is dangerous as it could lead to severe stages of disease for false negatives and panic in case of false positives. In interventional radiology, the use of AI computing and the ability to give decisions at a faster pace is difficult. Sometimes it happens that the algorithm enters into an infinite loop and the treatment process cannot be communicated [42]. In their research, F. Pesapane et al. analyzed compilations and provided myths and facts about why machine learning and deep learning cannot replace interventional radiologists. AI aims to gain human-level cognitive capabilities. However, the complete replacement of AI in place of radiologists is not reliable. The future of AI-based complete healthcare solutions may take decades, centuries, or never occur. Nevertheless, AI has the potential to perform interventional radiology along with diagnostic radiology. The holistic and exact human-like intelligence has not been achieved yet. Therefore, in the future, AI might play a big role in the medical sector to provide smart healthcare solutions. But the utilization of complete AI is the choice of the physician and patient considering the several advantages as well as limitations of AI in the healthcare sector [43].

5.9   CONCLUSION

This chapter focuses on the utilization of medical imaging techniques, such as X-ray, CT, PET, and MRI to develop a healthcare predictive model. The incorporation of advanced AI techniques such as machine learning, deep learning, residual network, and GANs on the big data of medical image modalities can lead to smart digital diagnosis tools. Therefore, a digital approach to smart healthcare solutions can be effectively developed. Early and faster diagnosis through digital pathology is a technological breakthrough. Experts can suggest treatment plans for remote healthcare services. The fusion of multimodal data to achieve reliable efficiency in healthcare prediction is explained in this chapter. The minimization of cost for diagnosis using 3D image reconstruction from 2D sliced radiographs will make healthcare solutions affordable and reachable to everyone. Smart digital healthcare solutions can be innovated for early diagnosis, classification of various diseases, predicting the severity of disease, and analyzing the progression of the disease with digital imaging techniques. In the future, the incorporation of explainable AI will aim to provide human-like cognitive interpretations and attempt to solve current-day AI limitations. There exists much potential for AI and medical images to provide digital diagnosis and smart healthcare solutions for remote and real-time tracking of health status.

REFERENCES

1. G. Choy, O. Khalilzadeh, M. Michalski, S. Do, A. E. Samir, O. S. Pianykh, J. R. Geis, P. V. Pandharipande, J. A. Brink, K. J. Dreyer, "Current applications and future impact of machine learning in radiology," *Radiology*, vol. 288, no. 2, pp. 318–328, 2018. https://doi.org/10.1148/radio l.2018171820

2. M. Avanzo, M. Porzio, L. Lorenzon, L. Milan, R. Sghedoni, G. Russo, R. Massafra, "Artificial intelligence applications in medical imaging: A review of the medical physics research in Italy," *Phys. Medica*, vol. 83, pp. 221–241, 2021. https://doi.org/10.1016/j.ejmp.2021.04.010

3. L.-Q. Zhou, J.-Y. Wang, S.-Y. Yu, G.-G. Wu, Q. Wei, Y.-B. Deng, X.-L. Wu, X.-W. Cui, C. F. Dietrich, "Artificial intelligence in medical imaging of the liver," *World J. Gastroenterol.*, vol. 25, no. 6, pp. 672–682, February 2019. https://doi.org/ 10.3748/wjg. v25.i6.672

4. J. C. Gore, "Artificial intelligence in medical imaging," *Magn. Reson. Imaging*, vol. 68, pp. A1–A4, 2020. https://doi.org/10.1016/j.mri.2019.12.006

5. X. Ou, X. Qin, B. Huang, J. Zan, Q. Wu, Z. Hong, L. Xie, "High-resolution X-ray luminescence extension imaging," *Nature*, vol. 590, no. 7846, pp. 410–415, 2021. https://doi.org/10.1038/s41586-021-03251-6

6. C. Krittanawong, "The rise of artificial intelligence and the uncertain future for physicians," *Eur. J. Intern. Med.*, vol. 48, pp. e13–e14, 2018. https://doi.org/10.1016/j.ejim.2017.06.017

7. M. H. Arnold, "Teasing out artificial intelligence in medicine: An ethical critique of artificial intelligence and machine learning in medicine," *J. Bioeth. Inq.*, vol. 18, no. 1, pp. 121–139, March 2021. https://doi.org/10.1007/s11673-020-10080-1

8. F. Coppola, L. Faggioni, M. Gabelloni, F. De Vietro, V. Mendola, A. Cattabriga, M. A. Cocozza, "Human, all too human? An all-around appraisal of the 'artificial intelligence revolution' in medical imaging," *Front. Psychol.*, vol. 12, pp. 1–15, 2021. https://doi.org/10.3389/fpsyg.2021.710982

9. "Differences between X-rays, CT scans & MRI's envision radiology." https://www.en vrad.com/difference-between-x-ray-ct-scan-and-mri#what-is-x-ray (accessed September 27, 2022).

10. "Computed tomography (CT)." https://www.nibib.nih.gov/scienceeducation/scienc-etopi cs/computed-tomography-ct (accessed September 27, 2022).
11. "Magnetic resonance imaging (MRI)." https://www.nibib.nih.gov/scienc eeducation/scienc e-topics/magnetic-resonance-imaging-mri (accessed September 27, 2022).
12. "MRI scans: Definition, uses, and procedure." https://www.medicalnewstoday.com/articl es/146309#side-effects (accessed September 27, 2022).
13. C. Lee, Z. Luo, K. Y. Ngiam, M. Zhang, K. Zheng, G. Chen, B. C. Ooi, W. L. J. Yip, "Big healthcare data analytics: Challenges and applications," in *Handbook of Large-Scale Distributed Computing in Smart Healthcare*. Cham: Springer International Publishing, pp. 11–41, 2017.
14. E. C. de Farias, C. di Noia, C. Han, E. Sala, M. Castelli, L. Rundo, "Impact of GAN based lesion-focused medical image super-resolution on the robustness of radiomic features," *Scient. Rep.*, vol. 11, no. 1, 2021. https://doi.org/10.1038/s41598-021-00898-z
15. Y. Xia, N. Ravikumar, J. P. Greenwood, S. Neubauer, S. E. Petersen, A. F. Frangi, "Super-resolution of cardiac MR cine imaging using conditional GANs and unsupervised transfer learning," *Med. Image Anal.*, vol. 71, p. 102037, 2021. https://doi.org/10.1016/j.media.2021.102037
16. J. Zhu, C. Tan, J. Yang, G. Yang, P. Lio, "Arbitrary scale super-resolution for medical images," *Int. J. Neural Syst.*, vol. 31, no. 10, p. 2150037, 2021. https://doi.org/10.1142/S0129065721500374
17. A. Ibrahim, S. Primakov, M. Beuque, H. C. Woodruff, I. Halilaj, G. Wu, T. Refaee, "Radiomics for precision medicine: Current challenges, future prospects, and the proposal of a new framework," *Methods*, vol. 188, pp. 20–29, 2021. https://doi.org/10.1016/j.ymeth.2020.05.022
18. T. Hu, M. Khishe, M. Mohammadi, G. R. Parvizi, S. H. Taher Karim, T. A. Rashid, "Real-time COVID-19 diagnosis from X-ray images using deep CNN and extreme learning machines stabilized by chimp optimization algorithm," *Biomed. Signal Process. Control*, vol. 68, p. 102764, 2021. https://doi.org/10.1016/j.bspc.2021.102764
19. P. L. Bartlett, "The sample complexity of pattern classification with neural networks: The size of the weights is more important than the size of the network," *IEEE Trans. Inf. Theory*, vol. 44, no. 2, pp. 525–536, 1998. https://doi.org/10.1109/18.661502
20. M. Chakraborty, S. V. Dhavale, J. Ingole, "Corona-Nidaan: Lightweight deep convolutional neural network for chest X-ray based COVID-19 infection detection," *Appl. Intell.*, vol. 51, no. 5, pp. 3026–3043, 2021. https//doi.org/10.1007/s10489-020-01978-9
21. D. Ardila, A. P. Kiraly, S. Bharadwaj, B. Choi, J. J. Reicher, L. Peng, D. Tse, "End-to-end lung cancer screening with three-dimensional deep learning on low-dose chest computed tomography," *Nat. Med.*, vol. 25, no. 6, pp. 954–961, 2019. https//doi.org/10.1038/s41591-019-0447-x
22. M. Kirienko, L. Cozzi, L. Antunovic, L. Lozza, A. Fogliata, E. Voulaz, A. Rossi, A. Chiti, M. Sollini, "Prediction of disease-free survival by the PET/CT radiomic signature in non-small cell lung cancer patients undergoing surgery," *Eur. J. Nucl. Med. Mol. Imaging*, vol. 45, no. 2, pp. 207–217, 2018. https://doi.org/10.1007/s00259-017-3837-7
23. S. A. Abdelaziz Ismael, A. Mohammed, H. Hefny, "An enhanced deep learning approach for brain cancer MRI images classification using residual networks," *Artif. Intell. Med.*, vol. 102, p. 101779, 2020. https://doi.org/10.1016/j.artmed.2019.101779
24. M. Hu, X. Qian, S. Liu, A. J. Koh, K. Sim, X. Jiang, C. Guan, J. H. Zhou, "Structural and diffusion MRI based schizophrenia classification using 2D pretrained and 3D naive convolutional neural networks," *Schizophr. Res.*, vol. 243, no. 2020, pp. 330–341, 2022. https://doi.org/10.1016/j.schres.2021.06.011

25. E. E. Bron, S. Klein, J. M. Papma, L. C. Jiskoot, V. Venkatraghavan, J. Linders, P. Aalten, "Cross-cohort generalizability of deep and conventional machine learning for MRI-based diagnosis and prediction of Alzheimer's disease," *NeuroImage Clin.*, vol. 31, 2021. https://doi.org/10.1016/j.nicl.2021.102712

26. E. Yee, D. Ma, K. Popuri, L. Wang, M. F. Beg, "Construction of MRI-based Alzheimer's disease score based on efficient 3D convolutional neural network: Comprehensive validation on 7,902 images from a multi-center dataset," *J. Alzheimer's Dis.*, vol. 79, no. 1, pp. 47–58, 2021. https://doi.org/10.3233/JAD-200830

27. R. Brookmeyer, E. Johnson, K. Ziegler-Graham, H. M. Arrighi, "Forecasting the global burden of Alzheimer's disease," *Alzheimer's Dement.*, vol. 3, no. 3, pp. 186–191, 2007. https://doi.org/.1016/j.jalz.2007.04.381

28. D. Zhang, Y. Wang, L. Zhou, H. Yuan, D. Shen, "Multimodal classification of Alzheimer's disease and mild cognitive impairment," *Neuroimage*, vol. 55, no. 3, pp. 856–867, 2011. https://doi.org/10.1016/j.neuroimage.2011.01.008

29. P. K. Chaudhori, R. B. Pachori, "FBSED based automatic diagnosis of COVID-19 using X-ray and CT images," *Comput. Biol. Med.*, vol. 134, 2021. https://doi.org/10.1016/j. compbiomed.2021.104454

30. M. Alshamrani, "IoT and artificial intelligence implementations for remote healthcare monitoring systems: A survey," *J. King Saud Univ. - Comput. Inf. Sci.*, vol. 34, no. 8, pp. 4687–4701, 2022. https://doi.org/10.1016/j.jksuci.2021.06.005

31. H. Rohmetra, N. Raghunath, P. Narang, V. Chamola, M. Guizani, N. R. Lakkaniga, "AI-enabled remote monitoring of vital signs for COVID-19: Methods, prospects and challenges," *Computing*, vol. 202, pp. 1–27. https://doi.org/10.1007/s00607-021 -00937-7

32. P. Dwivedi, M. K. Singha, "IoT based wearable healthcare system: Post covid-19," in *The Impact of the COVID-19 Pandemic on Green Societies*. Cham: Springer, pp. 305–321, 2021.

33. P. Hamet, J. Tremblay, "Artificial intelligence in medicine," *Metabolism*, vol. 69, pp. S36–S40, 2017. https/doi.org/10.1016/j.metabol.2017.01.011

34. R. H. Kassamali, B. Ladak, "The role of robotics in interventional radiology: Current status," *Quant. Imaging Med. Surg.*, vol. 5, no. 3, pp. 340–343, 2015. https.doi.org/10 .3978/j.issn .2223-4292.2015.03.15

35. M. K. K. Niazi, A. V. Parwani, M. N. Gurcan, "Digital pathology and artificial intelligence," *Lancet Oncol.*, vol. 20, no. 5, pp. e253–e261, 2019. https://doi.org/10.1016/S1 47020 45(19)30154-8

36. L. Browning, R. Colling, E. Rakha, N. Rajpoot, J. Rittscher, J. A. James, M. Salto-Tellez, D. R. J. Snead, C. Verrill, "Digital pathology and artificial intelligence will be key to supporting clinical and academic cellular pathology through COVID-19 and future crises: The PathLAKE consortium perspective," *J. Clin. Pathol.*, vol. 74, no. 7, pp. 443–447, 2021. https/doi.org/10.1136/jclinpath-2020-206854

37. M. I. A. Supriyanto, A. Fajar, R. Sarno, C. Fatichah, A. Fahmi, S. A. Utomo, F. Notopuro, "Slice reconstruction on 3D medical image using optical flow approach," *IEEE Asia Pacific Conf. Wirel. Mobile*, 2021, pp. 242–246, 2021. https/doi.org/10.110 9/APWiMob51111.2021.9435238

38. J. Van Houtte, E. Audenaert, G. Zheng, J. Sijbers, "Deep learning-based 2D/3D registration of an atlas to biplanar X-ray images," *Int. J. Comput. Assist. Radiol. Surg.*, vol. 17, no. 7, pp. 1333–1342, 2022. https/doi.org/10.1007/s11548-022-02586-3

39. M. Gurgitano, S. A. Angileri, G. M. Rodà, A. Liguori, M. Pandolfi, A. M. Ierardi, B. J. Wood, G. Carrafiello, "Interventional radiology ex-machina: Impact of artificial intelligence on practice," *Radiol. Med.*, vol. 126, no. 7, pp. 998–1006, 2021. https://doi.org/10 .1007/s11547021-01351-x

40. F. Pesapane, P. Tantrige, F. Patella, P. Biondetti, L. Nicosia, A. Ianniello, U. G. Rossi, G. Carrafiello, A. M. Ierardi, "Myths and facts about artificial intelligence: Why machine- and deep learning will not replace interventional radiologists," *Med. Oncol.*, vol. 37, no. 5, pp. 1–9, 2020. https/doi.org/.1007/s12032-020-01368-8

41. C. Chakraborty, S. B. Othman, F. A. Almalki, H. Sakli, "FC-SEEDA: Fog computing- based secure and energy efficient data aggregation scheme for internet of healthcare things," *Neural Comput. Appl.* 2023. https://doi.org/10.1007/s00521-023-08270-0

42. S. Ben Othman, A. A. Bahattab, A. Trad, H. Youssef, "PEERP: A priority-based energy-efficient routing protocol for reliable data transmission in healthcare using the IoT." *The 15th International Conference on Future Networks and Communications (FNC)*, Leuven, Belgium, 9–12 August 2020.

43. S. Ben Othman, F. A. Almalki, C. Chakraborty, H. Sakli, "Privacy-preserving aware data aggregation for IoT-based healthcare with green computing technologies," *Comput. Electr. Eng.*, vol. 101, 2022, p. 108025. https://doi.org/10.1016/j.compeleceng .2022.108025

6 Efficient and Fast Lung Disease Predictor Model

Abdelbaki Souid, Mohamed Hamroun,
Ben Othman Soufiene, and Hedi Sakli

6.1 INTRODUCTION

Pulmonary and thoracic diseases, infections, and cancers are a danger to human health. The World Health Organization reported about 3.23 million deaths worldwide from chronic obstructive pulmonary disease in 2019 [1], and the American Cancer Society Statistics Center states that each year, about 150,000 people die due to lung cancer, with an additional 200,000 new cases identified each year in the United States.

Overall, the chance that a man will develop a lung nodule or mass in his lifetime is about 1 in 15; for women, the risk is less (1 in 17). It is critical to acknowledge that lung cancer is one of the most common malignancies in the world leading to the deaths of thousands each year, caused by several factors, including smoking and chemical exposure [2].

According to the World Health Organization, approximately 4 million premature deaths occur due to illnesses such as pneumonia and asthma in low- and middle-income nations, where millions of people face uncontrolled surroundings and poverty. As a result, it is critical to discover a remedy that can combat the spread of such diseases and tumors. Many medical diagnostic methods have been employed to assist in addressing this condition, notably chest radiography, which is considered the primary tool in clinical practice for patients with nonspecific thoracic symptoms. Chest radiography, also known as a chest X-ray scan, is a low-cost procedure that is widely available in most healthcare facilities. The vast quantity of exams that must be interpreted is a well-established problem for the majority of radiologists to maintain diagnostic quality. Also, missed abnormality identification is also common, even among experienced radiologists [3–5].

COVID-19 can lead to severe lung infections, progressive lung damage, and breathing difficulties. Furthermore, the pandemic increased human susceptibility to illnesses related to COVID-19, such as pneumonia and some bacterial infections [6]. The idea of automated early detection of pulmonary diseases became more pressing than ever. Recently, with improvements to hardware acceleration and artificial intelligence, specifically deep learning methods, there has been an important boost in performance and largely superior results in many fields such as semantic segmentation

DOI: 10.1201/9781003366249-6

and object detection [7–9]. In the medical area, machine learning researchers are working on a variety of similar techniques to predict chest radiographs early [10–17].

The primary goal of this research is to investigate and address the challenge of recognizing eight lung malignancies. The model is composed of two major blocks: The first is a feature extraction module, which contains a pretrained CNN weight. The second block is in charge of using the new weight in identifying pathology percentages. This chapter is divided into sections starting with an introduction on the importance of the discussed topics. Section 6.2 reviews the past work on the classification problem, specifically with medical data. Section 6.3 presents the developed approach. The discussion, Section 6.4, dictates the outcome of the experiment that was carried out. A conclusion section loaded with perspectives of the presented work also addresses the weaker links of the work and how to improve them.

6.2 HISTORY OF COMPUTER-AIDED DETECTION ASSOCIATED WITH DEEP LEARNING

Computer-aided detection (CAD) dedicated to chest radiography exams has been established as an idea, and from the presented literature [12–17] there are promising results in the detection of several diseases such as nodule detection.

Many studies have been conducted in the medical field that incorporates artificial intelligence algorithms to help with diagnosis and provide reliable findings. However, healthcare facilities and skilled specialists are in short supply, particularly in rural areas and nations with economic problems. As a result of this, chest X-rays are generally used by medical experts in these regions to identify chest-related illnesses. However, for the sake of argument, these chest radiography exams are utilized in the identification of lung infections such as pneumonia, diagnosis is a very difficult process that must be performed by a handful of skilled radiologists [18]. To enhance pneumonia diagnosis, Han et al. [19] presented an ensembled model. The architecture achieves a maximum 95.6% accuracy score on the test data, the model was constrained to autonomously monitor the guided deformable registration in pulmonary regions and segmenting the region of interest (ROI). Zhang et al. [20] presented a method to obtain pixel-wise transcribed digitally reconstructed radiograph data and build a supervised cross-segmentation model in X-ray images. The Task Driven Generative Adversarial Network (TD-GAN) was used. It is challenging and time-consuming to close the gap in nodule annotations.

There are relatively few solutions that have addressed the 14 categories of disorders related to the chest for the multiclass challenge. Some employ an image descriptor capable of identifying deteriorated lung tissues in an X-ray exam. The work by Wang et al. [21] provided one of the main open-access chest X-ray datasets. The presented dataset has been implemented in numerous research articles and multiple artificial intelligence experiments; the bulk of the studies have risen the bar toward the expectation of deep learning from great results that use CNN architecture. Sivasamy and Subashini [22] utilized a deep learning approach to read chest X-rays and predict lung illnesses with 86.14% accuracy for the goal of using deep neural networks.

One-class detection of cardiothoracic illnesses is possible. The work presented by Rajpurkar et al. [23] demonstrated a 0.435 f1 binary CT scan pneumonia diagnosis classifier. There are also deep neural networks for detecting multiclass pulmonary diseases. A few studies employed cutting-edge methods and had favorable outcomes for one or two pulmonary illnesses that used meta-analysis, albeit they frequently had misclassification issues. Sahlol et al. [24] presented a novel hybrid approach for quick diagnosis and classification of the presence of tuberculosis within a chest radiograph. A transfer learning strategy was applied to a CNN architecture with previously trained weights on different dataset tasks to extract features from chest X-ray images. The metaheuristic artificial ecosystem-based optimization (AEO) method was employed as a prediction component to determine which of these features appeared to be the most relevant. The suggested method was evaluated on two publicly available datasets that help them to achieve substantial efficiency while lowering computational costs. The work of Souid et al. [25] presented a CNN to detect the presence of 14 pulmonary lesions on an X-ray exam. The outcome generalizes what lighter CNN can achieve concerning energy efficiency and prediction accuracy. In another application of transfer learning, Rajpurkar et al. [26] proposed a model to identify chest and pulmonary disorders. The trained model was tested using a single radiograph scan of the chest to calculate the likelihood of the 14 possible findings. The evaluation of these experiments revealed the best possible implementation with DenseNet-121 [27] achieving the highest test prediction accuracy. Table 6.1 is

TABLE 6.1
Recent related works to pathology detection from chest X-rays using deep learning methods

Reference	Aim	Used Dataset	Preprocessing technique and feature extraction	ML Technique	Accuracy
Chandra et al. [19]	Pneumonia detection from CXRs	RSNA Pneumonia Detection Challenge	Normalization and local binary features	ResNet Attention Deep learning	0.886
Wang et al. [21]	Developing a benchmark for ChestX-ray14 dataset	NIH ChestX-ray14		Multiple ImageNet CNN	0.742
A. Souid et al [25]	Detection of 14 lung pathologies from CXR	NIH ChestX-ray14	Radom oversampling, data cleaning	MobilenetV2 as FE Added layers	0.812
Rajpurkar et al. [26]	Detection 14 lung pathologies from chest X-ray	NIH ChestX-ray14	Weighted loss entropy	DenseNet 121	81.8%

a comparison of studies associated with ours concerning data availability and deep learning usage.

The presented work proposes a fast and efficient architecture for identifying multiple related pulmonary or thoracic findings using CNNs to address the unbalanced data using transfer learning and EfficientNet B1 [28] models for classification tasks to accurately estimate the existence of eight pulmonary classes with high sensitivity.

6.3 PROPOSED MODELS

6.3.1 DATASET PRESENTATION

The present research examines eight types of lung disorders. The ChestX-ray8 [29] is regarded as one of the most comprehensive open-source medical datasets comprising 108,948 frontal chest radiographs of 32,717 patients with multiple lung-related pathology labels. Later on, Wang et al. [29] expanded the ChestX-ray8 to include 112,120 scans and 14 pathology labels that were text mined. The use of the "No Finding" label was for samples that did not have to be specified with existing labels.

The dataset includes lung-related pathologies such as mass, nodule, pleural thickening, pneumonia, and pneumothorax, and others like "cardiomegaly". This dataset was burdened with several flaws, beginning with a huge class imbalance induced by a mismatched proportion of non-finding exam samples. A second issue was the large amount of uncommon pathology distribution, namely, pneumonia or hernia, by including a minority of data samples.

Our contribution starts with addressing these problems within the dataset. We combined this data source with two other datasets. The first added dataset was known as the optical coherence tomography (OCT) and chest X-ray dataset [30]. This dataset is divided into two sets: one for OCT and the second for chest X-rays. Our concern is reserved for the chest radiograph set. It contains 5,863 chest radiographs text mined as normal or pneumonia. By combining the presented data, we gain an increase in the number of samples of pneumonia pathology. The second dataset we considered was VinDr-CXR (VDC) [31]. The dataset consists of 18,000 X-ray exams in total. Also, the dataset's labels were mined using a natural processing model. Since the VDC shares some of its pathology labels with the ChestX-ray14, this dataset is extremely useful for balancing frequency distributions of certain classes.

There are still some drawbacks to this method. We cannot leverage the metadata contained in both due to major differences in metadata starting with the data type. The VDC dataset is in DICOM format, while the other two datasets are in JPEG format, which is a significant distinction that we cannot rely on. We previously mentioned the class correlation between VDC and ChestX-ray14, however, this was not for all of the specified diseases. Thus we had to choose between utilizing the entire dataset and training with 17 pathologies or lowering the number of classes.

This work chooses to acquire the following eight lung diseases in the presented work: atelectasis, cardiomegaly, consolidation, nodule/mass, pleural thickening, pneumothorax, pulmonary fibrosis, and pneumonia. In the next section, we will describe the novel method and the parameters used, and discuss the illustrated approach to avoid unbalanced data.

6.3.2 EFFICIENTNET FOR PULMONARY DETECTION

This section provides details of the steps of the presented approach. The approach starts with data cleaning, processing, and model implementation, then also detailing the model training specifics and the evaluation metrics used to quantify the pathology prediction task.

Our technique conforms to a unique methodology that begins with merging the dataset, then preprocessing the data and doing sanity checks before splitting it into three subdatasets: training, validation, and testing. As with typical machine learning models, we feed training and validation data into the model during training. The model is made up of two parts: a trained model weights and the transfer block. We analyze the model by computing the appropriate metrics until it is fit for final testing with foreign data.

6.3.3 DATA AUGMENTATION AND PROCESSING

First, we clean the needed data by identifying outliers, avoiding data leakage, and verifying the integrity of each class. The reformed dataset is then separated into three subsets, the large subset intended for the training phase, the second for validation, and the last tiny fraction for assessing the model's performance. Dataset augmentation is a useful approach for reducing model overfitting by increasing the amount of data training and adding various distortions and noise to the training data. On photographs, the presented method uses five data augmentation techniques: horizontal flip, brightness, contrast manipulation, random-sized cropping, and pixel value normalization to create pixel values ranging from 0 to 255.

To handle the imbalanced dataset, our method adds a positive weight and a negative weight to the cross-entropy loss in Equation 6.1:

$$L^w_{cross-entropy} - \left(w_{ps} \log\left(1 - f\left(x\right)\right) \right) \qquad (6.1)$$

In this case, positive weight w_{ps} was multiplied by the positive frequency $freq_s$ of each class to equal the negative weight w_{ng} that was also multiplied by negative frequency $freq_{ng}$:

$$w_{ps} \times freq_{ps} = w_{ng} \times freq_{ng} \qquad (6.2)$$

6.3.4 MODEL ARCHITECTURE

EfficientNet is capable of a wide range of image classification tasks. This makes it a good model for transfer learning [28]. Table 6.2 presents the network search architecture. The Mobile Inverted Bottleneck Conv (MB-Conv) Block, developed by Huang et al. [27], and depicted in Figure 6.1, is a major novel component. The

TABLE 6.2

The efficientNet conv network distribution

Level	Operation	Output size	Number of channels	Number of layers
1	Cv3*3	224,224	32	1
2	MBCv1, k3,3	112,112	16	1
3	MBCv6, k3,3	112,112	24	2
4	MBCv6, k5,5	56,56	40	2
5	MBCv6, k3,3	28,28	80	3
6	MBCv6, k5,5	14,14	112	3
7	MBCv6, k5,5	14,14	192	4
8	MBCv6, k3,3	7,7	320	1
9	Cv1,1/Pl/	FC, 7,7	1,280	1

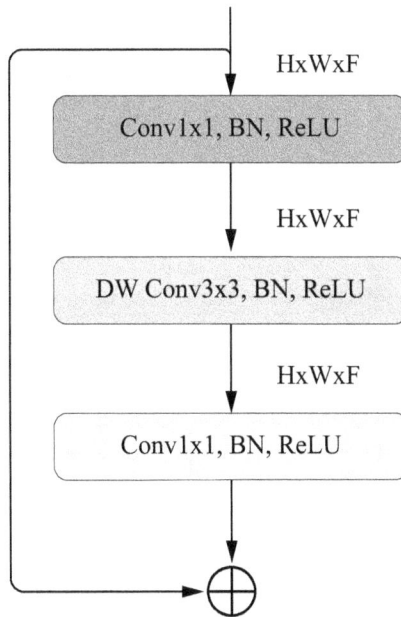

FIGURE 6.1 Depthwise conv. The kernel size is 1×1/3×3. Batch normalization is BN. H, W, and F are tensor forms of height, width, and depth. The multiplier for the number of repeated layers ranges from 1 to 4. (Adapted from the original EfficientNet research.)

EfficientNet conv network distribution is based on the idea of starting with a high parameter, compact baseline model, and progressively scaling each of its dimensions using a sequence of scaling factors.

Instead of developing a model from scratch, the usage of trained weights from the same tasks of different dataset models speeds up and improves the learning process. The presented method consists of two blocks, presented in Figure 6.1, by adding

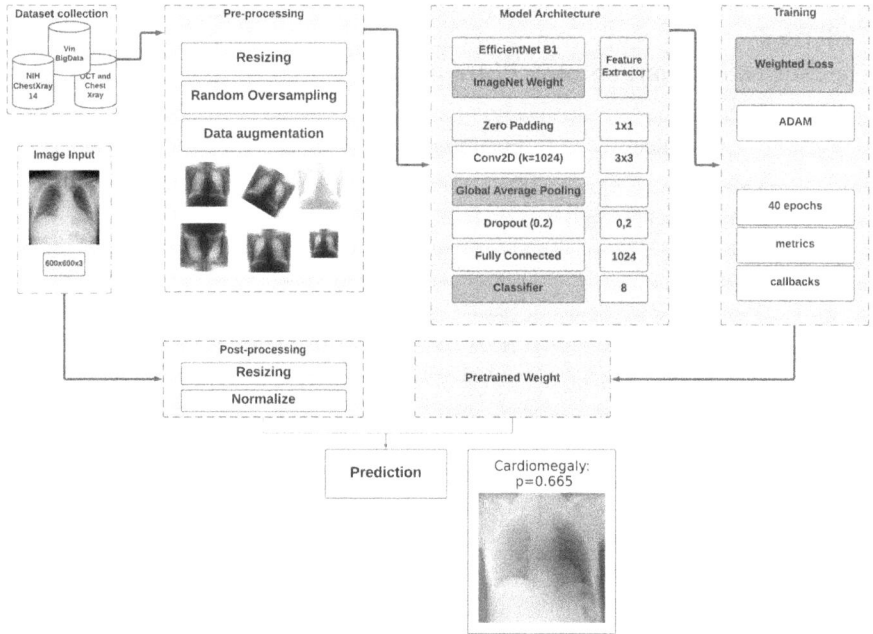

FIGURE 6.2   Proposed architecture: Input $224 \times 224 \times 3$, EfficientNet B1 ImageNet trained weights followed by a zero-padding; a conv layer (3, 3) kernel; and a GAP layer, dropout layer, dense layer with 1024, and a classifier layer with eight value vectors.

trained models on the ImageNet [32] dataset. To take full advantage of ImageNet weights, the transfer block starts with a zero-padding layer to assist and smooth the results, a conv layer with a 512 kernel and 33 stride size. Following the GAP (global average pooling) layer was a conditional dropout layer, a fully connected layer with 1024 output nodes, and an 8-output node classifier. The fundamental blocks are seen in Figure 6.2. Our dataset was separated into three parts: 70% for training, 20% for validation, and 10% for testing.

For the EfficientNet B1, our input size is (224,224, 3). We utilized "Adam" as the optimizing algorithm to create the model. The model training started with a learning rate of 1e–2 and is subsequently decreased to 1e–5.

The learning algorithm proceeded by freezing the weights of all layers of the model for 15 epochs with half the steps each epoch using trainable weights to fine-tune the model. The model was also tested with 0.5 thresholds to enhance accuracy and allow the model to generalize more.

6.4   EXPERIMENTAL RESULTS

The main metric is the receiver operating characteristic (ROC) to better assess the model's diagnostic performance. The test accuracy, area under the curve (AUC), sensitivity, and specificity for lung legion classification in chest radiography were evaluated.

$$Accuracy = \frac{TP + TN}{TP + FP + TN + FN} \tag{6.3}$$

$$Sensitivity = \frac{TP}{TP + FN} \tag{6.4}$$

$$Specificity = \frac{TN}{TN + FP} \tag{6.5}$$

The number of correctly recognized ailment samples is represented by TP (true positive), whereas the number of mistaken disease samples is represented by TN (true negative). The number of sickness samples in the sample that were mistakenly identified as disease-free is represented by FP (false positive), whereas the number of disease-free samples that were not classified as disease samples is marked as FN (false negative).

Both testing and training are done on a Google Colab [33] instance with one virtual GPU.

In this analysis, we identified a wide range of findings when compared to AUC values. This might be due to the random initialization of the models, as well as the stochastic nature of the optimizer, in addition to the loss function. The model was estimated using the residue test set. The graphical representation of the loss value versus the epoch for the three experiments is shown in Figure 6.3, where loss means training and validation loss signifies validation loss.

Based on the loss value, the EfficientNet B1 implies that incorporating more features enhances total model performance. The developed model's performance metrics were 0.265 in training and 0.245 in validation for loss and accuracy with a classwise accuracy of 76% to 95%, 81.5% for sensitivity, 80.8% for specificity, and

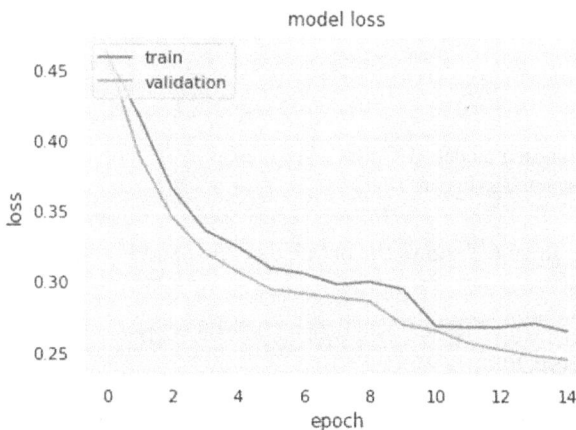

FIGURE 6.3 Loss value throughout the training stage. The dark gray curve denotes training loss, and the light gray curve denotes loss during validation.

TABLE 6.3

Evaluation metrics report for the EfficientNet B1

Pathology	Accuracy	Sensitivity	Specificity	AUC
Nodule/mass	0.771	0.713	0.776	0.835
Pleural thickening	0.744	0.786	0.742	0.841
Atelectasis	0.764	0.831	0.759	0.872
Consolidation	0.764	0.82	0.762	0.861
PT	0.792	0.809	0.791	0.882
Pneumothorax	0.824	0.879	0.822	0.925
Cardiomegaly	0.858	0.859	0.858	0.926
Pneumonia	0.951	0.825	0.954	0.963

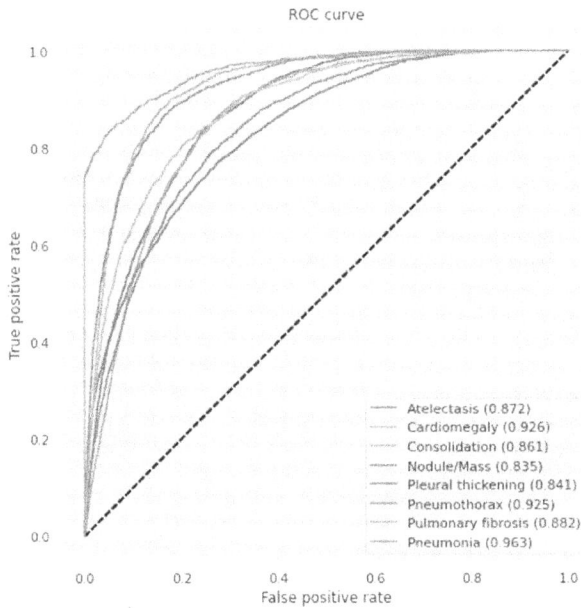

ROC curve

True positive rate

False positive rate

Atelectasis (0.872)
Cardiomegaly (0.926)
Consolidation (0.861)
Nodule/Mass (0.835)
Pleural thickening (0.841)
Pneumothorax (0.925)
Pulmonary fibrosis (0.882)
Pneumonia (0.963)

FIGURE 6.4 Proposed model AUC ROC. The greatest AUC for pneumonia was 0.963, and the lowest was for mass/nodule at 0.835.

0.888 for AUC. Table 6.3 shows the detailed results, and Figure 6.4 shows the ROC for the AUC.

6.5   DISCUSSION

To begin, we compared the obtained results to those of Rajpurkar et al. [26] and Wang et al. [29]. Whereas the DenseNet-121 has a superior individual AUC in three out of eight disease classes, EfficientNet B1 has a 30% improvement in more than three of them. Baltruschat et al. [34] are among those who have contributed to this

TABLE 6.4
AUC versus other methodologies

Pathology	Baltruschat et al. [34]	Rajpurkar et al. [26]	Wang et al. [29]	Proposed
Atelectasis	0.755	0.862	0.700	0.872
Cardiomegaly	0.875	0.831	0.810	0.926
Consolidation	0.749	0.893	0.703	0.861
Mass/nodule	0.821/0.758	0.909/0.892	0.693/0.669	0.835
Pleural thickening	0.761	0.798	0.669	0.841
Pneumothorax	0.846	0.944	0.799	0.925
Pulmonary fibrosis	0.818	0.806	0.786	0.882
Pneumonia	0.714	0.851	0.799	0.963
Avg	0.788	0.861	0.742	0,888

Notes: The comparison is based on eight diseases; the other technique contains more lung illnesses.

study. While our model was trained with fewer epochs, it nevertheless produced good results for six pathologies as well, a slightly higher average AUC of 0.888. The EfficientNet B1 is more general; three classes outperform the 0.9 AUC, and the GradCam Visualization is highly exact even at 224,224 image resolutions [35]. In comparison to prior novel studies, such as Wang et al. [29] that recorded an AUC of 0.745, Baltruschat et al. [34] with an AUC of 0.806, and Rajpurkar et al. [26] with an AUC of 0.812, the EfficientNet B1 produces exceptionally acceptable results. Table 6.4 shows the detailed results.

6.6   CONCLUSION

Based on the findings, our deep learning model might help radiologists refine the accuracy of their diagnosis for a wide range of pulmonary lesions. When expert radiologists are either overworked or unavailable in an emergency, a deep learning system, such as ours, can speed up scan explanations. Even though it can increase interpretation accuracy, our technique should only be used to augment pulmonary issue diagnosis.

Our research has several limitations. First, it did not extrapolate the entire dataset, which had over 15 pathologies. Also, this developed model was a feasibility study, thus we excluded expert comparisons from our analysis. The discrepancy between the AUC and the accuracy necessitates further examination, with the implementation of additional metrics. In the end, there were numerous strategies for dealing with the skewed dataset, and it was necessary to compare their efficiencies.

REFERENCES

1. "Chronic obstructive pulmonary disease (COPD)." https://www.who.int/news-room/fact-sheets/detail/chronic-obstructive-pulmonary-disease-(copd) (accessed March 30, 2022).

2. "Lung cancer statistics|How common is lung cancer?" https://www.cancer.org/cancer/lung-cancer/about/key-statistics.html (accessed March 30, 2022).

3. L. Monnier-Cholley, L. Arrivé, A. Porcel, K. Shehata, H. Dahan, T. Urban, M. Febvre, B. Lebeau, and J. M. Tubiana, "Characteristics of missed lung cancer on chest radiographs: A French experience," *European Radiology*, vol. 11, no. 4, pp. 597–605, Mar. 2001, doi: 10.1007/s003300000595.

4. P. K. Shah, J. H. M. Austin, C. S. White, P. Patel, L. B. Haramati, G. D. N. Pearson, M. C. Shiau, and Y. M. Berkmen, "Missed non-small cell lung cancer: Radiographic findings of potentially resectable lesions evident only in retrospect," *Radiology*, vol. 226, no. 1, pp. 235–241, Jan. 2003, doi: 10.1148/radiol.2261011924.

5. L. G. Quekel, A. G. Kessels, R. Goei, and J. M. van Engelshoven, "Miss rate of lung cancer on the chest radiograph in clinical practice," *Chest*, vol. 115, no. 3, pp. 720–724, Mar. 1999, doi: 10.1378/chest.115.3.720.

6. U. Z. Khuhawar, I. F. Siddiqui, Q. A. Arain, M. M. Siddiqui, and N. M. F. Qureshi, "On-ground distributed COVID-19 variant intelligent data analytics for a regional territory," *Wireless Communications and Mobile Computing*, vol. 2021, pp. 1–19, Dec. 2021, doi: 10.1155/2021/1679835.

7. M. T. T. Teichmann, and R. Cipolla, "Convolutional CRFs for semantic segmentation," *arXiv:1805.04777 [cs]*, May 2018, Accessed: Mar. 30, 2022. [Online]. http://arxiv.org/abs/1805.04777.

8. B. Gu, R. Ge, Y. Chen, L. Luo, and G. Coatrieux, "Automatic and robust object detection in X-ray baggage inspection using deep convolutional neural networks," *IEEE Transactions on Industrial Electronics*, vol. 68, no. 10, pp. 10248–10257, Oct. 2021, doi: 10.1109/TIE.2020.3026285.

9. Y. Pi, N. D. Nath, and A. H. Behzadan, "Convolutional neural networks for object detection in aerial imagery for disaster response and recovery," *Advanced Engineering Informatics*, vol. 43, p. 101009, Jan. 2020, doi: 10.1016/j.aei.2019.101009.

10. W. Sun, B. Zheng, and W. Qian, "Computer aided lung cancer diagnosis with deep learning algorithms," San Diego, California, United States, Mar. 2016, p. 97850Z, doi: 10.1117/12.2216307.

11. W. Sun, B. Zheng, and W. Qian, "Automatic feature learning using multichannel ROI based on deep structured algorithms for computerized lung cancer diagnosis," *Computers in Biology Medicine*, vol. 89, pp. 530–539, Oct. 2017, doi: 10.1016/j.compbiomed.2017.04.006.

12. N. Sakli, H. Ghabri, B. O. Soufiene, F. Almalki, H. Sakli, O. Ali, and M. Najjari, "ResNet-50 for 12-lead electrocardiogram automated diagnosis," *Computational Intelligence and Neuroscience*, vol. 2022, pp. 1–16, Apr. 2022, doi: 10.1155/2022/7617551.

13. S. Abdelbaki, S. Nizar, and S. Hedi, "Toward an efficient deep learning model for lung pathologies detection in X-ray images."

14. A. Souid, and H. Sakli, "Xception-ResNet autoencoder for pneumothorax segmentation," in 2022 *IEEE 9th International Conference on Sciences of Electronics, Technologies of Information and Telecommunications (SETIT)*, Hammamet, Tunisia, May 2022, pp. 586–590, doi: 10.1109/SETIT54465.2022.9875922.

15. J. G. Nam, E. J. Hwang, D. S. Kim, S.-J. Yoo, H. Choi, J. M. Goo, and C. M. Park, "Undetected lung cancer at posteroanterior chest radiography: Potential role of a deep learning–based detection algorithm," *Radiol Cardiothorac Imaging*, vol. 2, no. 6, p. e190222, Dec. 2020, doi: 10.1148/ryct.2020190222.

16. S. Schalekamp, B. van Ginneken, E. Koedam, M. M. Snoeren, A. M. Tiehuis, R. Wittenberg, N. Karssemeijer, and C. M. Schaefer-Prokop, "Computer-aided detection improves detection of pulmonary nodules in chest radiographs beyond the support by bone-suppressed images," *Radiology*, vol. 272, no. 1, pp. 252–261, Jul. 2014, doi: 10.1148/radiol.14131315.

17. C. S. White, T. Flukinger, J. Jeudy, and J. J. Chen, "Use of a computer-aided detection system to detect missed lung cancer at chest radiography," *Radiology*, vol. 252, no. 1, pp. 273–281, Jul. 2009, doi: 10.1148/radiol.2522081319.

18. T. Franquet, "Imaging of community-acquired pneumonia," *J Thorac Imaging*, vol. 33, no. 5, pp. 282–294, Sep. 2018, doi: 10.1097/RTI.0000000000000347.

19. Y. Han, C. Chen, A. Tewfik, Y. Ding, and Y. Peng, "Pneumonia detection on chest X-ray using radiomic features and contrastive learning," in 2021 *IEEE 18th International Symposium on Biomedical Imaging (ISBI)*, Nice, France, Apr. 2021, pp. 247–251, doi: 10.1109/ISBI48211.2021.9433853.

20. Y. Zhang, S. Miao, T. Mansi, and R. Liao, "Task driven generative modeling for unsupervised domain adaptation: Application to X-ray image segmentation," *arXiv:1806.07201 [cs]*, vol. 11071, pp. 599–607, 2018, doi: 10.1007/978-3-030-00934-2_67.

21. X. Wang, Y. Peng, L. Lu, Z. Lu, M. Bagheri, and R. M. Summers, "ChestX-ray: hospital-scale chest X-ray database and benchmarks on weakly supervised classification and localization of common thorax diseases," in L. Lu, X. Wang, G. Carneiro, and L. Yang (Eds.), *Deep Learning and Convolutional Neural Networks for Medical Imaging and Clinical Informatics*. Cham: Springer International Publishing, 2019, pp. 369–392, doi: 10.1007/978-3-030-13969-8_18.

22. J. Sivasamy, and T. S. Subashini, "Classification and predictions of lung diseases from chest X-rays using MobileNet," no. 0886, p. 8.

23. P. Rajpurkar, A. Park, J. Irvin, C. Chute, M. Bereket, D. Mastrodicasa, C. P. Langlotz, M. P. Lungren, A. Y. Ng, and B. N. Patel, "AppendiXNet: Deep learning for diagnosis of appendicitis from a small dataset of CT exams using video pretraining," *Sci Rep*, vol. 10, no. 1, p. 3958, Dec. 2020, doi: 10.1038/s41598-020-61055-6.

24. A. T. Sahlol, M. Abd Elaziz, A. T. Jamal, R. Damaševičius, and O. Farouk Hassan, "A novel method for detection of tuberculosis in chest radiographs using artificial ecosystem-based optimisation of deep neural network features," *Symmetry*, vol. 12, no. 7, p. 1146, Jul. 2020, doi: 10.3390/sym12071146.

25. A. Souid, N. Sakli, and H. Sakli, "Classification and predictions of lung diseases from chest X-rays using MobileNet V2," *Appl Sci*, vol. 11, no. 6, Art. no. 6, Jan. 2021, doi: 10.3390/app11062751.

26. P. Rajpurkar, J. Irvin, R. L. Ball, K. Zhu, B. Yang, H. Mehta, and T. Duan, "Deep learning for chest radiograph diagnosis: A retrospective comparison of the CheXNeXt algorithm to practicing radiologists," *PLoS Med*, vol. 15, no. 11, p. e1002686, Nov. 2018, doi: 10.1371/journal.pmed.1002686.

27. G. Huang, Z. Liu, L. van der Maaten, and K. Q. Weinberger, "Densely connected convolutional networks," *arXiv:1608.06993 [cs]*, Jan. 2018, Accessed: Mar. 29, 2022. [Online]. http://arxiv.org/abs/1608.06993

28. M. Tan, and Q. V. Le, "EfficientNet: Rethinking model scaling for convolutional neural networks," May 2019, doi: 10.48550/arXiv.1905.11946.

29. X. Wang, Y. Peng, L. Lu, Z. Lu, M. Bagheri, and R. M. Summers, "ChestX-ray8: Hospital-scale chest X-ray database and benchmarks on weakly-supervised classification and localization of common thorax diseases," May 2017, doi: 10.1109/CVPR.2017.369.

30. D. Kermany, "Labeled optical coherence tomography (OCT) and chest X-ray images for classification," *Mendeley*, Jan. 6, 2018, doi: 10.17632/RSCBJBR9SJ.2.

31. H. Q. Nguyen, K. Lam, L. T. Le, H. H. Pham, D. Q. Tran, D. B. Nguyen, and D. D. Le, "VinDr-CXR: An open dataset of chest X-rays with radiologist's annotations," *arXiv:2012.15029 [eess]*, Mar. 2022, Accessed: Apr. 1, 2022. [Online]. http://arxiv.org/abs/2012.15029

32. J. Deng, W. Dong, R. Socher, L.-J. Li, K. Li, and L. Fei-Fei, "ImageNet: A large-scale hierarchical image database," in *2009 IEEE conference on computer vision and pattern recognition*, Jun. 2009, pp. 248–255, doi: 10.1109/CVPR.2009.5206848.

33. T. Carneiro, R. V. M. D. Nóbrega, T. Nepomuceno, G. Bian, V. H. C. de Albuquerque, and P. Filho, "Performance analysis of Google Colaboratory as a tool for accelerating deep learning applications," *IEEE Access*, 2018, doi: 10.1109/ACCESS.2018.2874767.

34. I. M. Baltruschat, H. Nickisch, M. Grass, T. Knopp, and A. Saalbach, "Comparison of deep learning approaches for multi-label chest X-ray classification," *Sci Rep*, vol. 9, no. 1, Art. no. 1, Apr. 2019, doi: 10.1038/s41598-019-42294-8.

35. R. R. Selvaraju, M. Cogswell, A. Das, R. Vedantam, D. Parikh, and D. Batra, "Grad-CAM: Visual explanations from deep networks via gradient-based localization," Oct. 2016, doi: 10.1007/s11263-019-01228-7.

7 Artificial Intelligence Used to Recognize Fetal Planes Based on Ultrasound Scans during Pregnancy

Haifa Ghabri, Ben Othman Soufiene, and Hedi Sakli

7.1 INTRODUCTION

Medical imaging is critical in monitoring treatments, evaluating organ function, and identifying diseases. Ultrasound (US) images are among the medical images used to see numerous soft tissues (including the liver, spleen, pancreas, kidneys, and prostate) and detect anomalies such as malformations, tumors, blood clots, etc. [1].

Ultrasound is one of the most often-utilized imaging modalities, as it is affordable, does not require ionizing radiation, and can be conducted at the patient's bedside. It is well known for its application in pregnancy tests. Monitoring the growth of a fetus during pregnancy is critical, and in developing countries, monitoring of pregnant women is rare due to a lack of gynecologists, which can increase the mortality rate due to not paying attention to the fetus's development. Regular diagnosis is critical for pregnancy care. As a result, researchers are exploring novel ways for healthcare diagnosis and treatment.

The images of ultrasound scans appear immediately in the device's scan, therefore the doctor can usually provide rapid feedback. But due to low image quality, low contrast, and high variability, the doctor may not be able to interpret all the characteristics of the images, which is why the presence of a system that helps to make clinical decisions is essential.

The manual analysis of fetus development by doctors is tedious work. The presence of a system that helps sonographers in artificial intelligence (AI) advancements has illustrated the importance of the ability of automated diagnostic systems and their application in a variety of fields. The creation of intelligent systems in the health arena, as well as the processing of vast volumes of data and the generation of

DOI: 10.1201/9781003366249-7

meaningful outcomes from data, is of great significance. In the domain of health-care, computer-aided interpretation is becoming increasingly important. The burden of doctors has been reduced as a result of these technologies, while the efficiency and precision of diagnostics have risen [13].

AI plays an important role in the detection, classification, object detection, and tissue segmentation. With technological advancements, AI assists clinicians in making accurate diagnoses, making optimum judgments, selecting the best therapy, and making predictions based on models learned from thousands of medical imaging images. Several researchers have expressed the potential of AI in medicine [2, 3, 4].

Researchers have begun to build tools to help in the diagnosis of fetal development in order to reduce visual mistakes and compensate for manual interpretation. A sophisticated classifier, as well as a salient feature extractor capable of extracting relevant information from the data, are required for an effective decision support system. Deep learning approaches have been developed to solve these challenges and enhance detection rates.

The major goal of this work is to suggest a method for successfully monitoring fetal growth and assisting specialists in determining proper care. Our contribution is the application of a transfer-learning model with focal loss to recognize standard fetal planes, which will improve clinician productivity in detecting the presence of the fetus and its organs.

The content of this chapter is organized as follows. Section 7.2 examines related work in the literature, and Section 7.3 focuses on the suggested model and strategy. Section 7.4 discusses model training and parameters. The proposed model findings are discussed in Section 7.5. Section 7.6 concludes our proceedings and refers to our future work.

7.2   RELATED WORKS

In general, AI refers to intelligent systems that mimic human cognition and behavior. Machine learning (ML) is an area of AI that deals with processes that allow computers to learn from experience. Deep learning (DL) is an ML topic that involves artificial neural networks that learn through a hierarchy of concepts and are applied to enormous datasets.

AI is a significant development for the medical field since it is capable of evaluating complicated algorithms in treatment to improve diagnostic accuracy and classify pathologies and diseases. AI is a useful and effective tool for a variety of medical applications including the prediction of lung diseases from X-ray images [5], the detection of cardiovascular disease from a 12-lead electrocardiogram [6], and classification of breast cancer from ultrasound images [7]. Some research has employed ML techniques to classify, segment, and detect organs and pathologies from ultrasound images, but one of the primary drawbacks of ML is the usage of manual feature extraction, which needs a domain specialist. Many limitations have been overcome by deep learning introduced in recent years, and convolutional neural networks have established a new state of the art in ultrasound reconstruction, greatly outperforming the traditional baselines [18, 19, 20].

Many techniques treat fetal standard plane identification as a simple classification issue. A fetal facial is detected in the Yu et al. study [8] by a CNN-trained model. The method was evaluated on 2,418 images, with a mean AUC (area under the curve) of 0.99, precision of 0.96, accuracy of 0.96, and F1 of 0.97.

In the Qu et al. study [9], the CNN model was also utilized to automatically detect the fetal brain. The dataset contained 19,142 images that were modified and divided into five folds to test the technique. The CNN recorded the accuracy, precision, recall, and F1 values of 0.93, 0.93, 0.92, 0.93, and 0.93, respectively.

In the Kong et al. paper [10], a dense network is utilized to detect the fetal heart, fetal abdomen, fetal brain, and fetal facial. The testing set consisted of 5,678 US pictures, with precision of 0.98, recall of 0.98, and F1 of 0.98.

Similarly, Liang et al. [11] offer a DenseNet-based automated fetal standard plane categorization of the fetal heart, fetal abdomen, fetal brain, and coronal fetal facial. Their proposed model is trained alongside a placenta-transferring dataset to uncover and understand possible relationships between the datasets and maybe minimize overfitting. A test set of 4,455 photos is employed, with results of 0.99, 0.96, 0.99, and 0.95 for accuracy, recall, specification, and F1, respectively.

In the study by Montero et al. [12], a generative adversarial network (GAN) is utilized to enhance fetal brain classification using ResNet. The technique is validated using 2,249 pictures, yielding an AUC of 0.86, and accuracy and F1 of 0.81 and 0.80, respectively. Meng et al. [14] perform a cross-device categorization of six anatomical standard planes (heart, left ventricle, right ventricle, abdomen, femur, and lips). An enhanced feature alignment is applied to extract discriminative and domain-invariant features across domains. In the target domain, the average F1, recall, and precision values are 0.77, 0.77, and 0.78, respectively.

DL requires a significantly larger volume of data, and we can see that the number of records used to train a DL model is quite tiny. To confirm the efficacy of the suggested methodology, we combined four public databases in this study.

7.3   MATERIALS AND PROPOSED METHOD

Our study technique is as follows: Initially, our input data is an ultrasound image, which is then pre-processed. The following step is model training, in which deep learning is proposed to train the data to detect five planes of the fetus. Last, we evaluate our model results. Figure 7.1 summarizes the steps used in this study.

7.3.1 DATASET

A huge dataset [15] of routinely obtained maternofetal screening pictures from the United States is used in our work. It includes 12,400 2D images from 896 individuals, divided into six categories: maternal cervix, thorax, femur, abdomen, brain, and other. A specialist fetal doctor manually annotated the images. Figure 7.2 shows an example of each class in the suggested database. Figure 7.3 shows an overview of the dataset distribution where an issue of data imbalance and data scarcity is observed.

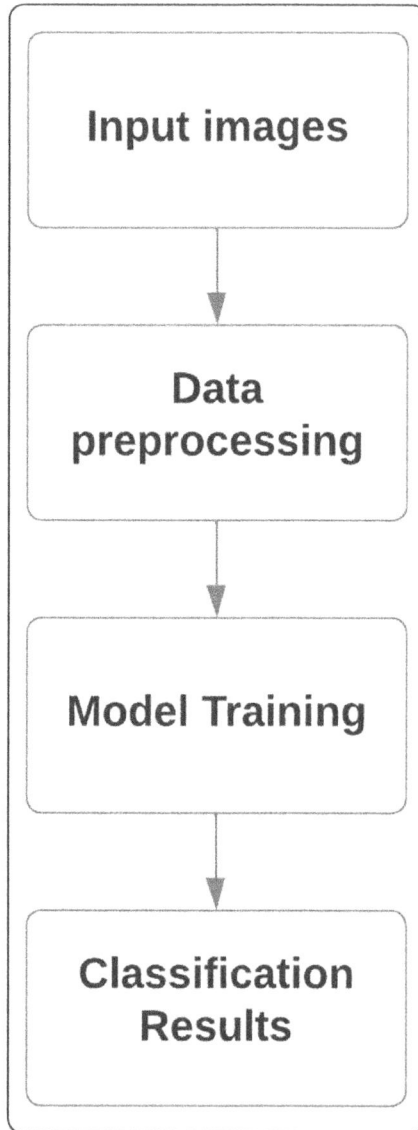

FIGURE 7.1 Our study's architecture.

7.3.2 PREPARING THE DATA

Due to the high presence of the class of images annotated as "other", we avoid over-fitting our proposed model.

The dataset utilized for this study contains 12,400 maternofetal images. After dropping "other" images, it becomes 8,187 images.

Fetal abdomen

Fetal brain

Fetal femur

Fetal thorax

Maternal cervix

Other

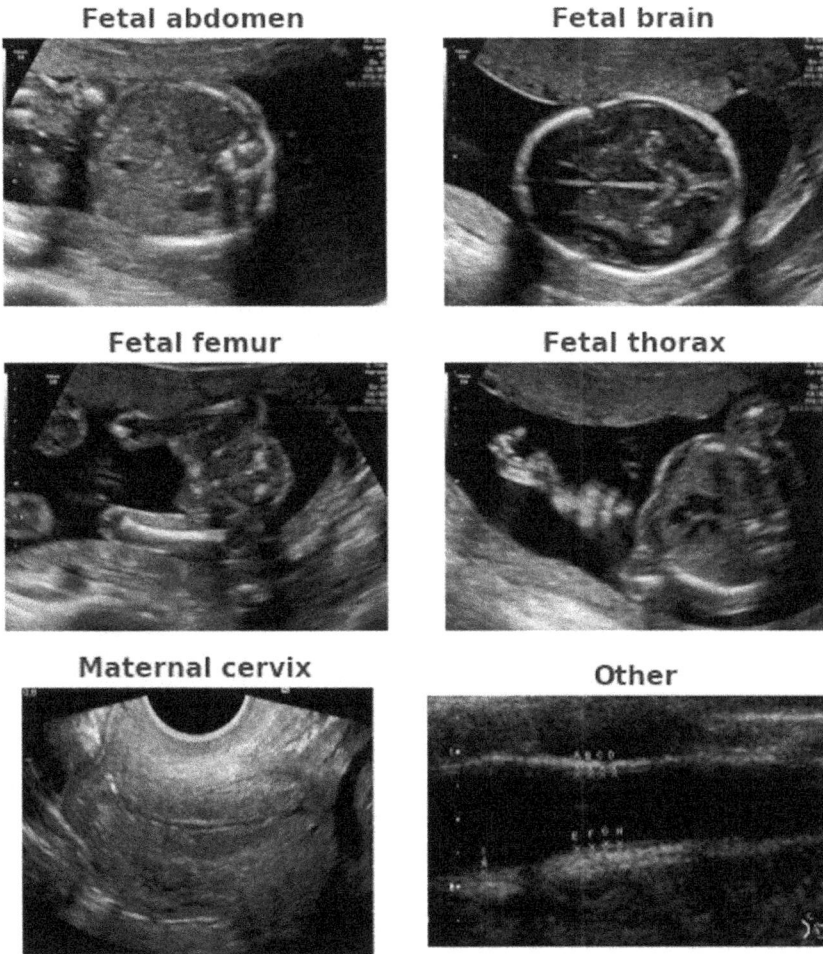

FIGURE 7.2   Samples from dataset classes.

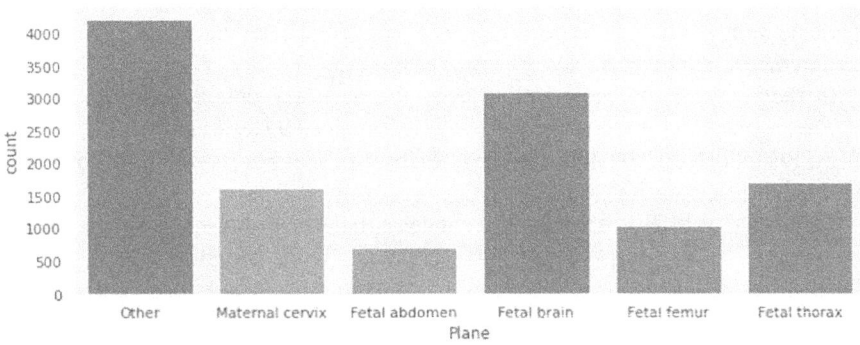

FIGURE 7.3   Data distribution.

We divided our dataset into two sets to train and test our proposed model: training–validation set and test set, with a ratio of 0.85:0.15. Training–validation was split into training and validation for training the model, with 5,567 and 1,391 images, respectively. The deep learning model requires a normalized input, which is why before training, the image input is resized to $256 \times 256 \times 3$ in height and width ($256 \times 256 \times 3$) for RGB color of the medical image.

7.3.3 MODEL ARCHITECTURE

The major goal of computer vision and deep learning is to develop stronger robust and efficient techniques with smaller models. EfficientNet produces better results by scaling depth, width, and resolution equally when the model is scaled down.

The pretrained model is used to automatically extract features and to improve the model's speed and stability. To augment the advantages of the pretrained weight, the features extracted are pooled using global average pooling. We apply dropout with a rate of 0.3 to reduce overfitting. Then to produce predictions of five classes, the dropout layer's output is transferred to the output layer with the softmax activation function.

Figure 7.4 illustrates the proposed model architecture.

7.3.4 MODEL TRAINING

The Adam optimizer is used as the optimization method with a learning rate of 0.001. Lin et al. [16] offer a focal loss function to solve the problem of imbalance between classes during training in object detection applications. To reduce class imbalance and let our model train in all dataset classes, we employ focal loss as the loss function demonstrating that the sparse-specific aspects of focal loss are equally applicable to classification problems with unbalanced datasets. Table 7.1 shows the optimal values of our deep neural network's hyperparameters.

7.4 RESULTS AND DISCUSSION

Our suggested model was trained with Google Colab [17]. Python 3.7 was used to implement the model. Each epoch took an average of 210 seconds to complete. This section discusses and evaluates the model findings.

In the training and validation phases, the accuracy obtained is 98.83% and 96.76%, respectively. In terms of precision, we obtained 99.09% and 97.20%, respectively. Recall achieves 98.43% and 96.30%, respectively. For loss, 0.0101 and 0.0702 were achieved for each phase.

The use of transfer learning with a model initially with ImageNet weight causes the model to become disordered from one epoch to the next until it stabilizes in the final epochs. This effect can be seen clearly in the first epochs (epochs 1–7).

Figures 7.5, , and show the model's accuracy, precision, and recall, respectively. We note that the model gradually converges after the 7th iteration, reaching a stable accuracy precision and recall at the 14th iteration.

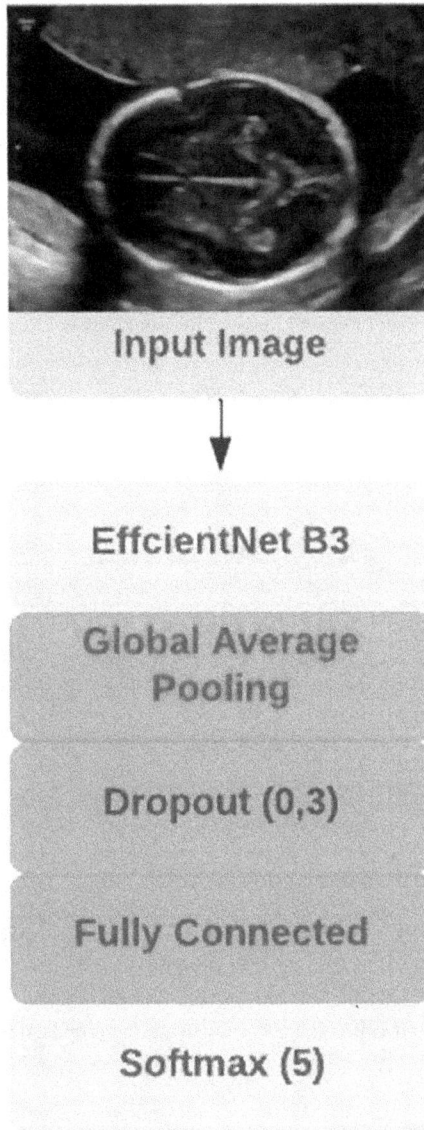

FIGURE 7.4 The proposed model architecture.

Figure 7.8 shows the model's loss, and we can see that after the 7th iteration, the model gradually converges to a low loss at the 14th iteration.

EfficientNetB3 had better classification performance than other studies cited in the literature. Table 7.2 compares our study to others presented in the related works section in terms of recall, precision, and accuracy.

TABLE 7.1

Hyperparameters used for the neural network

Hyperparameter	Optimized value
Optimizer	Adam
Epoch	14
Batch	16
Learning rate	0.001
Loss function	Focal loss
Input image size	$256 \times 256 \times 3$

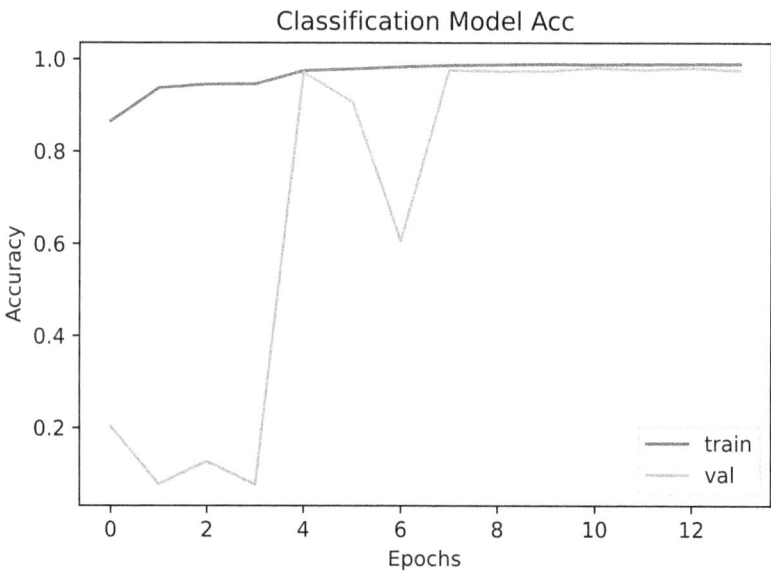

FIGURE 7.5   Training and validation accuracy using the proposed model.

7.5   CONCLUSION

We present a transfer-learning model with focal loss to classify five standard fetal planes using data from 12,400 maternofetal images. Our research focuses on the usage of focal loss and how critical it is to enhance model performance while dealing with imbalanced data. The proposed model achieves 98.83% and 99.09% in terms of accuracy and precision. These results show the efficacy of the proposed model compared to the values achieved in other studies.

EfficientNet will be used in future work as a platform to diagnose pregnant women and assist gynecologists.

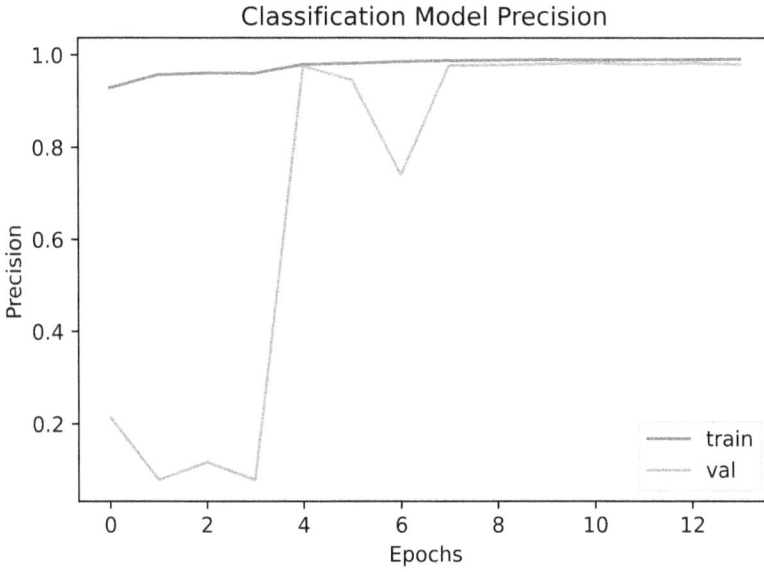

FIGURE 7.6 Training and validation precision using the proposed model.

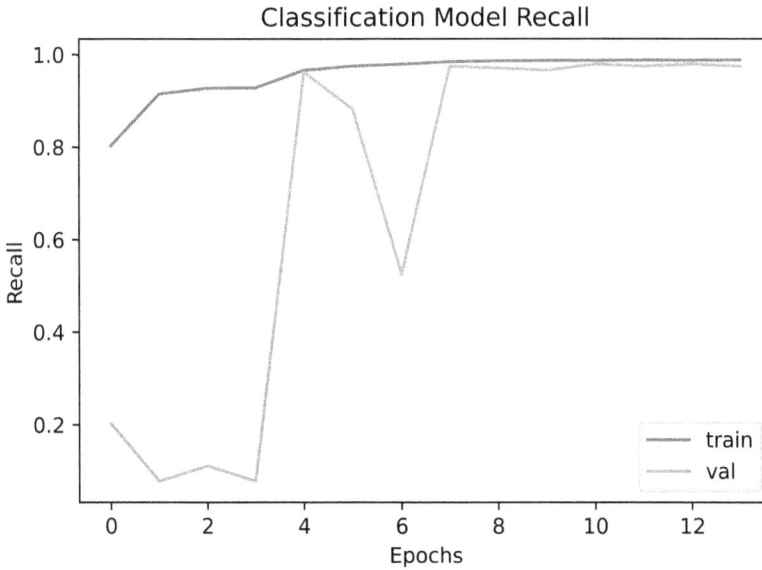

FIGURE 7.7 Training and validation recall using the proposed model.

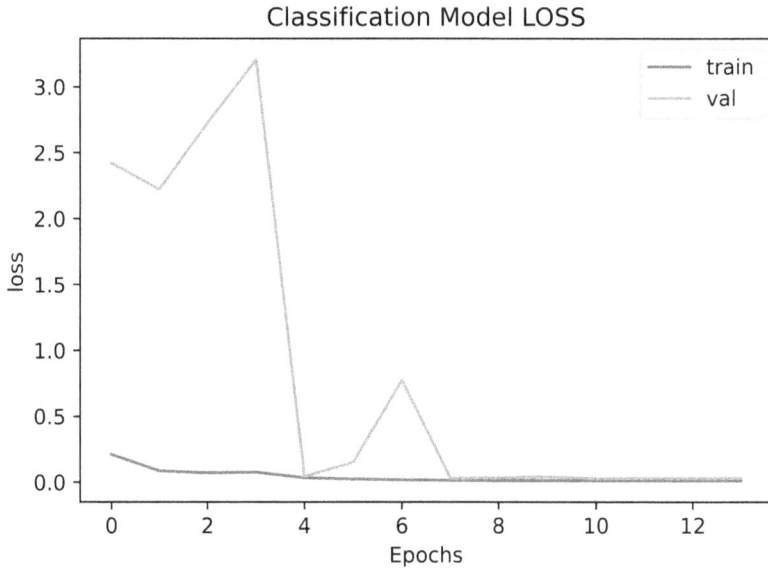

FIGURE 7.8   Training and validation loss using the proposed model.

TABLE 7.2
Comparison of studies in terms of accuracy (Acc), precision (Pre), and recall (Rec)

Reference	Number of images	Model	Classes	Acc (%)	Pre (%)	Rec (%)
Qu et al. [9]	15,314	CNN	1	93	93	92
Kong et al. [10]	17,036	DenseNet	4	—	98	98
Liang et al. [11]	17,840	DenseNet	5	99	—	96
Montero et al. [12]	6,498	ResNet	1	81	—	—
Our work	12,400	Transfer Learning: EfficientNet	5	98.83	99.09	98.43

REFERENCES

1. P. Zaffino, S. Moccia, E. De Momi, M. F. Spadea, A Review on Advances in Intra-Operative Imaging for Surgery and Therapy: Imagining the Operating Room of the Future. *Ann. Biomed. Eng.*, 48(8), Aug. 2020, 21712191. https://doi.org/10.1007/s10439 -020-02553-6.
2. W. Khan, N. Zaki, M. M. Masud, A. Ahmad, L. Ali, N. Ali, L. A. Ahmed, Infant Birth Weight Estimation and Low Birth Weight Classification in United Arab Emirates Using Machine Learning Algorithms. *Sci. Rep.*, 12(1), July 2022, Art. no. 1. https://doi.org/10 .1038/s41598-022-14393-6.

3. C. F. Baumgartner, K. Kamnitsas, J. Matthew, T. P. Fletcher, S. Smith, L. M. Koch, B. Kainz, D. Rueckert, SonoNet: Real-Time Detection and Localisation of Fetal Standard Scan Planes in Freehand Ultrasound. *IEEE Trans. Med. Imaging*, 36(11), Nov. 2017, 2204–2215. https://doi.org/10.1109/TMI.2017.2712367.

4. L. J. Salomon, Z. Alfirevic, F. Da Silva Costa, R. L. Deter, F. Figueras, Tet al Ghi, P. Glanc, ISUOG Practice Guidelines: Ultrasound Assessment of Fetal Biometry and Growth. *Ultrasound Obstet. Gynecol.*, 53(6), 2019, 715–723. https://doi.org/10.1002/uog.20272.

5. A. Souid, N. Sakli, H. Sakli, Classification and Predictions of Lung Diseases From Chest X-Rays Using MobileNet V2. *Appl. Sci.*, 11(6), Jan. 2021, Art. no. 6. https://doi.org/10.3390/app11062751.

6. N. Sakli, Haifa Ghabri, Ben Othman Soufiene, Faris Almalki, Hedi Sakli, Obaid Ali, Mustapha Najjari, ResNet-50 for 12-Lead Electrocardiogram Automated Diagnosis. *Comput. Intell. Neurosci.*, 2022, Apr. 2022, e7617551. https://doi.org/10.1155/2022/7617551.

7. A. S. Becker, M. Mueller, E. Stoffel, M. Marcon, S. Ghafoor, A. Boss, Classification of Breast Cancer From Ultrasound Imaging Using a Generic Deep Learning Analysis Software: A Pilot Study. *Br. J. Radiol.*, Dec. 2017, 20170576. https://doi.org/10.1259/bjr.20170576.

8. Z. Yu, E.-L. Tan, D. Ni, J. Qin, S. Chen, S. Li, B. Lei, T. Wang, A Deep Convolutional Neural Network-Based Framework for Automatic Fetal Facial Standard Plane Recognition. *IEEE J. Biomed. Health Inform.*, 22(3), May 2018, 874–885. https://doi.org/10.1109/JBHI.2017.2705031.

9. R. Qu, G. Xu, C. Ding, W. Jia, M. Sun, Standard Plane Identification in Fetal Brain Ultrasound Scans Using a Differential Convolutional Neural Network. *IEEE Access*, 8, 2020, 83821–83830. https://doi.org/10.1109/ACCESS.2020.2991845.

10. P. Kong, D. Ni, S. Chen, S. Li, T. Wang, B. Lei, Automatic and Efficient Standard Plane Recognition in Fetal Ultrasound Images Via Multi-Scale Dense Networks. In A. Melbourne, R. Licandro, M. DiFranco, P. Rota, M. Gau, M. Kampel, R. Aughwane, P. Moeskops, E. Schwartz, E. Robinson, A. Makropoulos (Eds.), *Data Driven Treatment Response Assessment and Preterm, Perinatal, and Paediatric Image Analysis*, Vol. 11076. Springer International Publishing, Cham, 2018, pp. 160–168. https://doi.org/10.1007/978-3-030-00807-9_16.

11. J. Liang, R. Huang, P. Kong, S. Li, T. Wang, B. Lei, SPRNet: Automatic Fetal Standard Plane Recognition Network for Ultrasound Images. In Q. Wang, A. Gomez, J. Hutter, K. McLeod, V. Zimmer, O. Zettinig, R. Licandro, E. Robinson, D. Christiaens, E. A. Turk, A. Melbourne (Eds.), *Smart Ultrasound Imaging and Perinatal, Preterm and Paediatric Image Analysis* (Vol. 11798). Springer International Publishing, Cham, 2019, pp. 3846. https://doi.org/10.1007/978-3-030-32875-7_5.

12. A. Montero, E. Bonet-Carne, X. P. Burgos-Artizzu, Generative Adversarial Networks to Improve Fetal Brain Fine-Grained Plane Classification. *Sensors*, 21(23), 2021, 7975.

13. U. R. Acharya, H. Fujita, S. L. Oh, U. Raghavendra, J. H. Tan, M. Adam, A. Gertych, Y. Hagiwara, Automated Identification of Shockable and Non-Shockable Life-Threatening Ventricular Arrhythmias Using Convolutional Neural Network. *Future Gener. Comput. Syst.*, 79, Aug. 2017. https://doi.org/10.1016/j.future.2017.08.039.

14. Q. Meng, D. Rueckert, B. Kainz, Unsupervised Cross-Domain Image Classification by Distance Metric Guided Feature Alignment. In *Medical Ultrasound, and Preterm, Perinatal and Paediatric Image Analysis*. Springer, Cham, 2020, pp. 146–157.

15. X. P. Burgos-Artizzu, D. Coronado-Gutiérrez, B. Valenzuela-Alcaraz, E. Bonet-Carne, E. Eixarch, F. Crispi, E. Gratacós, Evaluation of Deep Convolutional Neural Networks for Automatic Classification of Common Maternal Fetal Ultrasound Planes. *Sci. Rep.*, 10(1), 2020, 10200. https://doi.org/10.1038/s41598-020-67076-5.

16. T.-Y. Lin, P. Goyal, R. Girshick, K. He, P. Dollar, Focal Loss for Dense Object Detection, p. 9.

17. T. Carneiro, R. V. Medeiros Da Nobrega, T. Nepomuceno, G.-B. Bian, V. H. C. De Albuquerque, P. P. R. Filho, Performance Analysis of Google Colaboratory as a Tool for Accelerating Deep Learning Applications. *IEEE Access*, 6, 2018, 61677–61685. https://doi.org/10.1109/ACCESS.2018.2874767.

18. C. Chakraborty, S. B. Othman, F. A. Almalki, H. Sakli, FC-SEEDA: Fog Computing-Based Secure and Energy Efficient Data Aggregation Scheme for Internet of Healthcare Things. *Neural Computing & Applications*, 2023. https://doi.org/10.1007/s00521-023-08270-0.

19. Soufiene Ben Othman, Abdullah Ali Bahattab, Abdelbasset Trad, Habib Youssef, PEERP: A Priority-Based Energy-Efficient Routing Protocol for Reliable Data Transmission in Healthcare Using the IoT. *The 15th International Conference on Future Networks and Communications (FNC)*, Leuven, Belgium, 9–12 August 2020.

20. Soufiene Ben Othman, Faris A. Almalki, Chinmay Chakraborty, Hedi Sakli, Privacy-Preserving Aware Data Aggregation for IoT-Based Healthcare With Green Computing Technologies. *Computers and Electrical Engineering*, 101, 2022, 108025. https://doi.org/10.1016/j.compeleceng.2022.108025.

8 Artificial Intelligence Techniques for Cancer Detection from Medical Images

*Rabiaa Tbibe, Ben Othman Soufiene,
Chinmay Chakraborty, and Hedi Sakli*

8.1 INTRODUCTION

The word "cancer" describes a wide range of diseases in which cells develop and multiply in an uncontrolled manner, killing other healthy cells in the body. One of the hallmarks of cancer is the rapid development of abnormal cells that spread beyond their normal limits, which can then penetrate organs and destroy healthy tissue, and then invade nearby parts of the body and spread to other organs [1]. There are more than a hundred forms of cancer, including brain and other types of tumors, lung cancer, colon cancer, skin cancer, oral cancer, breast cancer, and prostate cancer [2].

Cancer symptoms vary from case to case depending on the organ affected by the disease. These symptoms include feeling very tired; losing weight for no apparent reason; changes in the skin, such as redness, swelling, a darkening of the color, or the appearance of lumps under the skin and obvious changes in a mole or wart; persistent cough; constant pain in the joints and muscles of the body; abnormal discharge or bleeding; high temperature; changes in bowel or bladder working patterns; and indigestion or discomfort after eating.

The transformation of a normal cell into a cancerous cell occurs in multiple stages, and this transformation usually takes place from a precancerous lesion to a malignant tumor. These changes are caused by the interaction between the individual's genetic factors and some external factors. Table 8.1 shows the differences between adenomas and cancerous tumors.

The incidence of cancer increases significantly with age, likely due to the increase in the risk of developing certain cancers with age, the accumulation of cancer risks, and the decrease in the effectiveness of cellular repair mechanisms as a person gets older. Alcohol and tobacco usage are two leading factors in cancer.

DOI: 10.1201/9781003366249-8

TABLE 8.1

Differences between adenomas and cancerous tumors

Adenomas	Cancerous tumors
Usually one specific block	Usually a branched and indeterminate mass
Outside shape of the tumor is round or oval	Outside is irregular and uneven
No side effects	Accompanied by side effects
Slow growing	Fast growing
Usually surrounded by a membrane outside the tumor	Not surrounded by a membrane outside the tumor
No ability to spread	Able to spread
Often do not recur after removal	Tumor recurrence possible after removal
Often not fatal	Fatal

Over many years, medical devices, smart health networks, and artificial intelligence-based disease prevention systems have made significant contributions to improving global health, and have now matured to the point where they can be used as a substitute in many fields.

An early and accurate cancer diagnosis is critical to promoting long-term patient survival and saving millions of lives; if the cancer is diagnosed in its early stages, it can likely be cured, but if the diagnosis is delayed, the tumor can grow deeper and spread to other parts of the body.

This chapter focuses on some recent studies based on automated and computer-aided detection systems with artificial intelligence that aim to develop modern methods for detecting cancers through medical images.

8.2   MEDICAL IMAGING TESTS FOR CANCER DETECTION

An imaging exam allows medical professionals to view what is happening inside the body. These exams expose the body to various sources of energy to pick up images that depict the structure and function of the inside organs so that medical professionals may spot any alterations that may be brought on by conditions like cancer.

Medical imaging is usually the first step to fighting the spread of cancer via identifying cancer in its earliest stages, finding out what stage the cancer is in, predicting if the tumor is potentially cancerous, and identifying if the cancer returned after treatment [3].

Various types of scans are used to obtain images of what is going on inside the body, including computed tomography (CT), X-ray, mammography, magnetic resonance imaging (MRI), and ultrasound. Typical imaging methods used to fight cancer are listed in Table 8.2.

TABLE 8.2
Types of scans

Imaging method	Application	Advantages	Disadvantages
X-ray	Low-radiation dosages are used in X-rays to provide images of the tissues, bones, and organs. X-rays may be taken of any part of the body to look for a tumor or cancer.	• The amount of radiation used is safe. • It produces an image for immediate review [4].	• Sometimes X-ray does not diagnose the disease because of noise in the image or blurring images [4].
CT scan	On a CT scan, any aspect of the body, including bones, muscles, fat, and organs, can be seen.	• CT scans are a lot more detailed than X-rays [1].	• High radiation dosages are involved. • Radiation is harmful and can result in cancer.
MRI	An MRI is often used to look at the heart, brain, liver, pancreas, male and female reproductive organs, and other soft tissues.	• Accurate method of disease detection.	• Involves long-term side effects.
Thermography	Thermography, commonly known as thermal imaging, is an infrared imaging technique to track and record temperature changes on the skin's surface.	• Results are available in real time and require little or no processing.	• Only a skilled individual can interpret the findings. • Images are difficult to read due to low quality and low resolution [5].
Mammography	A mammogram is an X-ray exam of the breast that is used to detect the early signs of breast cancer in women who have breast problems such as a lump, pain, or nipple discharge.	• The most effective technique for breast cancer. • It uses low levels of X-rays for imaging.	• Risk of false alarm. • Reading the mammogram twice leads to an increase in the detection cost [5].
Microscopy	It is a tool to see objects that are too small to see with naked eye. It has the capacity to investigate the 3D interior of living cells and organisms.	• Microscopy in image analysis provides quantitative support for improving characterizations of various diseases [6].	• Vacuum environment [1].

(Continued)

TABLE 8.2 CONTINUED
Types of scans

Imaging method	Application	Advantages	Disadvantages
Ultrasound	Medical ultrasound, also called sonography, is a technology that observes events inside the human body by using high-frequency sound waves [1].	• It's safe to use on pregnant individuals. • Quick.	• Quality and interpretation of the image highly depends on the skill of the person doing the scan [5].
Nuclear medicine imaging	These scanners take pictures after a radioactive tracer (called a radionuclide) is put into the blood. A radionuclide scan is another name for this kind of scan.	• Detects the disease at an early stage. • Provides a crystal-clear image.	• Involves long-term side effects.

8.3   ARTIFICIAL INTELLIGENCE AND MEDICAL IMAGING

The manual classification of images is a challenging and time-consuming task. This task is highly susceptible to interobserver variability and human errors. Manual classification results in extremely poor critical outcomes, thus markedly increasing the workload of radiologists. In addition, medical care costs that are relevant to imaging quickly increase [3]. Therefore, new diagnostic techniques are needed. Currently, computer-aided diagnosis is one of several important research areas in medical imaging and diagnostic radiology. It helps doctors diagnose diseases with a high degree of efficiency, while reducing examination time and cost, as well as avoiding unnecessary biopsy procedures.

The techniques used in computer-aided diagnosis have undergone significant technological advancement over the last few decades. Initially, image-based computer-aided diagnosis systems used traditional machine learning approaches that required human researchers to design meaningful image features, which would then be fed into a trainable prediction algorithm such as a classifier. Computer-aided diagnosis using advances in artificial intelligence, and especially deep learning techniques, has overcome this obstacle by discovering, in a trainable manner, the informative features that optimally represent the data for the specific task [7].

The best outcomes thus far for image analysis have been obtained using convolutional neural networks (CNNs). These networks are a type of model consisting of multiple layers of simple computational nodes but with complex connections that mimic the workings of the human visual cortex, allowing more than high-level features to be learned [8].

In this context, artificial intelligence approaches, and especially deep learning techniques, offer unprecedented interest and success in medical imaging due to advances in the development of algorithms. These algorithms can surpass human performance in object recognition tasks in medical images and act as a wonderful aid to clinicians, and thus contribute to the automatic detection of cancer [9].

8.4 RECENT ARTIFICIAL INTELLIGENCE TECHNIQUES FOR CANCER DETECTION BASED ON MEDICAL IMAGING

In this section, we will focus on modern techniques based on artificial intelligence on medical images to detect cancers.

8.4.1 LUNG CANCER

One of the main causes of cancer-related deaths among individuals worldwide is lung cancer. Unfortunately, this cancer is often detected at an advanced stage when few treatment options are left.

Lung cancers are divided into two types: small-cell lung cancer and non-small-cell lung cancer. Non-small-cell lung cancer is more common because lung nodules cannot be detected.

The most effective way to prevent lung cancer is early detection and diagnosis, which is a complex process due to the overlap of all lung cells. Usually, computed tomography, X-rays, and MRI scans are used to diagnose lung cancer. These techniques are expensive and time-consuming, and, unfortunately, they detect the disease in its advanced stages, which reduces the patient's recovery rate and increases the risk of death. Image processing and data mining with the help of artificial intelligence methods can provide enhanced early detection.

Primakov et al. [10] presented a deep learning-based approach that can automatically detect lung tumors through a CT scan. This work can be summarized in three basic steps as shown in Figure 8.1:

1. Image preprocessing – CT scan images were collected for pretreatment of 1,414 patients and then processed to reduce heterogeneity and noise and improve images and contrast.
2. Lung isolation – The main part of this step is to accurately determine the axis of the spine and indicate the locations of the bones to extract only the lung image and thus identify the cells affected by tumors.
3. Tumor detection and segmentation using a convolutional neural network.

Although this model has an accuracy of 94.4%, it is not capable of detecting all tumors, as it is limited to detecting and segmenting primary non-small-cell lung cancer tumors.

In another study, researchers designed a chest CT-based methodology capable of binary classification (healthy lung or injured lung) [11]. This study uses 3D AlexNet

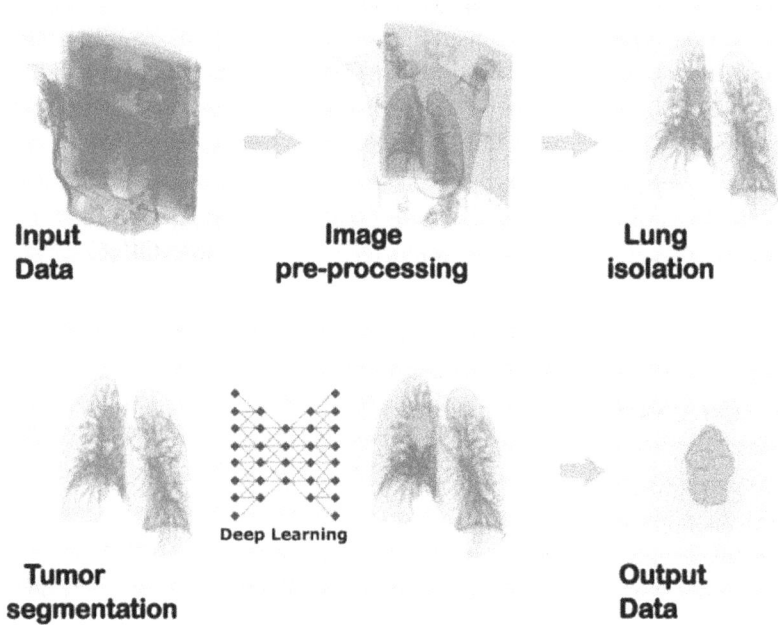

FIGURE 8.1 Proposed workflow.

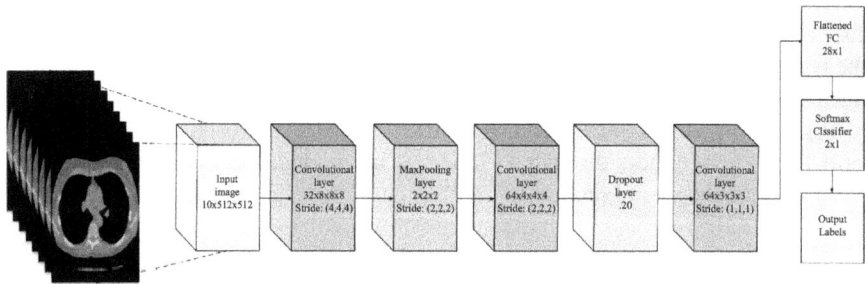

FIGURE 8.2 The 3D CNN architecture for lung cancer classification.

variants of Inception and Inception-ResNet to classify lung defects, a new method of its kind. Figure 8.2 shows the structure of this method. This proposed method achieved a rating accuracy of 97.17, however, the data set used in this work does not suffice to say that this method is very reliable and can be adopted and applied within hospitals.

Researchers have also tested new lung cancer detectors using machine learning techniques followed by CNN, SVM (support vector machine), and KNN (K-nearest neighbor) classification [12, 13]. All these methods are theoretically successful, but their efficacy has not been proven in practice.

8.4.2 BRAIN CANCER

A brain tumor is an abnormal growth in brain cells that causes damage to various blood vessels and nerves in the human body [14]. Brain tumors include gliomas, ependymomas, pineal gland tumors, and pituitary adenomas. Early diagnosis of a brain tumor will increase the patient's survival rate. Until now, MRI images were the most widely used diagnosis method for brain cancer.

MRI contrast agents play a very important role in disease diagnosis. This increases the demand for these new MRI techniques with improved sensitivity and superior functionality.

Different MRI methods produce different types of tissue contrast images. Thus, they provide accurate information on the structure of the cancer and allow the diagnosis and segmentation of tumor cells.

A method based on combining a CNN and a hybrid semantic network has been proposed for tumor region segmentation [15]. The classification used in the proposed work includes MRI and CT images. In the proposed architecture, shown in Figure 8.3, brain images are first segmented using a semantic segmentation network that contains a series of convolution layers and pooling layers. The tumor is then classified as a meningioma, glioma, or pituitary tumor using a CNN model trained on 22 layers of the GoogLeNet architecture. The overall accuracy of this method

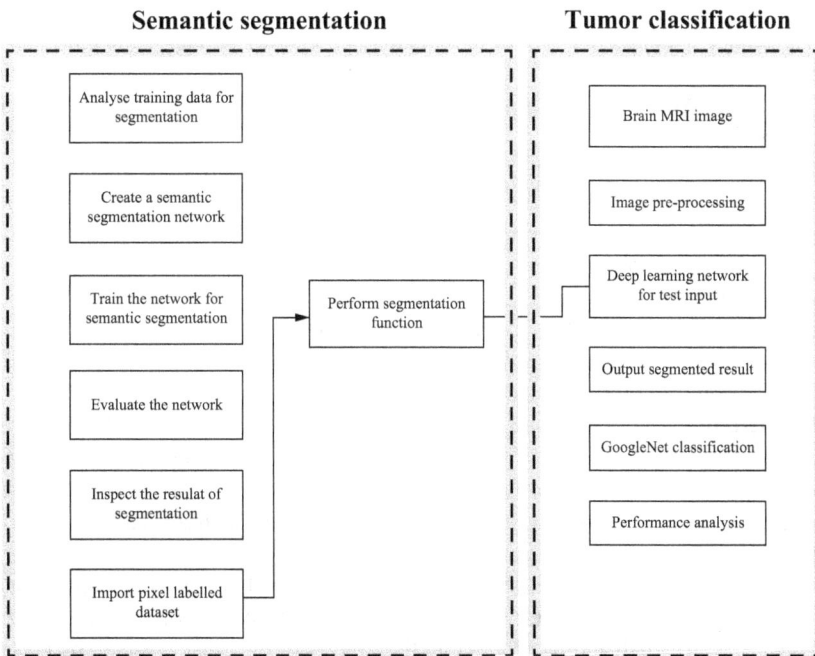

FIGURE 8.3 Overall flow diagram of the proposed work.

was 99.57%, 99.78%, and 99.56% for meningioma, glioma, and pituitary adenoma, respectively.

Addeh et al. presented an intelligent method based on a radial function neural network (RBFNN) and a CNN for MRI scans to determine brain tumor detection [16]. The proposed method is centered on four main units: segmentation, feature extraction, classification, and learning algorithm. In the segmentation module, the GrabCut method is applied to segment the tumor area. In the feature extraction module, a CNN is used to extract new deep features from segmented images that cannot be seen or discovered by a human expert. The accuracy of this work is 99.6%.

Also, a machine learning technique to identify and classify neoplastic or non-tumorous areas by MRI of the brain has been proposed [17]. In the first stage, the skull is manually removed from the image to gain time by removing the unwanted region, and mean filtering is used to filter out the noise factor. Then, the Chan-Vese technique is used to divide the active tumor by selecting the exact initial point. In the next step, tumor region features are extracted using a gray-level co-occurrence matrix. Finally, a two-class classifier is implemented using an SVM and then its performance is validated with KNN.

All research has proven that MRI is the ideal solution to detect brain cancer because it represents a safe solution compared to other imaging methods, which represent a danger in terms of radiation to the brain.

8.4.3 BREAST CANCER

Breast cancer is a malicious tumor that begins in the breast tissues. This malignancy may spread to distant sections of the body or may spread straight into surrounding surroundings. Although women are nearly always the ones who get this sort of cancer, men can also get it.

Recent functions involving examinations have generated a great deal of interest in the use of computational techniques to aid in the detection and diagnosis of breast cancer among other malignancies. This attention is focused on mammography; this specific mammography method is a straightforward but useful tool for predicting breast cancer at an early stage.

Researchers have adopted X-rays for early detection of breast cancer through image processing using contrast-limited adaptive histogram equalization (CLAHE) and separation of tumor tissues through segmentation [18].

Furthermore, an SVM classifier was used to classify features extracted from mammograms into two categories (normal and abnormal). This method achieved an accuracy of 98.95% for normal mammography and 98.01% for abnormal mammography. This method is theoretically good but requires a larger data set to verify its promising results.

In another study, Jahangeer et al. created a new method for early detection of breast cancer using mammograms [19]. First, the mammogram images are entered, and then they are analyzed by processing the images of the areas affected by cancer. The filtered images are then hashed using a new technology formed on the integration of deep learning technologies of the VGG-16 network and string hybrid networks,

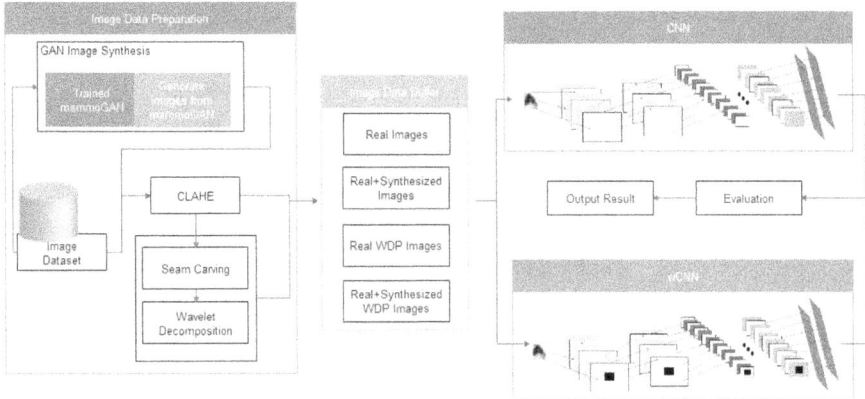

FIGURE 8.4 The proposed architecture.

as shown in Figure 8.4. In this method, the classification is performed according to the classification of the new gradient descent decision tree. This method can not only detect cancer but also predict the level of disease severity using a gradient regression decision tree classifier and a stable learning path that is used for ease of convergence. The accuracy value of the proposed hybrid VGG-16 and series network segmentation technique was 96.45, and the accuracy value of the proposed gradient descent decision tree classification technique was 95.15.

A technique for automatically determining whether a mammogram is normal or abnormal – the diverse features-based breast cancer detection (DFeBCD) system – has been proposed [20]. Four different sets of features are employed. Among these, features based on statistical measures, local binary patterns, and taxonomic indices are static. The proposed DFeBCD dynamically extracts the fourth set of features from mammography images using a highway network-based deep CNN.

Chouhan et al. used two classifiers – SVM and the Emotional Learning Inspired Ensemble Classifier (ELiEC) – on these distinguishing features using the IRMA mammography dataset. This method has been activated on 838 images, and their accuracy ranges between 91% and 93%.

8.4.4 Prostate Cancer

Prostate cancer is the second most common type of cancer and the leading cause of death among men worldwide. There are 1.1 million new cases diagnosed each year, according to the World Health Organization. It is an abnormal and uncontrollable growth of cells in the prostate gland. This type of cancer is often slow growing and can be treated successfully and effectively when detected in its early stages.

Soufiene et al. [21] designed a new method for detecting prostate cancer based on MRI under the name of ProCDet. This method was pretrained on ImageNet and it consists of three principal modules, as shown in Figure 8.5:

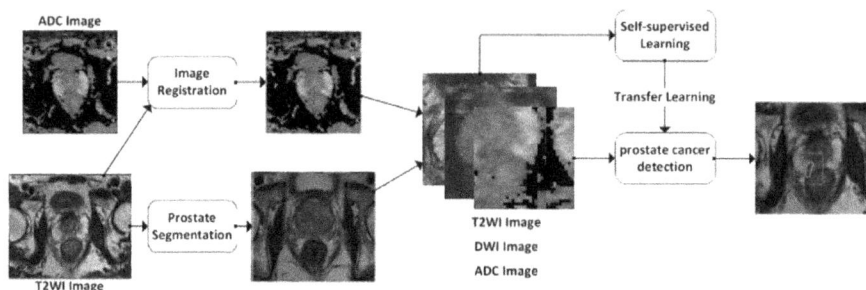

FIGURE 8.5   The ProCDet method.

- The registration of prostate MRI images finds the spatial relationship between the different sequences.
- Segmentation of the prostate creates a prostate segmentation network based on the attention mechanism to segment the prostate and eliminate background noise.
- With the segmentation of prostate cancer lesions, a 3D prostate cancer lesion segmentation network is used to pinpoint the precise site of prostate cancer.

To solve the problem of limited data volume, the researchers worked to create their own data set, and this model achieved an accuracy of 91.82%.

Likewise, Soufieneet al. [22] introduced the PROMETEO model, which is a computer-aided diagnosis system based on deep learning for prostate cancer detection. This system has the advantage of being able to analyze whole-tissue images of slides that were first sampled and preprocessed using different filters. In the first stage, it removes the useless areas of tissue. The patches are then used as inputs to a custom CNN, which reports on malicious areas on the heatmap. The effect of applying the stain normalization process to the patches is then analyzed to reduce color contrast between different scanners. After training the network, an accuracy of 99.98% was achieved.

Table 8.3 provides a summary of the aforementioned methods.

8.5   CONCLUSION

Doctors consider different cancer treatments, such as targeted and immunological radiation and chemotherapy, to make the appropriate treatment decision according to the type and location of the cancer, the stage of the infection, and the degree of severity based on clinical examination and various radiographs.

Over time, therapeutic strategies in the war against cancer have changed, as treatment is no longer the only effective weapon, but it is necessary to detect cancer early; predict the course of the disease; and provide evidence about whether the cancerous tumor is slow, aggressive, or resistant to treatment. Artificial intelligence has

TABLE 8.3
Comparative table of detection models

Reference	Cancer type	Image type	Accuracy
Primakov et al. [10]	Lung cancer	CT scan	94.4%
Neal Joshua et al. [11]	Lung cancer	CT scan	97.17%
Xu et al. [12]	Lung cancer	CT scan	95.96%
Mahima et al. [13]	Lung cancer	CT scan	98.06%
Ruba et al. [15]	Brain cancer	MRI + CT scan	99.56%
Addeh et al. [16]	Brain cancer	MRI images	99.6%
Budati et al. [17]	Brain cancer	MRI images	99.75%
Mavra et al. [18]	Breast cancer	X-ray images	98.01%
Jahangeer et al. [19]	Breast cancer	Mammograms	95.15%
Chakraborty et al. [20]	Breast cancer	Mammograms	93%
Soufiene etal. [21]	Prostate cancer	MRI images	91.82%
Soufiene et al. [22]	Prostate cancer	CT scan	99.98%

changed the rules of the game in the diagnostic process, as it can read several slides of samples from several patients within minutes and detect and distinguish diseased cells.

It is true that artificial intelligence will not replace doctors, but it is an important assistant, especially with the lack of radiologists and the struggle against time to diagnose tumors and save the lives of patients. Human specialists require access to patient histories, whereas the artificial intelligence model only needs images to do its job.

REFERENCES

1. Charnpreet Kaur and Urvashi Garg, Artificial Intelligence Techniques for Cancer Detection in Medical Image Processing: A Review, *Materials Today: Proceedings*, 2021, ISSN 2214-7853, doi: 10.1016/j.matpr.2021.04.241.
2. G.M. Cooper, *The Cell: A Molecular Approach*. 2nd edition. Sunderland, MA: Sinauer Associates; 2000. The Development and Causes of Cancer. Available from: https://www.ncbi.nlm.nih.gov/books/NBK9963
3. A. R. M. Al-shamasneh and U. H. Binti Obaidellah, Artificial Intelligence Techniques for Cancer Detection and Classification: Review Study, *European Scientific Journal*13(3), 2017, 342. doi: 10.19044/esj.2017.v13n3p342.
4. A.T. Chikhalekar, Analysis of Image Processing for Digital X-Ray, *International Research Journal of Engineering and Technology*, 3(5), 2016, 1364–1368.
5. F. Sadoughi, Z. Kazemy, F. Hamedan, L. Owji, M. Rahmanikatigari, T. Azadboni, Artificial Intelligence Methods for the Diagnosis of Breast Cancer by Image Processing: A Review, *Breast Cancer: Targets and Therapy*, 10, 2018, 219–230.
6. F. Xing, Y. Xie, H. Su, F. Liu, and L. Yang, Deep Learning in Microscopy Image Analysis: A Survey, 2017, 1–19.

7. E. Al-Daoud, Cancer Diagnosis Using Modified Fuzzy Network, *Universal Journal of Computer Science & Engineering Technology*, 1(2), 2010, 73–78.

8. H. Suzuki, T. Yoshitaka, T. Yoshio, and T. Tada, Artificial Intelligence for Cancer Detection of the Upper Gastrointestinal Tract, *Digestive Endoscopy*, 33(2), 2021, 254–262. doi: 10.1111/den.13897.

9. Omer F. Ahmad, Antonio S. Soares, Evangelos Mazomenos, Patrick Brandao, Roser Vega, Edward Seward, Danail Stoyanov, Manish Chand, and Laurence B. Lovat, Artificial Intelligence and Computer-Aided Diagnosis in Colonoscopy: Current Evidence and Future Directions, *The Lancet Gastroenterology & Hepatology*, 4(1), 2019, 71–80. doi: 10.1016/S2468-1253(18)30282-6.

10. S. P. Primakov, A. Ibrahim, J. E. van Timmeren et al. Automated Detection and Segmentation of Non-Small Cell Lung Cancer Computed Tomography Images, *Nature Communications*, 13, 2022, 3423. doi: 10.1038/s41467-022-30841-3.

11. Eali Stephen Neal Joshua, Debnath Bhattacharyya, Midhun Chakkravarthy, and Yung-Cheol Byun, 3D CNN with Visual Insights for Early Detection of Lung Cancer Using Gradient-Weighted Class Activation, *Journal of Healthcare Engineering*, 2021, 2021, Article ID 6695518, 11 pages. doi: 10.1155/2021/6695518.

12. Yeguo Xu, Yuhang Wang, and Navid Razmjooy, Lung Cancer Diagnosis in CT Images based on Alexnet Optimized by Modified Bowerbird Optimization Algorithm, *Biomedical Signal Processing and Control*, 77, 2022, 103791. doi: 10.1016/j.bspc.2022.103791.

13. S. Mahima, S. Kezia, and E. Grace Mary Kanaga, Deep Learning-Based Lung Cancer Detection. In: Peter, J.D., Fernandes, S.L., Alavi, A.H. (eds) *Disruptive Technologies for Big Data and Cloud Applications. Lecture Notes in Electrical Engineering*, vol 905. Springer, Singapore, 2022.

14. M. Masood T. Nazir, M. Nawaz, A. Mehmood, J. Rashid H.-Y. Kwon, T. Mahmood, and A. Hussain, A Novel Deep Learning Method for Recognition and Classification of Brain Tumors from MRI Images. *Diagnostics*, 11, 2021, 744. doi: 10.3390/diagnostics11050744.

15. T. Ruba, R. Tamilselvi, M. P. Beham, and N. Aparna. Accurate Classification and Detection of Brain Cancer Cells in MRI and CT Images using Nano Contrast Agents. *Biomedical and Pharmacology Journal*, 13(3), 2020.

16. Abdoljalil Addeh and Moshtagh Iri, Brain Tumor Type Classification Using Deep Features of MRI Images and Optimized RBFNN, *ENG Transactions*, 2, 2021, 1–7.

17. A. K. Budati and R. B. Katta, An Automated Brain Tumor Detection and Classification from MRI Images Using Machine Learning Techniques with IoT, *Environment, Development and Sustainability*, 24, 2022, 10570–10584. doi: 10.1007/s10668-021-01861-8

18. Mehmood Mavra, et al. Machine Learning Enabled Early Detection of Breast Cancer by Structural Analysis of Mammograms, *Computers, Materials and & Continua*, 67, 2021, 641–657.

19. G. S. B. Jahangeer and T. D. Rajkumar, Early Detection of Breast Cancer Using Hybrid of Series Network and VGG-16, *Multimedia Tools and Applications*, 80, 2021, 7853–7886. doi: 10.1007/s11042-020-09914-2

20. C. Chakraborty, S. B. Othman, F. A. Almalki, et al. FC-SEEDA: Fog Computing-Based Secure and Energy Efficient Data Aggregation Scheme for Internet of Healthcare Things, *Neural Comput & Applic*, 2023. doi: 10.1007/s00521-023-08270-0

21. Soufiene Ben Othman, Abdullah Ali Bahattab, Abdelbasset Trad, and Habib Youssef, PEERP: A Priority-Based Energy-Efficient Routing Protocol for Reliable Data Transmission in Healthcare using the IoT. In *The 15th International Conference on Future Networks and Communications (FNC)*, 2020, Leuven, Belgium.
22. Soufiene Ben Othman, Faris A. Almalki, Chinmay Chakraborty, and Hedi Sakli, Privacy-Preserving Aware Data Aggregation for IoT-Based Healthcare with Green Computing Technologies, *Computers and Electrical Engineering*, 101, 2022, 108025. doi: 10.1016/j.compeleceng.2022.108025

9 Handling Segmentation and Classification Problems in Deep Learning for Identification of Interstitial Lung Disease

Tapas Pal, Biswadev Goswami,
and Rajesh P Barnwal

9.1 INTRODUCTION

Medical images from computed tomography (CT), MRI, fluoroscopy, angiography, and mammograms provide some of the most important and life-saving data for the diagnosis of disease and treatment. The age-old process of reviewing the images manually has been successful in saving countless lives. But the effectiveness of this diagnosis is limited to radiologists and clinical specialists. This means that traditional image interpretation is extremely subjective and offline [19].

According to medical experts, one in four patients receive false-positive data from image review. This could be because of a fatigued reviewer and the complexity of medical images. Even though false positives are better than false negatives in terms of fatality, they can lead to unnecessary follow-ups and in some cases painful invasive treatments. These challenges originated the need for further improvement in medical image-related jobs. Computer-based image processing and disease diagnosis is already widely implemented in Europe under the National Health Service (NHS). And these systems have been successful in reducing the average reporting time for critical patients from 11.2 days to 2.7 days [33].

Deep learning–based image processing can be helpful in the following ways:

- Fast and robust – Artificial intelligence (AI) can assess large amounts of data in a very short time, which is very important in many critical time-sensitive cases.

DOI: 10.1201/9781003366249-9

- Automation of radiological analysis – Primary and common analyses can be automated, so radiologists can be free to do important research-based activity. It can also improve decision-making and diagnostic accuracy.
- Minimizing human error – Different humans have varying abilities and perceptions. The objective nature of AI can eliminate natural cognitive bias, vision-related differences, and presumptions.

Even after showing very promising results, AI-based methods are far from becoming an automatic panacea. In deep learning models, training is a main challenge. In traditional computer vision tasks, image annotation is relatively simple, for example, labeling of cat, man, and lion. Deep learning applications in medical images require a good amount of very minutely labeled and annotated data. Labeling medical images requires considerable domain knowledge and experience. Automated decision-making can replace expert radiologists [39].

This chapter enlightens the developed and upcoming technologies of computer-based medical image processing. In addition, the chapter presents the following:

- Explicit knowledge of and common research problems on how computer science is taking part in different image-based disease diagnosis and their challenges.
- A careful description of different methods related to deep learning and image analysis in the medical domain.
- Some examples are given to show the time and cost efficiency of intelligent computer-based medical image processing over manual efforts for medical image labeling by experts.
- The main focus is on deep learning methods and an emerging lung disease, interstitial lung disease (ILD).
- It draws attention to the crucial intervention of computer-based techniques in image segmentation and classification. The evolution in this field has been discussed to show the future path of success in computer-based disease diagnosis and treatment.
- In the end, the chapter will discuss some gaps in existing studies and scopes for image-based ILD detection.

9.2   WHAT IS ILD?

ILD stands for interstitial lung disease. It can be defined as diffuse parenchymal disorders that impair the gas exchange function of the lungs by disrupting the alveolar walls [1]. The prevalence of ILD is 81 in 10 million males and 67 in 10 million females. ILD patients present with dyspnea, cough, abnormal chest imaging, and impaired pulmonary function test results. ILDs can be classified as known causes and unknown causes. Connective tissue disease; environmental, occupational, drug, and radiation induced; and smoking-related disease are some examples of known causes of ILD. Unknown causes of ILD are idiopathic pulmonary fibrosis, eosinophilic ILD, and vasculitis [1].

9.2.1 Diagnosis of ILD

Diagnosis of ILD is done by careful patient history, physical examination, pathology testing, imaging, bronchoscopy, and thoracoscopic biopsy. The initial assessment of pattern and parenchymal distribution concerns the associated features [1]:

- Pleural effusion
- Mediastinal lymphadenopathy

Predominant parenchymal abnormalities are:

- Reticular or linear
- Small nodules
- Linear or nodular opacity
- Consolidation opacity
- Ill-defined borders
- Silhouetting of normal structure
- Obliteration of normal structures like diaphragm intrapulmonary blood vessels

Apart from dominant findings, some additional radiographic changes are also key to diagnosing and staging ILD. These are:

- Prominent changes in upper lung zones found in sarcoidosis, silicosis, coal worker's pneumonia
- Calcified pleural plaques with interstitial opacity in asbestos-related ILDs
- Pleural thickening and pleural effusion in connective tissue disorders

Invasive diagnosis is painful and often avoided in aged and advanced-stage patients. Medical study shows 90% to 95% of ILD patients present with abnormal radiographic images. In many ILDs, the clinical context and characteristic features of high-resolution computed tomography (HRCT) images are enough to establish the diagnosis. Proper interpretation and classification of images, specially HRCT, require highly efficient domain experts.

9.2.2 Different Image Patterns in CT Images for ILD Diagnosis

We can observe different image patterns in the CT image of lungs for the different stages of development of ILD. Following are the few types of symptoms that can be observed in CT images for ILD patients:

Emphysema – It is the condition of the lungs when air sacs get damaged, narrowed, or collapsed. People who smoke for a long time or inhale polluted air may develop emphysema.

Ground glass opacity – It is the condition of the lungs when some portion of the lungs develop a hazy area that creates opacity in the lungs, but the bronchial structures can still be seen.

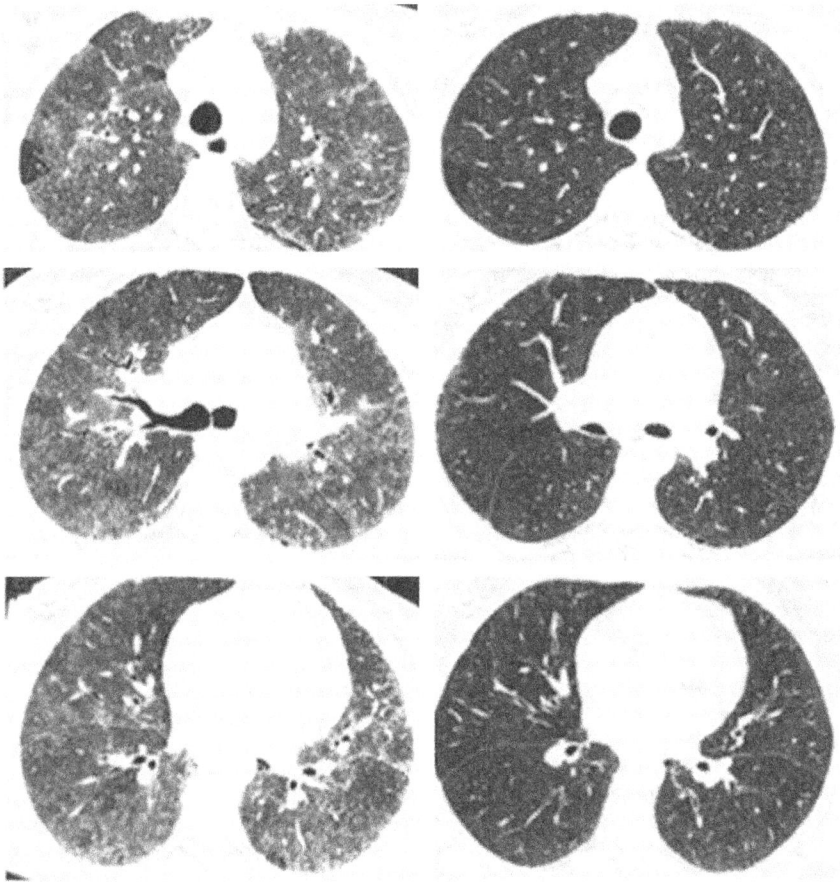

FIGURE 9.1 Various patterns of ILD [2].

Reticular – Reticulation is the condition of lungs when intralobular septa may thicken and appear as several linear opacities that form a mesh.

Honeycomb – Honeycombing indicates damaged and fibrotic lung tissue that contains many cystic air spaces with thick fibrous walls. The pattern looks like a honeycomb. Honeycombing represents the worst situation of the lungs.

The pattern of each symptom for ILD patients is described in Figure 9.1.

9.3 ROLE OF COMPUTER-BASED DISEASE DIAGNOSIS USING MEDICAL IMAGES

Image-based disease diagnosis is largely dependent on image acquisition and image interpretation. Different medical imaging tools have been developed substantially in the last decade. X-ray, different CT, and MRI are providing radiological images with much higher resolution. The field of medical image interpretation is also being explored rapidly. The most popular machine learning application in this field is computer vision. Computer vision uses a traditional machine learning approach that depends heavily on expert-crafted features. With the advancement of image acquisition tools, a large variety of image data is available. A large variation of data and the varied craft of images make traditional learning unreliable. Deep learning methods are evolving and gaining the ability to handle large and complex data. Computer-based techniques play vital roles in processing medical images, diagnosis with the help of computers, better segmentation and interpretation of the medical images, guided therapy, and disease analysis (seeFigure 9.5 Table 9.1). Using computer-based techniques improves the ability of doctors to diagnose disease and risk analysis more accurately. It gives some predictions that are very helpful even when domain expert doctors are not available.

These techniques can be grossly classified into two types:

- Conventional machine learning algorithms, such as k-nearest neighbor (KNN), neural networks (NNs; Figure 9.2), and decision trees
- Contemporary algorithms, such as convolutional neural networks (CNNs; Figure 9.3), extreme learning models (ELMs), and generative adversarial networks (GANs; Figure 9.4) [3]

This chapter presents the latest research works on deep learning methods that are bringing some revolutionary and evolutionary changes in the treatment of very common and morbid diseases like ILD.

9.4   CLASSIFICATION AND SEGMENTATION METHODS FOR IDENTIFICATION OF ILD

For the identification of ILD patterns and to propose the direction of diagnosis of the disease, the deep learning modules can be used for classification or segmentation processes.

Classification – Classification (Figure 9.6) is a predictive model where a class label is predicted for a given input data. The application of classification in ILD is mainly for the identification of a patient with the help of learned symptoms of ILD.

Segmentation – Segmentation (Figure 9.6) is the method of segregating input data into several groups. With the help of segmentation, one can localize each ILD pattern in the image of a patient's lung.

9.4.1   CLASSIFICATION OF ILD THROUGH CT IMAGES

Lung CT image classification can be a single-label classification or multilabel classification. As shown in Figure 9.7, in deep learning techniques, the image for ILD classification can be processed in one of three ways: patch based, slice based, and voxel based.

TABLE 9.1

Brief introduction and comparison of different deep learning–based models

Model	Features	Merits	Demerits
Convolution neural network (CNN) [4]	Convolution filters transform 2D datasets into 3D. Convolutional architecture explicitly assumes that the input is the image. This presumption helps in reducing the parameters in the network (Figure 9.3).	The learning time of this model is very fast yet efficient.	For classification purposes, CNN requires a good number of labeled datasets.
Recurrent neural network (RNN) [5]	This neural network forms the cyclic connection between neurons. Recurrent neural networks can learn sequential events very well. The different types are LSTM, BLSTM, MDL-STM, and HLSTM.	This model is very effective in tasks related to natural language processing (NLP) and shows high accuracy in speech and character recognition.	The greatest problem of this network is the vanishing gradient. Learning the sequences is a very time-consuming job.
Deep reinforcement learning [6]	It learns the task by trial and error. The machine is trained with real-life facts, then it makes a series of decisions.	This model rectifies the errors during the training process. This model can be applied to a specific context for best result.	It cannot be applied to a simple problem with many solutions. It requires plenty of data with many computations.
Deep Boltzmann machine (DBM) [7]	This method uses more hidden layers and connections between nodes are undirected (Figure 9.5).	This model requires fewer labeled data for training. As it is based on probabilistic methods, it can be applied in recognition-related jobs.	Adjusting the weight and time required for the probability of data is the main challenge of the DBM.
Deep belief network (DBN) [8]	A DBN is a network technique based on the hybrid generative graph-based model. The top two layers have no direction afterwards the layers are directed and linked to the lower layer.	Due to the unsupervised probabilistic deep learning nature, it can be employed in image recognition tasks.	The data model is quite complex and the training requires huge data and expensive hardware.

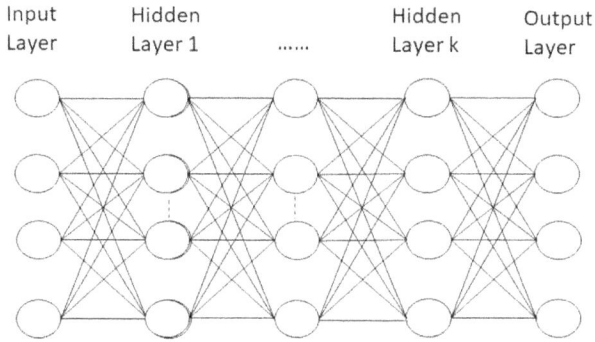

FIGURE 9.2 Architecture depicting a deep learning neural network (input, output, and k-hidden layers).

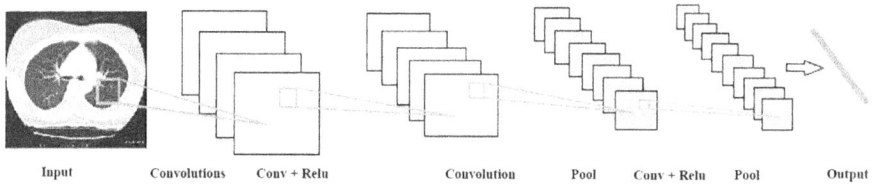

FIGURE 9.3 Steps for CNN-based lung image analysis.

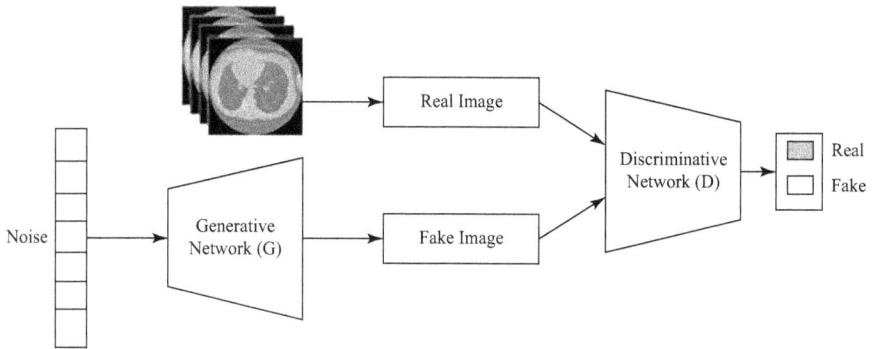

FIGURE 9.4 Architecture of a generative adversarial network (GAN).

- Patch based – A patch is the small subsection of a 2D image. An image is comprised of more than one patch of equal size. Patch size is chosen by the programmer. Patch-based classification can work in two different modes: one patch in one decision (OPOD) and all patches in one decision (APOD) [9].

- Slice based – A slice of a CT image is the cross-sectional representation of the body or any organ of the body. It is the 2D representation of the CT image [10].
- Voxel based – Whereas pixel means "picture elements" and it is a 2D representation of a point, voxel means "volume elements" and it provides graphical information of a point in 3D space [11].

From Figure 9.7, one can observe that the patch-based method mainly relies on different patches in the image of the lungs, whereas the slide-based method uses the 2D cross-sectional representation of any slice of the CT image for classification tasks. Whereas in the voxel-based method, each voxel of the lung is 3D volumetric information for classification of the CT image as healthy or otherwise based on the detected features.

9.4.1.1 Recent Works on Automated Classification of ILD Using Deep Learning

Some recent works, published from 2016 to 2022, on lung image classifications are presented in Figure 9.8 Tables 9.2 and .

9.4.2 Segmentation in CT Images for ILD

Medical image segmentation is ideally similar to the concept of image segmentation in which some specific organs are extracted from 2D or 3D medical images acquired from different imaging instruments like CT, MRI, PET, X-ray, or PET/CT depending on the organ. This can be done in a manual, semiautomatic, or fully automatic manner. Fully automatic segmentation is the latest research trend and a huge area of improvement. Again, this fully automatic segmentation is grossly categorized in two ways: (1) intensity-based segmentation and (2) shape-based segmentation [6].

Intensity-based segmentation is one in which the voxels inside an organ consist of near-equivalent gray values where interorgan gray values are different. The intensity

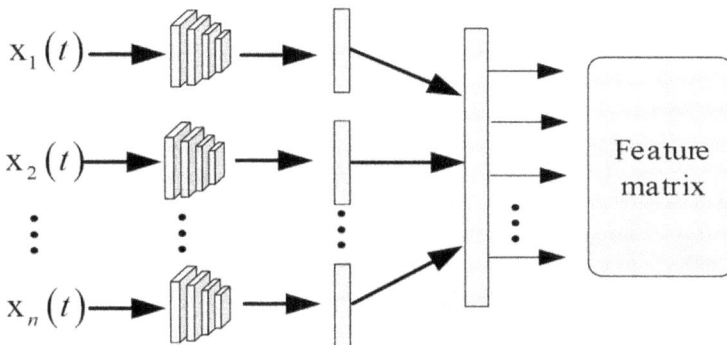

FIGURE 9.5 Multichannel CNN.

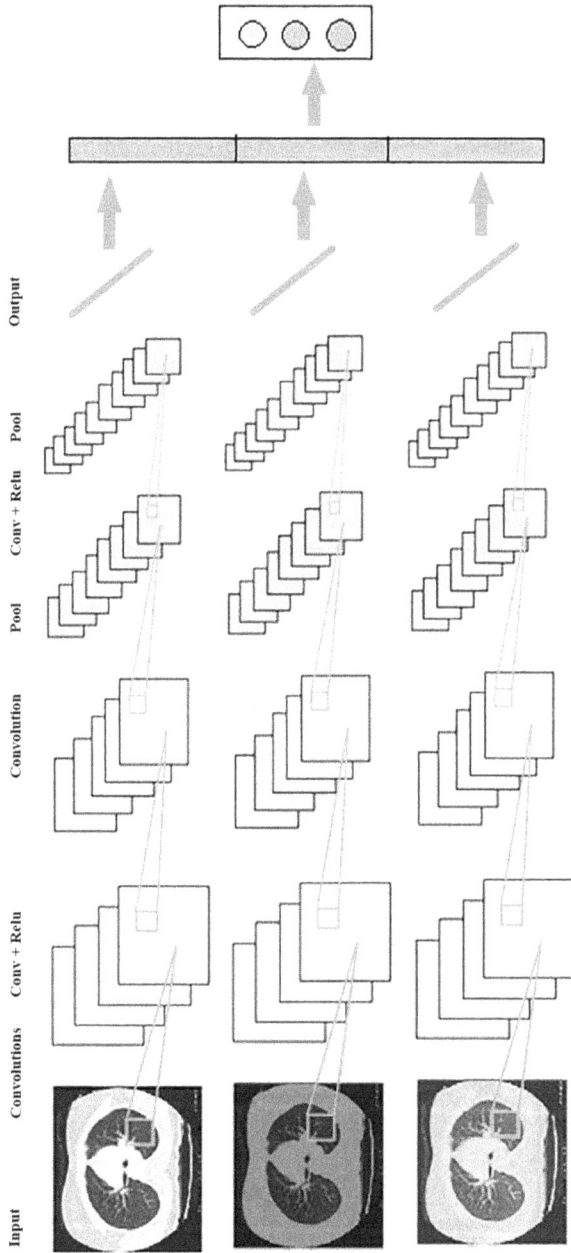

FIGURE 9.6 Architecture of CNN model for classification and segmentation.

(A) Patch-Based   (B) Slice-Based   (C) Voxel-Based

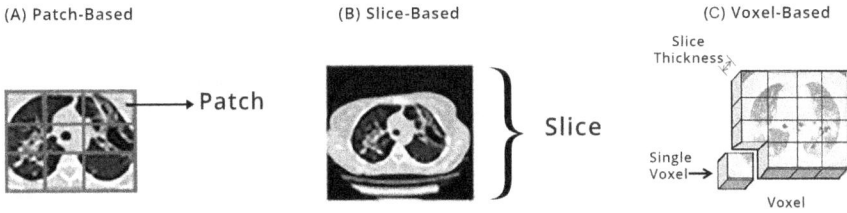

FIGURE 9.7 Different approaches for handling images in the classification of ILD using deep learning.

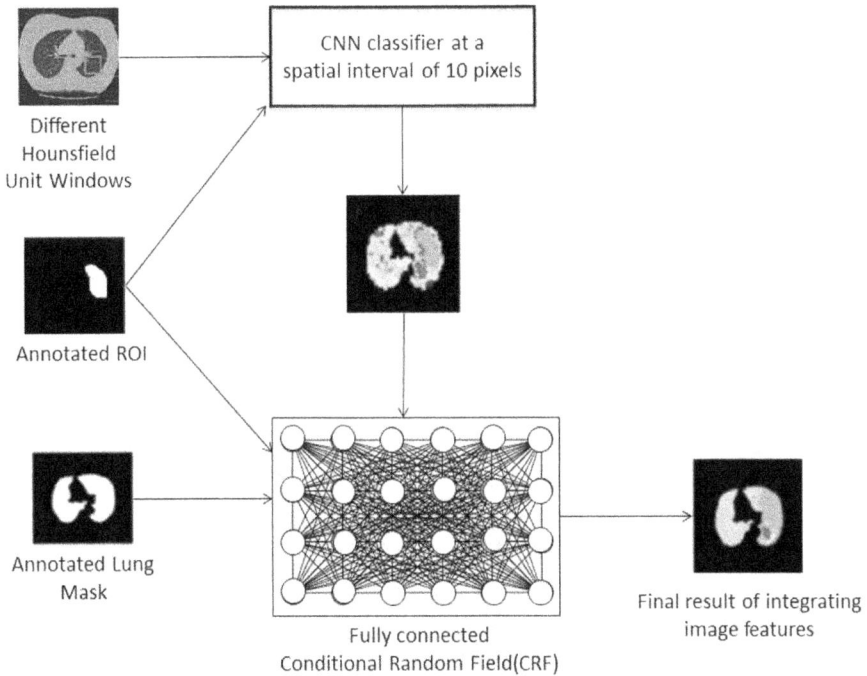

FIGURE 9.8 Integrating image features, unary prediction, and hard constraints [10].

difference in intraorgan voxels is hardly recognizable by the eye, but computers can easily track it.

Traditional medical image segmentation requires handcrafted image feature extraction like line, edge detection, and models to find the image gradient along organ boundaries such as graph cuts and active contours.

The lung segmentation is usually classified based on (a) threshold, (b) region, (c) shape, (d) neighboring anatomy, and (e) machine learning.

TABLE 9.2
Some of the recent works on the classification of ILD

Reference	Year	Publisher	Dataset	Classification using region of interest selection by experts/automatic
[12]	2017	Springer	MedGift ILD Database, CT Emphysema Database	Comparative study of classification
[13]	2019	Hindawi BioMedical Research International	MedGIFT	Classification/segmentation (radiologist helped identify the ROI)
[14]	2017	Springer	Databases of LIDC-IDRI	Classification (radiologist helped identify the ROI)
[15]	2019	Multidisciplinary Digital Publishing Institute (MDPI)	Kaggle lung CT images and Data Science Bowl	Classification (expert's intervention not needed for finding the ROI)
[10]	2017	Arxiv	University Hospitals of Geneva (HUG)	Segmentation and classification (expert's intervention not needed for finding the ROI)
[9]	2017	Elsevier	LIDC, DICOM	Classification (expert's intervention not needed for finding the ROI)
[16]	2019	Springer	University Hospitals of Geneva (HUG) database, a texture classification benchmark Kylberg Texture Dataset (KTD)	Classification (lung area annotated by experts)
[11]	2020	Nature	COPD Gene study dataset, www.ncbi.nlm.nih.gov	Classification (training point selected by two pulmonologists)
[17]	2019	Elsevier	ILD dataset	Classification (expert's intervention not needed for finding the ROI)
[18]	2021	IEEE Transaction	Datasets are available at https://github.com/yadavpa1/Lung-GAN	Classification (expert's intervention not needed for finding the ROI)

TABLE 9.3
Objectives, proposed methods, results, and metrics used by publications included in Table 9.2

Reference	Objective	Proposed method	Results	Metrics
[12]	Comparative study to classify the five patterns of lung diseases, namely, healthy, emphysema, fibrosis, ground glass and micronodules. Comparison between the performance of random forest, SVM, and CNN.	1. Patch extraction: 20x20 mm with overlap of 80% with a resolution of 1 mm/pixel. Patches were extracted from labeled ground truth regions. 2. Then two forms of classifier, random forest and SVM, were used. 3. Random forest and SVM worked using two metrics separately: (i) intensity metrics of first order and (ii) texture metrics that include gray-level run length matrix, gray-level co-occurrence matrix (GLCM), Law's texture filters, fractal dimension, and neighborhood gray-tone difference matrix (NGTDM). 4. First-order features alone, texture features alone, and combination of these have been tested. 5. CNN model is used for classification and Adam adaptive gradient descent algorithm is used with learning rate of 0.001. Amazon Web Services (AWS) was used for implementation.	The accuracy was 98.2, 79.0, and 69.9 for training, validation, and test case, respectively.	Accuracy mean, standard deviation, confusion matrix.
[13]	Automatic segmentation of lungs ROI by fusing radiomics and U-Net deep learning features.	1. At first the lung image's contour was handcrafted by experts. 2. The medical image is denoised. 3. Texture is extracted GLCM for different angles: 0°, 45°, 90° and 135°. 4. The same denoised image is given as input to the U-Net and deep features are extracted. 5. Texture features and deep features are fused to form the segmentation contour. 6. If the resultant segmentation contour and handcrafted contour are the same, then the contour is the final contour as well as the ROI, otherwise again the GLCM will be used with different angles to find texture features and the same procedure will be followed as described from steps 3 to 6. A Wiener filter was used to reduce Gaussian noise.	They claimed that their model DSC is 89.42%, which is higher than GLCM (82.47) and U-Net (85.83). Also, the SEN of their model is 94.99, which is higher than GLCM (93.08) and U-Net (92.94).	DSC (dice similarity coefficient). SEN (sensitivity).
[14]	Identifying the malignancy risk in lung nodules.	1.ROI extraction: a. Drawing outline to nodule by many radiologists. b. Filling the contour of the nodule that was identified by radiologists. c. Extracting the overlapped area of different contours. 2. Finding the nodule's morphological characteristics and shape in ROI. 3. Finding the pulmonary HOG (histogram of oriented gradients) feature. 4. Finding the LBP (local binary pattern) characteristics of pulmonary nodules. 5. The nodule ROI, LBP image of the nodule, and HOG image of the same nodule are passed to three different CNN channels. 6. The classification result of each channel is used for predicting the likelihood of nodules to be malignant.	The claimed accuracy is 91.75 and AUC (area under curve) is 0.9702.	Accuracy and AUC (area under curve).

(Continued)

TABLE 9.3 CONTINUED
Objectives, proposed methods, results, and metrics used by publications included in Table 9.2

Reference	Objective	Proposed method	Results	Metrics
[15]	To diagnose lung disease and increase the accuracy of diagnosis.	They proposed two 3D CNN architectures. The first CNN uses softmax as its primary classifier. The second CNN used a radial basis function (RBF)-based SVM as its classifier. The results of both 3D CNN architecture were compared for performance analysis.	The 3D CNN, which used an RBF-based SVM classifier, showed the better result with an accuracy rate of 91.81% and specificity of 94.23%.	Accuracy, sensitivity, precision, and specificity.
[10]	1. Automatic labeling incorporation in lung image. 2. ILD detection without manual ROI. 3. Detecting multiple ILD patterns using multilabel classification. 4. Segmenting the ILD area of different ILD patterns: healthy, emphysema, ground glass, fibrosis, and micronodules.	1. 32×32 patches from lung images were resized to 224×224 and passed to three different CNN channels for the different HU variant. This results in initial classification of lung images as healthy, emphysema, ground glass, fibrosis, micronodules. 2. Multilabel predictions on the same slice: Fisher vector CNN (FV-CNN) is implemented to localize targeted ILD patterns by activating feature maps at different network depths. The multivariate linear regression is used for training of the unordered features. 3. (a) Multilabel classified image and ground truth labels by radiologists were used as hard constraints of conditional random field (CRF). Fully connected CRF was used for propagating ILD labels from manual drawn regions to whole lung slices. (b) The fully connected CRF results in multiclass image segmentation and labeling. The whole process is depicted in Figure 9.8.	The AUC score for ground glass, reticular, honeycomb, and emphysema were 0.982, 0.972, 0.893, and 0.993, respectively.	Precision, recall, confusion matrix, F-score. and AUC.
[9]	Classifying ILD using "hybrid kernel-based SVM (HK-SVM)" and comparing the result with other classifiers like ANN, CNN, and KNN.	The paper described the functionality of different well-known classifiers and concluded that HK-SVM gives the better result.	Accuracy of ANN, KNN, CNN, and HK-SVM are 57.50%, 72.94%, 84.14%, and 90.52%, respectively.	Precision, recall rate, confusion matrix, accuracy and F-score.
[16]	Here, they suggested two-stage transfer learning to classify ILD patterns more accurately.	They proposed a new CNN architecture with two-stage transfer learning. Lung annotation was done by the experts. Some textures were extracted from unannotated areas of the lungs. These patterns were similar to ILD patterns. The first learning was from unlabeled textures of unannotated areas of CT slices. This was unsupervised learning. The second learning phase was from the intermediate domain dataset from the CNN intermediate layer. It is supervised learning. In this way CNN was trained using two-stage transfer learning (TSTL). They built a deep convolutional autoencoder (DCAE), which was used to enhance the performance of the CNN network. DCAE finds the texture properties of patches. A local discriminator was used for tuning the network by the help of auxiliary patches. A global discriminator was used for finding target patches that have ILD properties. In this way, lungs were classified for different ILD textures. The unsupervised part is depicted in Figure 9.8.	The performance for TSTL–DCAE is 0.9810, 0.9654, and 0.9786 for three different datasets. The result is claimed as better in comparison to other existing classifiers.	Confusion matrix, F1 score, and performance accuracy.

(Continued)

TABLE 9.3 CONTINUED
Objectives, proposed methods, results, and metrics used by publications included in Table 9.2

Reference	Objective	Proposed method	Results	Metrics
[11]	Finding all eight patterns of ILD. The patterns are normal parenchyma, five interstitial patterns (linear scar, reticular, ground glass, nodular, subpleural), and two emphysematous patterns (paraseptal and centrilobular).	Training points were placed manually on CT images by two pulmonologists. During training-point plotting, the entire volume of the lungs was considered. Here, a total of seven CNN models were used to classify the ILD patterns. Final classification was done by assembling the result of each CNN and using an optimal prediction outcome. The specialty of the work was that contextual information was concatenated with the final classification steps. Axial, sagittal, and coronal slices (three orthogonal planes) were considered for the CNN. Hence it was a 3D architecture. Practically, the classifiers classify the whole voxel instead of the slice.	Results presented achieved the geometric mean (GM) of 93.5%, specificity (SP) of 98.4%, sensitivity (SN) of 88.9%, and balanced accuracy (BA) of 93.61%.	AUC, SN, SP, GM, and BA.
[17]	Combining Riesz wavelet-based approach and deep learning-based approach to predict the five ILD classes in a better way.	1. Each patch was selected from the spatial domain of the CT image. 2. The feature space of the patch was created by ten filter responses, a histogram of Hounsfield units (HUs) and the number of air pixels in the patch. 3. Riesz order 5 was selected after several experiments. 4. After the final Riesz vector was developed, a softmax was generated from the Riesz feature vector. The softmax classifies the 5 ILD classes as shown in Figure 9.8. 5. A separate deep learning (DL) architecture was used to classify the 5 ILD patterns for each patch. 6. The feature vectors from the Riesz wavelet-based approach and DL-based approach were combined to predict ILD classes by forming a separate softmax classification.	The claimed accuracy of the model was 78.1% and AUC performance was 0.931.	Accuracy, AUC, confusion matrix.
[18]	To classify healthy lungs or lungs affected by any disease versus the lungs affected by some other disease. For example, tuberculosis (TB) vs. healthy lungs, COVID-19 vs. pneumonia, and pneumonia vs. normal. The classification is done by unsupervised learning using unlabeled data.	A multilayer generative adversarial network (GAN) architecture was used to learn textures of different lung diseases, including pneumonia, TB, and COVID-19. The learning features were used to train two modules: random forest and support vector classification (SVC). These were called base learners. The output of the two base learners was passed as input to a meta-classifier. The meta-classifier predicted the final classification result using logistic regression. The combination of multiple classifiers formed a stack of classifiers and the architecture gave better results as claimed in the paper.	Claimed accuracy is up to 99.5%.	Confusion matrix, F1 score, accuracy.

9.4.2.1 Methods for Segmentation of ILD Patterns

Various approaches to segmenting an ILD pattern in CT images of lungs are available in the literature. Table 9.4 describes some of the approaches that have been proposed and published in recent years. From the table, it is clearly shown that machine learning-based automatic segmentation is versatile and effective in all kinds of lung ailments.

Lung segmentation has the following challenges:

- In abnormal lungs, parenchyma nodules and blood vessels need to be segmented with lung parenchyma.
- Lung parenchyma is required to be separated from bronchus regions that are often confused with lung tissue.

TABLE 9.4
Description of various methods for segmentation of ILD in CT image

Segmentation method	Application	Merits	Demerits
Thresholding	Segments the well-defined structure, tumors, cavities, and nodules.	Very basic computation, inexpensive, and fast.	Does not consider attenuation variations and pathologic changes.
Region based	Normal structure, regions with nominal noise, and abnormality.	Fast computing and works well with clear attenuation variation.	Fails to segment the moderate to high abnormality level. Fails when pathogenic conditions impair adjacent structure.
Shape based	Abnormal condition of shape due to pathogenesis.	High accuracy when the shape of a particular pathogenesis is well defined.	Difficult to assure and create representative training features. Performance is highly dependent on training data.
Neighboring anatomy-guided methods	Very efficient for pleural effusion identification and classification.	Works well with cases where attenuation-based matrices fail.	Expensive computation. Fails when opacity prevails through intraregions.
Machine learning	All kinds of pathologic conditions specially ground glass opacity, consolidation, and honeycombing.	Efficient in ill-defined pathogenic condition and diffused changes in all regions, ground glass opacity, septal lines, and honeycomb.	Computationally expensive; separations of pathologic conditions are not well defined.

Many image analysis techniques are already in use for automatically separating lung parenchyma from CT images. The dominating techniques use thresholding [10, 16]. These techniques use contrast information of images as per published reviews [20]. A proposed stepwise segmentation is as follows [21]:

1. Extraction of the lung region by gray-level thresholding
2. Separation of lung lobes by dynamic programming
3. Postprocessing by morphological operation for smoothing the irregular boundaries

Nowadays, deep learning techniques are getting huge interest for medical image segmentation-related research due to frugal learning and the ability for fast and accurate learning. Havaei et al. [22] showed improvements in automatic brain tumor segmentation using deep learning over traditional methods.

With the introduction of a fully convolutional network (FCN) [23], the CNN architecture for dense prediction without fully connected layers revolutionized the job of segmentation, which is much faster than any classical method. Fully connected layers lose object detailing in pooling layers. So FCN used the concepts of encoder–decoder for spatial dimension reduction and then upsampling.

Another breakthrough in lung image segmentation was the introduction of U-Net architecture in 2015 [24], which is also based on FCN architecture. U-Net is an association of convolution layers in the contracting path and the expansive path deconvolution layers.

Guet al. [25] proposed a context encoder network. In this model, a context extractor was designed for the segmentation work where the images are given as input of the feature encoder module, and the ResNet-34 block is pretrained from ImageNet datasets to replace the U-Net encoder block. The context extractor generates high-level semantic feature maps that include a dense atrous convolution (DAC) and a residual multikernel pooling (RMP) block. Extracted semantic features are given as input into the feature decoder module, which augments the feature size.

The conventional local convergence filter can work with low-contrast medical images. This has been further improved by the FCN of U-Net. This comparison has been shown using lung nodule segmentation [26].

9.4.2.2 Recent Works on Automated Segmentation of ILD Patterns Using Deep Learning

This section presents some recent works between 2016 to 2022. Tables 9.5 and summarize the used datasets and proposed methods for lung image segmentation using deep learning.

9.5 DISCUSSION

In automated classification, overlapping futures are very confusing. For this reason, we can see the training accuracy is good [12], but test accuracy decays. In some studies, only a particular texture is classified [13], but ILDs include a wide variety

TABLE 9.5

Some of the recent works on the segmentation of lung images

Reference	Year	Publisher	Dataset
[27]	2018	Elsevier	LIDC-IDRI
[28]	2018	International Conference on Networking and Network Applications	MedGIFT
[29]	2020	Elsevier	LUNA16, VESSEL12, and HUG-ILD
[30]	2018	Springer Nature	LIDC-IDRI, MICCAI-2018, ASU-Mayo, Data Science Bowl
[31]	2019	IEEE 8th Joint International Information Technology and Artificial Intelligence Conference (ITAIC 2019)	University Hospitals of Geneva (HUG)
[32]	2019	Elsevier	Lung Image Database Consortium (LIDC), DICOM Image Library, and Medical College Hospital

of diseases with variable features. Nodule regions of interest (ROIs) can be hand-crafted before using them with CT images in multichannel CNN (Figure 9.5) [14]. Handcrafted regions of interest require expert intervention. The use of preexisting CNN architecture [15] in raw images has shown misclassification in 11.47% and 13.60% of samples. The comparison by Pang et al. is based on different deep architectures, but strategies like slice-based or voxel-based classification are not compared [9]. Some researchers have found that accuracy is not the same for all classes of ILDs [17]. Though the GAN is used for classification, it is still a gray area with many limitations and needs to be explored more for better results [18].

In many segmentation-related studies, the generation of masks is done by manual and mathematical models [27], whereas in other studies, the masks are taken from available datasets [29]. Separate methods and manual annotation are time-consuming and require a domain expert. But computer-aided systems are meant to relieve medical experts. In some research, several deep layers are used [28]. Deep layers are computationally expensive. The optimization is compromised to achieve the desired accuracy if complex layers are used. Medical images have very low contrast if separate costly techniques are not used like CT with contrast. The available images of secured datasets vary in size also. But some research [30] is carried out on good-quality images only. Even if the data pretreatments [31] are done, it is at the cost of mathematical straightforwardness. In most, diagnosis-related findings are required to be extracted. Isolated findings fail to provide clinical decisions. For example, patchy consolidation [32] is only the general feature of lungs that cannot isolate TB.

Other aspects like centrilobular small nodules and branching linear opacities are not considered.

9.6   RESEARCH GAPS AND FUTURE RESEARCH DIRECTIONS

Finding ILD using deep learning without experts is a promising research area. Many researchers are involved in this area by realizing the novelty of the work. We have found that many researchers reached the state of the art in the classification and segmentation model for analyzing different patterns found in ILD. Still, some challenges remain. The majority of the work is dependent on experts or radiologists who help with either handcrafting the region of interest or selecting training points. Also, lungs can have multiple patterns. Classifying only a single ILD pattern does not produce accurate results. So multilabel classification is needed for ILD detection. Very few papers used multilabel classification for ILD detection. Deep learning is a data-hungry model. Accuracy depends on the availability of a big volume of data. But acquiring the correct amount of data is a problem for medical imaging. Labeling of data is also a huge issue. Hence, a pure unsupervised learning approach should be focused more on this case, but from the literature review, very few papers focus on this area. Only classifying or segmenting the patterns is not sufficient; the location of the pattern in the lungs plays a crucial role in finding the exact subtype of ILD. The patient case history is also very important for the diagnosis of ILD. So, there is a need for a context-based deep learning model for making accurate decisions.

9.7   CONCLUSION

From all the data and ideas gathered in this chapter, it is clear that the application and research on medical imaging and deep learning are progressing at lightning speed. Deep learning has opened a new horizon in the field of medical image-based diagnosis and treatment after more than 100 years since it was first started with the invention of X-ray by Wilhelm Rontgen. Deep learning is rapidly automating many challenges that were thought to be unsolvable by computing. But many problems remain. Deep learning models are mostly black boxes. Even though the mathematical calculations are straightforward, the output generated is extremely complicated. Immense data are fed into the models, but understanding how the models work is a bit complicated and many researchers work without knowing the details. Medical professionals often exclude many parameters and accept some parameters depending on an instant thinking process and human-dependent perception. These decisions depend on the real-world situation and interpersonal information exchange between patient and doctor. The legal implications and software black boxes are also hard to rely on for medical professionals. Many software black boxes do not have a solid theoretical base. HIPAA guidelines protect the personal health information of patients. This issue majorly restricts researchers from acquiring the enormous data required for deep learning. Real-life disease data is not static. It is increasing and changing. Legal data restrictions are another barrier for these data-hungry software.

TABLE 9.6

Objectives, proposed methods, results, and metrics used by publications included in Table 9.5

Ref	Objective	Proposed Method	Results	Metrics
[27]	Segmentation of lung parenchyma by modifying the training process of U-Net.	1. Ground truth taken by manual segmentation. 2. Cropping the lung to keep the required area only. 3. U-Net system is trained with input images and with their exact masks. 4. An image is given as input for generating that particular mask as output in test phase. 5. The mask of a particular image is applied for segmenting the important area that is lung parenchyma.	Dice coefficient index is treated as similarity metrics and used for efficiency calculation. The result from the proposed network is compared with the manually segmented ground truth. Dice coefficient index achieved 0.9502.	Dice coefficient.
[28]	Lung parenchyma segmentation, candidate nodule detection, and classification.	1. A raw lung CT slice is processed with threshold erosion and dilation to get lung masks. HU value of CT ranges from −2048 to 400. A 1000 value for the air and 400 indicates the bone. Based on experiments, the window range is helpful in finding the ROI. The mask for parenchyma is constructed by baseline value of −400. This mask is usually bigger than the real lung mask because the binary value of CT is changing. Erosion and dilation method are used to fix the binary lung mask. 2. The training of 3D U-Net is improved with GAN. 3. Contextual CNN is used for classification of benign and malignant nodules.	Calculated dice coefficient of the ground truth, with respect to the segmented result. Then minimized it. Total loss is calculated as total pixelwise loss and dice loss after generation of mask through U-Net. Then the probability function of classification is calculated to find the probable malignancy. If this result is more than 0.5, then it is malignant.	Dice coefficient, loss function, probability.
[29]	Methodology for lung CT segmentation consists of three stages, namely, training stage, testing stage, and postprocessing stage.	1. Lung masks are taken from the datasets. 2. Outlining manually by expert for ground truth. 3. Implementation of Residual U-Net for the semantic segmentation applied on lung CT images. Thus the advantages of both residual and U-Net architecture is achieved.	Accuracy calculated using soft dice loss function, recall ratio, and Jaccard index. Mean accuracy is more than 95% in all databases.	Dice coefficient (DSC), recall Jaccard index (JI)

(Continued)

TABLE 9.6 CONTINUED

Objectives, proposed methods, results, and metrics used by publications included in Table 9.5

Ref	Objective	Proposed Method	Results	Metrics
[30]	Proposed UNet++ with an average IoU gain of 3.9 and 3.4 points more in comparison to U-Net and wide U-Net, respectively. The model segments successfully colon polyp, liver, and lung nodule.	UNet++ shares the feature of UNET. The difference lies in redesign of skip pathways connecting two subnetworks that also use deep supervision.	Set side by side U-Net, wide U-Net, and UNet++ with respect to the number parameters and perfection in segmentation for the purpose of segmenting lung nodule, segmenting polyp in colon, segmenting liver, and cell nuclei. Without deep supervision U-Net++ can achieve a significant increase in performance between U-Net and wide U-Net, resulting in betterment of 2.8 and 3.3 points in IoU (intersection over union). UNet++ used with deep supervision gives 0.6 points better result with respect to non-deep supervision UNet++.	Intersection over union (IoU %).
[31]	Improvement over segmentation-based algorithm for detection of lung nodule. Here, the ResNet and U-Net are used for segmentation. Then the classification network is trained based on segmented nodules for categorization of suspected regions of lung nodule.	1. The data pretreatment is done in three ways: (i) association, (ii) data enhancement, and (iii) coordinate transform association. 2. Identical residual module used in U-Net (just adding 1×1 before and after CNN) for proper resizing. 3. Output segments are compared with dice coefficients and masks are selected. 4. Then actual segmentation was done by U-Net. 5. Multiclassification network used for nodule classification. 6. The work shows effectiveness of combining multiple classification networks. The VGG, Inception, and DenseNet classification networks are compared. Finally, the effect of combining multiclass networks are also investigated.	Accuracy checked by recall and precision. The accuracy is more in U-Net block segmentation.	Recall and precision.

(Continued)

TABLE 9.6 CONTINUED

Objectives, proposed methods, results, and metrics used by publications included in Table 9.5

Ref	Objective	Proposed Method	Results	Metrics
[32]	Proposed MR U-Net method for segmenting TB affected regions from normal regions in lungs CT images.	1. First, the CT images are resized and intensity enhanced as those are taken from different data sources. 2. Multires block replaces conv. block of UNet++ with 3×3, 5×5, and 7×7 filters in parallel. 3. Next, the 5×5 and 7×7 filters are replaced with the 3×3 filters. 4. Last, the adder operation is carried on with the three 3×3 filters in a parallel form and a 1×1 filter.	The accuracy is calculated in the form of system accuracy and detection accuracy from which recall and precision have been calculated.	Recall rate, precision.

BIBLIOGRAPHY

1. M. Gao, Z. Xu, L. Lu, A. P. Harrison, R. M. Summers and D. J. Mollura, "Multi-label deep regression and unordered pooling for holistic interstitial lung disease pattern detection," in International Workshop on Machine Learning in Medical Imaging, 2016.

2. M. Gao, Z. Xu, L. Lu, A. P. Harrison, R. M. Summers and D. J. Mollura, "Holistic interstitial lung disease detection using deep convolutional neural networks: Multi-label learning and unordered pooling," *arXiv preprint arXiv:1701.05616*, pp. 1–21, 2017.

3. A. Krizhevsky, I. Sutskever and G. E. Hinton, "ImageNet classification with deep convolutional neural networks," *Communications of the ACM*, vol. 60, no. 6, pp. 84–90, 2017.

4. W. Zaremba, I. Sutskever and O. Vinyals, "Recurrent neural network regularization," vol. 60, *arXiv preprint arXiv:1409.2329*, pp. 84–90, 2014.

5. B. A. Skourt, A. E. Hassani and A. Majda, "Lung CT image segmentation using deep neural networks," *Procedia Computer Science*, vol. 127, p. 109–113, 2018.

6. P. Jeyaraj and E. Nadar, "Deep Boltzmann machine algorithm for accurate medical image analysis for classification of cancerous region," *Cognitive Computation and Systems*, vol. 1, no. 3, pp. 85–90, 2019.

7. A. Khatami, A. Khosravi, T. Nguyen, C. Lim and S. Nahavandi, "Medical image analysis using wavelet transform and deep belief networks," *Expert Systems with Applications*, vol. 86, pp. 190–198, 2017.

8. A. O'Neil, M. Shepherd, E. Beveridge and K. Goatman, "A comparison of texture features versus deep learning for image classification in interstitial lung disease," in *Annual Conference on Medical Image Understanding and Analysis*, 2017.

9. T. Pang, S. Guo, X. Zhang and L. Zhao, "Automatic lung segmentation based on texture and deep features of HRCT images with interstitial lung disease," *BioMed research international*,vol. 2019 2019. https://doi.org/10.1155/2019/2045432

10. H. Wang, T. Zhao, L. Li, H. Pan, W. Liu, H. Gao, F. Han, Y. Wang, Y. Qi and Z. Liang, "A hybrid CNN feature model for pulmonary nodule malignancy risk differentiation," *Journal of X-ray Science and Technology*, vol. 26, no. 2, pp. 171–187, 2018.

11. H. Polat and H. D. Mehr, "Classification of pulmonary CT images by using hybrid 3D-deep convolutional neural network architecture," *Applied Sciences*, vol. 9, no. 5, p. 940, 2019.

12. M. Ajin and L. Mredhula, "Diagnosis of interstitial lung disease by pattern classification," *Procedia Computer Science*, vol. 115, pp. 195–208, 2017.

13. S. Huang, F. Lee, R. Miao, Q. Si, C. Lu and Q. Chen, "A deep convolutional neural network architecture for interstitial lung disease pattern classification," *Springer*, vol. 58, no. 4, pp. 725–737, 2020.

14. D. Bermejo-Peláez, S. Y. Ash, G. R. Washko, R. S. J. Estépar and M. J. Ledesma-Carbayo, "Classification of interstitial lung abnormality patterns with an ensemble of deep convolutional neural networks," *Scientific Reports*, vol. 10, no. 1, pp. 1–15, 2020.

15. R. Joyseeree, S. Otalora, H. Muller and A. Depeursinge, "Fusing learned representations from riesz filters and deep CNN for lung tissue classification," *Medical Image Analysis*, vol. 56, pp. 172–183, 2019.

16. P. Yadav, N. Menon, V. Ravi and S. Vishvanathan, "Lung-GANs: Unsupervised representation learning for lung disease classification using chest CT and x-ray images," *IEEE Transactions on Engineering Management*vol. 70, no. 8, pp. 2774–2786, 2023.10.1109/TEM.2021.3103334.

17. B. Skourt, A. E. Hassani and A. Majda, "Lung CT image segmentation using deep neural networks," *Procedia Computer Science*, vol. 127, pp. 109–113, 2018.

18. C. Zhao, J. Han, Y. Jia and F. Gou, "Lung nodule detection via 3D U-Net and contextual convolutional neural network," in *International Conference on Networking and Network Applications (NaNA)*, 2018.

19. A. Khanna, N. D. Londhe, S. Gupta and A. Semwal, "A deep Residual U-Net convolutional neural network for automated lung segmentation in computed tomography images," *Biocybernetics and Biomedical Engineering*, vol. 40, no. 3, pp. 1314–1327, 2020.

20. Z. Zhou, M. R. Siddiquee, N. Tajbakhsh and J. Liang, "UNet++: A nested U-Net architecture for medical image segmentation," *Deep Learn Med Image Anal Multimodal Learn Clin Decis Support*, 2018. doi: 10.1007/978-3-030-00889-5_1

21. H. Cheng, Y. Zhu and H. Pan, "Modified U-Net block network for lung nodule detection," in *8th Joint International Information Technology and Artificial Intelligence Conference (ITAIC)*, 2019.

22. M. Ramkumar, D. Jayakumar and R. Yogesh, "Multi res U-Net based image segmentation of pulmonary tuberculosis using CT images," in *7th International Conference on Smart Structures and Systems (ICSSS)*, 2020.

23. C. V. Broaddus, J. Ernst, K. E. Talmadge, L. Stephen, S. F. Kathleen, S. M. Lynn, R. Stapleton and M. B. Gotway, "Murray and Nadal's Textbook of Respiratory Medicine," in *Murray and Nadal's Textbook of Respiratory Medicine*, 7th ed. Elsevier Health Sciences, 2021.

24. A. O'Neil, M. Shepherd, E. Beveridge, and K. Goatman, "Comparison of Texture Features Versus Deep Learning for Image Classification in Interstitial Lung Disease," Springer, 2017.

25. T. Pang, S. Guo, X. Zhang, and L. Zhao, "Automatic lung segmentation based on texture and deep features of HRCT images with interstitial lung disease," in *Hindawi Bio Medical Research International*, 2019.

26. H. Wang, T. Zhao, L.C. Li, H. Pan, W. Liu, H. Gao, F. Han, Y. Wang, Y. Qi, and Z. Liang, *A Hybrid CNN Feature Model for Pulmonary Nodule Malignancy Risk Differentiation*. Springer, 2017.

27. Huseyin Polat and Homay Danaei Mehr, "Classification of Pulmonary CT Images by Using Hybrid 3D-Deep Convolutional Neural Network Architecture," MDPI, 2019.

28. M. Ajin, *Diagnosis Of Interstitial Lung Disease By Pattern Classification*. Elsevier, 2017.

29. S. O. H. M. A. RanveerJoyseeree, *Fusing Learned Representations from Riesz Filters and Deep CNN for Lung Tissue Classification*. Elsevier, 2019.

30. N. V. R. S. PoojaYadav, "Lung-GANs: Unsupervised Representation Learning for Lung Disease Classification using Chest CT and X-ray Images," *IEEE Transaction*, vol. 70, no. 8, pp. 2774–2786, 2023. doi: 10.1109/TEM.2021.3103334.

31. I. J. Goodfellow, J. Pouget-Abadie, M. Mirza, B. Xu, D. Warde-Farley, S. Ozair, A. Courville and Y. Bengio, "Generative adversarial network," *Communications of the ACM*, vol. 63, no. 11, pp. 139–144, 2020.

32. J. Li, M. Erdt, F. Janoos, T.-c. Chang and J. Egger, "Medical image segmentation in oral-maxillofacial surgery," *Computer-Aided Oral and Maxillofacial Surgery*, pp. 1–27, 2021.

33. K. Nakagomi, A. Shimizu, H. Kobatake, M. Yakami, K. Fujimoto and K. Togashi, "Multi-shape graph cuts with neighbor prior constraints and its application to lung segmentation from a chest CT volume," *Med. Image Anal*, vol. 17, no. 1, pp. 62–77, Jan 2013.

34. S. Hu, E. A. Hoffman and J. M. Reinhardt, "Automatic lung segmentation for accurate quantitation of volumetric X-ray CT images," *IEEE Transactions on Medical Imaging*, vol. 20, no. 6, pp. 490–498, June 2001.

35. M. Havaei, A. Davy, D. Warde-Farley, A. Biard, A. Courville, Y. Bengio, C. Pal, P.-M. Jodoin and H. Larochelle, "Brain tumor segmentation with deep neural networks," *Medical image analysis*, vol. 35, pp. 18–31, 2017.

36. J. Long, E. Shelhamer and T. Darrell, "Fully convolutional networks for semantic segmentation," in *IEEE Conference on Computer Vision and Pattern Recognition*, 2015.

37. O. Ronneberger, P. Fischer and T. Brox, "U-Net: Convolutional networks for biomedical image segmentation," in *International Conference on Medical Image Computing and Computer-Assisted Intervention*, 2015.

38. Z. Gu, J. Cheng, H. Fu, K. Zhou, H. Hao, Y. Zhao, T. Zhang, S. Gao and J. Liu, "CE-Net: Context encoder network for 2d medical image segmentation," *IEEE Transactions on Medical Imaging*, vol. 38, no. 10, pp. 2281–2292, 2019.

39. J. Rocha, A. Cunha and A. M. Mendonça, "Conventional filtering versus u-net based models for pulmonary nodule segmentation in CT images," *Journal of Medical Systems*, vol. 44, no. 4, pp. 1–8, Mar. 2020.

10 Computer Vision Approaches in Radiograph Image Analysis

A Targeted Review of Current Progress, Challenges, and Future Perspectives

Abdelbaki Souid, Ben Othman Soufiene, and Hedi Sakli

10.1 INTRODUCTION

Computer vision (CV) is the wide field concerned with giving computers the ability to process, analyze, and recognize visual content, such as videos and multidimensional images. CV is common across a wide range of applications, including oil and gas [1–3], oceanography and agriculture [4], medical analysis [5–9], and robotic surgery [10, 11]. The primary types of computer vision tasks are image classification, object identification and recognition from images, and image segmentation [12]. Image classification challenges are among the most typical CV issues [13, 14], These are commonly deployed, notably in the medical industry, and are frequently expressed as standard supervised machine learning (ML) tasks [15], where a label is a set of characteristics X (typically derived from an image) that is used to predict a certain result y.

Researchers have devised several methods for extracting low-level and high-level features from photos [16]. Corner points, edges, color intensity, and scale-invariant features, such as SIFT and SURF, are examples of typical features [18, 19]. The scientific community was drawn to SURF in particular because these characteristics are invariant to picture scale, rotation, posture, and lighting, which were previously regarded as major issues in CV and medical imaging. ML models are trained to utilize these attributes to perform supervised classification tasks. By using machine learning, computers are able to learn from historical observations without having to

DOI: 10.1201/9781003366249-10

to explicitly program them [17]. Instead, heuristics can be designed to account for the infinite combinations of features within observations. Among the most common methods of machine learning are the support vector machine (SVM) [18] and methods based on ensembles, such as random forests (RFs) [19] and artificial neural networks (ANNs) [20]. SVM was the most used way for dealing with computer vision problems including classification, object identification, and object tracking. One significant downside of this technique is that the performance of the chosen ML model would be largely dependent on the quality of the extracted picture characteristics.

A classic example is developing an automated diagnosis/classification system for 27 cardiovascular illnesses based on electrocardiogram (ECG) signal readings [21, 22]. Based on a collection of chest X-ray pictures from different pathology patients, a classification algorithm to classify patients as either lung pathology infected or normal (healthy) was suggested. It should be emphasized that in all of these cases, the main job is to determine whether the input data (ECG signal or picture) includes a certain ailment from a list of recommended classes, which is referred to as a multiclass classification issue.

The quality of these characteristics is frequently affected by factors such as light and object orientation inside an image sample, as well as noise and other relevant aspects. Handcrafted features in ML-based deployed solutions may be significantly less successful than outcomes from controlled data.

Deep learning breakthroughs have evolved and improved over time, focusing mostly on one method known as convolutional neural networks (CNNs). CNNs are the most common deep learning architecture because of their unique ability to harness the spatial and temporal relationship between image attributes that must be decoded to extract the meaningful information hidden in images [23–25].

Machine learning and deep learning advancements have resulted in substantial success in the medical sphere; for example, in ophthalmology, there have been two important areas where machine learning and new deep learning systems have been utilized. First, artificial intelligence (AI) algorithms have been demonstrated to reliably predict diabetic retinopathy in recent studies, including preregistered prospective clinical trials [26–29]; glaucoma [26, 30]; age-related macular degeneration (AMD) [26, 31, 32]; retinopathy of prematurity (ROP) [33]; and refractive error, as measured by digital fundus photography [34]. Several cardiovascular risk factors [35] were also appropriately predicted using fundus images. Second, various retinal illnesses, such as neovascular AMD, early stages of AMD, and diabetic macular edema (DME), have been discovered [36] utilizing optical coherence tomography (OCT) [37, 38].

In this chapter, we concentrate on deep learning computer vision in the literature linked to pneumology and cardiology, as well as recent developments and important problems, with an emphasis on the most prevalent computer vision tasks (classification, segmentation, and object detection). The following are the primary contributions of the study:

- We present an in-depth critical technical examination of the most recent advances in medical image analysis and comprehension. We also present a comprehensive evaluation of existing work on the subject that covers the

previously presented medical field with sophisticated vision tasks, such as medical picture classification and segmentation.
- There is an in-depth discussion and evaluation of various applications that utilize medical images and deep learning applications and approaches with discussion and assessment of publicly available medical datasets.

The remainder of this work is structured as follows: Section 10.2 discusses the most recent advances in medical pneumology image analysis, with an emphasis on critical tasks such as categorizing, segmenting, and identifying structures and regions of interest. We also provide a list of the numerous medical datasets that are available in the public domain to serve the researcher in the field of radiological pneumology. Section 10.3 focuses on cardiology applications and the possible datasets that are available to the general public to work with, presenting a fantastic chance to speed up research and development in this field. Section 10.4 concludes with findings and future directions.

10.2   OVERVIEW OF MACHINE LEARNING FOR RADIOLOGICAL PNEUMOLOGY

In this section, we will review the literature focusing on artificial intelligence for lung pulmonary, splitting it into subsections based on the type of work being done (image-level prediction, segmentation, data generation, domain adaptation). We will also address the public datasets that have been or are still in use to develop these models (Table 10.1). Some works that have an equal emphasis on artificial intelligence for lung pulmonary in Tables 10.2 and 10.3. Only research that quantitatively analyze their outcomes was included in the segmentation and localization categories.

10.2.1   Datasets

This section contains an overview of the public dataset encountered in the literature examined in this study, in addition to any others that are known to us; Table 10.1 contains specifics. Each dataset is given an acronym that is utilized in Table 10.1 to specify which one was utilized in the work indicated.

Based on the work provided in [39], we begin by presenting the ChestX-ray14 (C14) dataset, which includes 112,120 chest X-rays (CXRs) from 30,805 patients [40]. The National Institutes of Health in the United States collects chest radiographs. The photos are delivered as 8-bit grayscale with a dimension of 1024×1024 pixels. Also, this dataset was text mining labeled by radiology reports, revealing the existence of 14 distinct abnormalities. In 2019 CheXpert (XP) was presented as a dataset containing 224,316 CXRs from 65,240 patients [41]. Between October 2002 and 2017, CXRs were collected at Stanford Hospital. The images were distributed in their original resolution as 8-bit grayscale images. A rule-based labeler was used to automatically label radiology reports, showing the presence, absence, ambiguity, or omission of 12 pathologies, as well as the existence or absence of support devices. The PadChest

TABLE 10.1

Datasets for the study

	Studies (S) Images (I) Patients (P)	PoV	Label annotation			Dataset format	Labeling
			Types	Labels	Studies		
Chest X-ray14 [40] (C14)	P: 31K I: 112K	AP-PA	CL BB	14 8	112K 983	PNG	RP RI
CheXpert [41] (XP)	P: 65K S: 188K I: 224K	AP-PA	CL	14	224K	JPEG	RP RI
PadChest [42] (PC)	P: 67K S: 110K I: 160K	AP-PA	CL	193	110K DICOM	DICOM	RIR
PLCO [43] (PL)	P: 25K I: 89K	AP-PA	CL BB	22 17	89K 89K	DICOM	RI
Open I [44] (O)	P: 3,955 I: 7,910	AP-PA	R		3,955	JPEG	RI
Ped-Pneumonia [37] (PP)	I: 5,856	AP-PA	CL	2	5,856	JPEG	RI
VinBigData [45] (VD)	P: I: 18K	AP-PA	CL BB	15	18K	DICOM	RI
SIIM–ACR [47] (SI)	I: 16K P: 16K	AP-PA	SE	1	16K	DICOM	RI
CXR14 Rad Labels [46] (CR)	P: 1,709 S: 4,473	AP-PA	CL BB	14	4,473	JPEG	RI

(*Continued*)

TABLE 10.1 CONTINUED
Datasets for the study

	Studies (S) Images (I) Patients (P)	PoV	Label annotation			Dataset format	Labeling
			Types	Labels	Studies		
(LIDC-IDRI) [49] (LI)	P: 1,709 S: 4,374	CT	CL SE	1	4,374	DICOM	
LungCT-Diagnosis [50]	P: 61 I: 4,682	CT	SE CL	1	4,682	DICOM	
COVID-CXR [48] (CC)	P: 449 I: 866	AP-PA	CL BB SE			PNG+JPEG	RI

Notes: Values greater than 10,000 are rounded and abbreviated with the letter K, which stands for thousand (i.e., 10K for 10,000).

Abbreviations: RP, report parsing; RIR, radiologist interpretation of reports; RI, radiologist interpretation of chest X-rays; RCI, radiologist cohort agreement on chest X-rays; LT, laboratory tests types of annotations; BB, bounding box; CL, classification; R, report; SE, segmentation; PoV, position of view.

TABLE 10.2
Relevant work to the image classification task

Reference	Method	Dataset
Tang et al. [52]	Abnormality detection, multiple networks compared to radiologist labeling.	C14, O, PP, RP
Souid et al. [51]	Detection of 8 lung pathologies including pneumothorax, pneumonia, and mass/nodule using transfer learning.	C14, VD, XP
Wu et al. [56]	COVID-19 image [57], RSNA [58], USNLM-NLM(MC) [59]. The models achieved 95% accuracy and 90% recall for NASNet Large for 4 classes.	C
Chadaga et al. [60]	Using feature extraction methodologies and traditional ML classifiers, the accuracy, specificity, and sensitivity attained were 95.95%, 95.13%, and 96%, for only the first dataset.	5,644 patients for a blood test
Stephen et al. [61]	The database provided by Melendez et al. [59]. CNN achieves 94% training accuracy. The ensemble model obtained an accuracy of 96.4% with a recall of 99.62%.	Private CXR
Mittal et al. [62]	Various capsule network designs are evaluated for pediatric pneumonia detection.	PP
Chouhan et al. [53]	Part of the data comes from the data collective of Cohen et al. [48]. Computed tomography calculated opacification percentage (median [interquartile]: 3.6% [0.5%, 12.1%] versus 8.7% [2.7%, 21.2%]; P < .01).	Part of C14

TABLE 10.3
Pulmonary segmentation models

Reference	Method	Dataset
Wang et al. [63]	UNet design with dense connections.	PR
Cardenas et al. [70]	Given a lung-segmented chest radiograph scan with patches, U-Net for bone suppression is used.	PR
Mortani Barbosa et al. [71]	CNN trained on CT projection pictures to quantify airspace illness.	PR
Larrazabal et al. [72]	Autoencoder denoising as postprocessing to enhance segmentation.	PR
Xue et al. [73]	Cascaded U-Net with faulty segmentations and sample selection.	PR
Souid et al. [69]	Xception–Resnet autoencoder to segment pneumothorax masks.	SIIM–ACR
Gu et al. [74]	Unique CAD system that uses a 3D feature set to detect lung nodules in lung CT images.	LD

(PD) dataset has 160,868 chest radiographs from 109,931 investigations and 67,000 patients [42]. CXRs were collected at San Juan Hospital in Spain from 2009 to 2017. The photographs are stored in full resolution as 16-bit grayscale images. Physicians manually classified 27,593 records. A recurrent neural network was trained using these labels and then used to label the rest of the dataset from the reports. There were 174 observations, 19 diagnoses, and 104 anatomic sites extracted from the reports. The Prostate, Lung, Colorectal, and Ovarian (PLCO) Cancer Screening Trial provided another dataset (PL) [43]. This study's lung arm contains 185,421 CXRs from 56,071 patients. The National Institutes of Health distributes a standard set of 25,000 patients and 88,847 frontal CXRs. This dataset includes 22 pulmonary and thorax pathologies labels with four levels of abnormalities and their locations. The Open-I (O) dataset includes 7,910 CXRs from 3,955 scans and 3,955 patients [44]. The pictures are supplied in the form of anonymized DICOM images. The Ped-Pneumonia (PP) collection includes 5,856 pediatric chest radiograph images [37]. The X-rays were obtained from China's Guangzhou Women and Children's Medical Center. The photos are presented as 8-bit grayscale images of varying resolutions. The labels include bacterial and viral pneumonia as well as normal. The VinDr-CXR (VD) [45] dataset consists of 18,000 chest radiographs. The text was mined using 14 illness picture labels and partitioned into training and test sets. Because the VinDr-CXR uses parts of the ChestX-ray 14's lung diseases, CXR14-Rad-Labels (CR) provide annotations for some of the ChestX-ray14 data [46]. It consists of four labels representing 4,374 studies and 1,709 patients. Three radiologists agreed to collect these labels. These radiologists were selected out of a pool of 11 radiologists for the validation portion (2,412 studies from 835 patients) and 13 radiologists for the test portion (2,412 studies from 835 patients) (1,962 studies from 860 patients). Individual labels for each radiologist, as well as agreement labels, were supplied. The SIIM–ACR (SI) dataset was made available for a Kaggle competition on pneumothorax identification and segmentation [47]. Although the competition organizers have not validated the data sources, researchers have discovered that at least some (perhaps all) of the photos are from the ChestX-ray14 collection. They are sent as DICOM files with a resolution of 1024 × 1024. In affirmative circumstances, pixel segmentations of the pneumothorax are shown. At the time of writing, the COVID-CXR (CV) collection had 930 CXRs (the dataset remains in continuous development) [48]. CXRs are collected from a variety of locations using various methods, including screen pictures from papers studying COVID-19. The labels that are provided vary depending on the information available from the source of the photograph. Images are sent as 8-bit PNG or JPEG files with no specified resolution.

LIDC-IDRI stands for the Lung Image Database Consortium Image Collection and Image Database Resource Initiative [49]. This dataset (abbreviated LI for this study) consists of four labels representing 4,374 studies and 1,709 patients. Several radiologists reached an agreement to acquire these labels. For the validation split, radiologists were chosen from a group of 11 labels (2,412 studies from 835 patients) and 13 for the test split (2,412 studies from 835 patients) (1,962 studies from 860 patients). Distinctive labels for each radiologist, as well as agreement labels, were supplied. The LungCT-Diagnosis dataset is freely accessible from The Cancer

Imaging Archive (TCIA) and was last updated in 2014. In 2012 [50], 61 patients were covered. The number of scans in DICOM format was 4,682, with a size of 2.5 GB and a CT modality and slice thickness ranging from 3 to 6 mm. Metadata such as patient data and tumor slices are also included in this dataset. It also displays the number of tumor slices for each patient.

10.2.2 DEEP LEARNING FOR MEDICAL PNEUMOLOGY

10.2.2.1 Image-Level Prediction Task

Predicting a label (classification) or a continuous value (regression) done by evaluating a whole image is referred to as image-level prediction. Classification labels include pathology (e.g., pneumonia, emphysema), information such as the patient's gender, and picture orientation. Regression values might indicate a pathology's severity score or other information such as the subject's age.

Studies recapped in Table 10.2 have scan-level forecasts. The majority of these studies employ off-the-shelf deep learning models to predict pathology, metadata, or a set of labels supplied with the dataset. Predicting the labels of the ChestX-ray14 dataset is the most widely researched image-level prediction challenge, as demonstrated in the work by Souid et al. [51], which analyzes the performance of several techniques to classify eight illness categories from the ChestX-ray14 dataset and VinBigData. The work presented by Tang et al. [52] examines the effectiveness of several deep learning models for recognizing abnormal cases on multiple public chest X-ray datasets. Another often-researched condition is pneumonia. Transfer learning is a technique of reusing trained neural network weights to train the model on a new dataset, by altering and retraining just the classification layer of the model. The modified CNN consumes all of the architectural advantages of the basic CNN. The work by Chouhan et al. [53] also employed transfer learning with five neural nets to build an ensemble model to detect pneumonia. Chhikara et al. [54] utilized models such as the InceptionV3 architecture, integrating dropout layer, pooling, and dense layers at the network's outputs. The work by Chen et al. [55] addresses the use of trained models such as Inception ResNet, NASNet, and others.

10.2.2.2 Segmentation

One of the most often investigated themes in CXR analysis is segmentation, which consists of literature focusing on anatomical detection, oddities, or unexpected artifacts. Table 10.3 summarizes the segmentation literature evaluated for this investigation. On chest radiographs, many computer-aided diagnostic systems rely on anatomical segmentation of the heart, lungs, clavicles, or ribs. To increase performance and efficiency, designating the region of interest for future image processing operations is generally the first step [63–65]. Furthermore, depending on form or area data, segmentation may be used to quantify clinical characteristics. The cardiothoracic ratio, for example, a clinically utilized parameter to assess heart enlargement (cardiomegaly), may be determined directly from heart and lung segmentation [66, 67]. Surprisingly, just a few studies looked at abnormality segmentation. Hurt et al. [68] focused on the segmentation of pneumonia. Souid et al. [69], on the other hand, developed a mechanism for segmenting the pneumothorax. It is important to note that these studies made use of freshly available challenge datasets (hosted by Kaggle), specifically RSNA pneumonia and SIIM–ACR.

In general, studies that approached this as a localization problem (i.e., via bounding-box type annotations) dominated the determination of anomalous sites on CXR rather than the accurate delineation of abnormalities by segmentation.

The research by Larrazabal et al. [72] integrated noise removal autoencoders, which were taught to generate anatomically realistic segmentations from the original predictions.

10.3 OVERVIEW OF MACHINE LEARNING FOR MEDICAL CARDIOLOGY

Cardiologists make patient-care choices based on data loads. They typically have greater exposure to quantitative data about patients than other specialties. Regardless of some possible drawbacks, it is critical that machine learning approaches be used to make data-driven decisions. The road to machine learning-based clinical decision support tools is still lengthy, with numerous obstacles ahead. With the advent of fuzzy logic in signal interpretation, intriguing prospects emerge in this approach, enabling an uncertainty-aware mapping of linguistic concepts to numeric intervals. Table 10.4 shows the cardiology deep learning solution.

Koulaouzidis et al. [75] based their work on machine learning in cardiac/coronary computer tomography (CCT). The coronary artery calcium (CAC) score is a relatively recent approach for detecting and stratifying coronary atherosclerosis. Coronary calcium in chest CT images is frequently not recorded or measurable. Eng et al. [76] invented a new algorithm to automate this score on non-gated chest CT. The model gained sensitivity and positive predictive scores for predicting the CAC score; about 94% for sensitivity and close to 100% for CAC. This was in strong

TABLE 10.4
Summary of the work in medical cardiology

Reference	Method	Dataset
Eng et al. [76]	Coronary artery calcium scoring system from CT scan.	Private
Pickhardt et al. [77]	DI model capable of predicting congenital heart disease from CT scan and echocardiogram.	Private
Zeleznik et al. [78]	Machine learning models for cardiovascular disease screening utilizing imaging biomarkers.	Private
Kim et al. [80]	On a chest radiograph, a deep learning system separates the heart area from the lungs.	—
Arnaout et al. [81]	Distinguishes between a healthy heart and a heart with congenital problems with excellent accuracy and may enable automated screening of congenital heart disorders.	107,823 fetal ultrasound images

accord with physicians' visual ratings. The work of Pickhardt et al. [77] proposed a deep learning model that predicts future cardiovascular events with good accuracy, based on numerous biometrics acquired from 9,223 CT images of patients. Similarly, work by Zeleznik et al. [78] confirmed that using such algorithms in clinical practice may allow for opportunistic screening of cardiovascular disease using imaging biomarkers. Because chest radiographs are widely used as an early diagnostic tool for a wide range of cardiovascular diseases, they provide a suitable modality to investigate with deep learning. Using chest radiographs, an algorithm identified the maker of a cardiac rhythm device with 99.6% accuracy [79]. Deep learning techniques were also used to diagnose valvular heart disease. The work of Kim et al. [80] explored a deep learning method that separates the heart area from the lungs on a chest radiograph. This area is then utilized to define the cardiovascular boundaries and detect the carina in order to test for valvular heart disease symptoms.

Deep learning algorithms can improve access to healthcare. However, they have the potential to exacerbate preexisting inequities. The data about which AI algorithms are trained, as well as the labels associated with them, are extremely important. Hence, biases against underrepresented groups in training data may persist [82]. Biases can be decreased by increasing the amount of data available for training and hence the number of data collection facilities. A mixed methodology will be used to choose algorithms and training data, allowing diverse professionals to contribute input to eliminate biases in the technology's design [83].

10.4   CONCLUSION

The promise of machine learning and deep learning models to transform how we live and operate in medicine. It is expected that the area will evolve fast in the coming decades, but various hurdles must be overcome before AI can be widely adopted in healthcare facilities. Many strategies have been detailed in an attempt to decipher the deep learning systems' "black box" aspect, but further work is needed. Also, it is very beneficial to build more accurate algorithms to stratify patients into distinct risk groups and treatment arms in order to give personalized medication to the global population.

This chapter also identified important hurdles and constraints to expanding the practical implementation of AI-powered solutions across a larger range of medical applications. Data was revealed to be the primary building component in the construction of various solutions. There is a lot of evidence in the literature that good performance can always be achieved with good data.

REFERENCES

1. Elyan E, Jamieson L, Ali-Gombe A. 2020. Deep Learning for Symbols Detection and Classification in Engineering Drawings. *Neural Networks*. 129:91–102. doi:10.1016/j. neunet.2020.05.025
2. Moreno-García CF, Elyan E, Jayne C. 2019. New Trends on Digitisation of Complex Engineering Drawings. *Neural Computing & Applications* 31(6):1695–1712. doi:10.1007/s00521-018-3583-1

3. Moreno-García CF, Elyan E, Jayne C. 2017. Heuristics-Based Detection to Improve Text/Graphics Segmentation in Complex Engineering Drawings. In: Boracchi G, Iliadis L, Jayne C, Likas A, editors. *Engineering Applications of Neural Networks* [Internet]. Vol. 744. Cham: Springer International Publishing; [accessed 2022 Oct 5]; p. 87–98.

4. Ali-Gombe A, Elyan E, Jayne C. 2017. Fish Classification in Context of Noisy Images. In: Boracchi G, Iliadis L, Jayne C, Likas A, editors. *Engineering Applications of Neural Networks* [Internet]. Vol. 744. Cham: Springer International Publishing; [accessed 2022 Oct 5]; p. 216–226.

5. Schwab E, Gooßen A, Deshpande H, Saalbach A. 2020. Localization of Critical Findings in Chest X-Ray without Local Annotations Using Multi-Instance Learning [Internet]. [accessed 2022 Oct 5]. http://arxiv.org/abs/2001.08817

6. Pomponiu V, Nejati H, Cheung N-M. 2016. Deepmole: Deep neural networks for skin mole lesion classification. In: *IEEE International Conference on Image Processing (ICIP)* [Internet]. Phoenix, AZ: IEEE; [accessed 2022 Oct 5]; p. 2623–2627.

7. Esteva A, Kuprel B, Novoa RA, Ko J, Swetter SM, Blau HM, Thrun S. 2017. Dermatologist-Level Classification of Skin Cancer with Deep Neural Networks. *Nature*. 542(7639):115–118. doi:10.1038/nature21056

8. Levine AB, Schlosser C, Grewal J, Coope R, Jones SJM, Yip S. 2019. Rise of the Machines: Advances in Deep Learning for Cancer Diagnosis. *Trends in Cancer*. 5(3):157–169. doi:10.1016/j.trecan.2019.02.002

9. Schlemper J, Oktay O, Schaap M, Heinrich M, Kainz B, Glocker B, Rueckert D. 2019. Attention Gated Networks: Learning to Leverage Salient Regions in Medical Images. *Medical Image Analysis*. 53:197–207. doi:10.1016/j.media.2019.01.012

10. Vyborny CJ. 1994. Can Computers Help Radiologists Read Mammograms? *Radiology*. 191(2):315–317. doi:10.1148/radiology.191.2.8153298

11. Gumbs AA, Frigerio I, Spolverato G, Croner R, Illanes A, Chouillard E, Elyan E. 2021. Artificial Intelligence Surgery: How Do We Get to Autonomous Actions in Surgery? *Sensors*. 21(16):5526. doi:10.3390/s21165526

12. Gonzalez RC, Woods RE, Masters BR. 2009. Digital Image Processing, Third Edition. *Journal of Biomedical Optics*. 14(2):029901. doi:10.1117/1.3115362

13. Szegedy C, Wei Liu, Yangqing Jia, Sermanet P, Reed S, Anguelov D, Erhan D, Vanhoucke V, Rabinovich A. 2015. Going Deeper with Convolutions. In: *IEEE Conference on Computer Vision and Pattern Recognition (CVPR)* [Internet]. Boston, MA: IEEE; [accessed 2022 Oct 5]; p. 1–9.

14. Krizhevsky A, Sutskever I, Hinton GE. 2017. ImageNet classification with deep convolutional neural networks. *Communications of ACM*. 60(6):84–90. doi:10.1145/3065386

15. Bishop CM. 2016. *Pattern Recognition and Machine Learning*. 1st edition 2006 (corrected at 8th printing 2009). New York: Springer.

16. Lowe DG. 2004. Distinctive Image Features from Scale-Invariant Keypoints. *International Journal of Computer Vision*. 60(2):91–110. doi:10.1023/B:VISI.0000029664.99615.94

17. Bay H, Tuytelaars T, Van Gool L. 2006. SURF: Speeded Up Robust Features. In: Leonardis A, Bischof H, Pinz A, editors. *Computer Vision – ECCV 2006* [Internet]. Vol. 3951. Berlin, Heidelberg: Springer; [accessed 2022 Oct 5]; pp. 404–417.

18. Hearst MA, Dumais ST, Osuna E, Platt J, Scholkopf B. 1998. Support vector machines. *IEEE Intelligent Systems and Their Applications*. 13(4):18–28. doi:10.1109/5254.708428

19. Breiman L. 2001. [No title found]. *Machine Learning*. 45(1):5–32. doi:10.1023/A:1010933404324

20. Amato F, López A, Peña-Méndez EM, Vaňhara P, Hampl A, Havel J. 2013. Artificial Neural Networks in Medical Diagnosis. *Journal of Applied Biomedicine*. 11(2):47–58. doi:10.2478/v10136-012-0031-x

21. Sakli N, Ghabri H, Soufiene BO, Almalki FarisA, Sakli H, Ali O, Najjari M. 2022. *Res*Net-50 for 12-Lead Electrocardiogram Automated Diagnosis. In Maleh Y, editor. *Computational Intelligence and Neuroscience.* 2022:1–16. doi:10.1155/2022/7617551

22. Souid A, Sakli N, Sakli H. 2021. Classification and Predictions of Lung Diseases from Chest X-rays Using MobileNet V2. *Applied Sciences.* 11(6):2751. doi:10.3390/app11062751

23. Yang D, Martinez C, Visuña L, Khandhar H, Bhatt C, Carretero J. 2021. Detection and Analysis of COVID-19 in Medical Images Using Deep Learning Techniques. *Scientific Reports.* 11(1):19638. doi:10.1038/s41598-021-99015-3

24. Li C, Chen H, Li X, Xu N, Hu Z, Xue D, Qi S, Ma H, Zhang L, Sun H. 2020. A Review for Cervical Histopathology Image Analysis Using Machine Vision Approaches. *Artificial Intelligence Review.* 53(7):4821–4862. doi:10.1007/s10462-020-09808-7

25. Yu C, Helwig EJ. 2022. The Role of AI Technology in Prediction, Diagnosis and Treatment of Colorectal Cancer. *Artificial Intelligence Review.* 55(1):323–343. doi:10.1007/s10462-021-10034-y

26. Ting DSW, Cheung CY-L, Lim G, Tan GSW, Quang ND, Gan A, Hamzah H, Garcia-Franco R, San Yeo IY, Lee SY, et al. 2017. Development and Validation of a Deep Learning System for Diabetic Retinopathy and Related Eye Diseases Using Retinal Images From Multiethnic Populations With Diabetes. *JAMA.* 318(22):2211. doi:10.1001/jama.2017.18152

27. Gulshan V, Peng L, Coram M, Stumpe MC, Wu D, Narayanaswamy A, Venugopalan S, Widner K, Madams T, Cuadros J, et al. 2016. Development and Validation of a Deep Learning Algorithm for Detection of Diabetic Retinopathy in Retinal Fundus Photographs. *JAMA.* 316(22):2402. doi:10.1001/jama.2016.17216

28. Abràmoff MD, Lou Y, Erginay A, Clarida W, Amelon R, Folk JC, Niemeijer M. 2016. Improved Automated Detection of Diabetic Retinopathy on a Publicly Available Dataset Through Integration of Deep Learning. *Investigative Ophthalmology & Visual Science.* 57(13):5200. doi:10.1167/iovs.16-19964

29. Gargeya R, Leng T. 2017. Automated Identification of Diabetic Retinopathy Using Deep Learning. *Ophthalmology.* 124(7):962–969. doi:10.1016/j.ophtha.2017.02.008

30. Li Z, He Y, Keel S, Meng W, Chang RT, He M. 2018. Efficacy of a Deep Learning System for Detecting Glaucomatous Optic Neuropathy Based on Color Fundus Photographs. *Ophthalmology.* 125(8):1199–1206. doi:10.1016/j.ophtha.2018.01.023

31. Burlina PM, Joshi N, Pekala M, Pacheco KD, Freund DE, Bressler NM. 2017. Automated Grading of Age-Related Macular Degeneration From Color Fundus Images Using Deep Convolutional Neural Networks. *JAMA Ophthalmol.* 135(11):1170. doi:10.1001/jamaophthalmol.2017.3782

32. Grassmann F, Mengelkamp J, Brandl C, Harsch S, Zimmermann ME, Linkohr B, Peters A, Heid IM, Palm C, Weber BHF. 2018. A Deep Learning Algorithm for Prediction of Age-Related Eye Disease Study Severity Scale for Age-Related Macular Degeneration from Color Fundus Photography. *Ophthalmology.* 125(9):1410–1420. doi:10.1016/j.ophtha.2018.02.037

33. Brown JM, Campbell JP, Beers A, Chang K, Ostmo S, Chan RVP, Dy J, Erdogmus D, Ioannidis S, Kalpathy-Cramer J, et al. 2018. Automated Diagnosis of Plus Disease in Retinopathy of Prematurity Using Deep Convolutional Neural Networks. *JAMA Ophthalmol.* 136(7):803. doi:10.1001/jamaophthalmol.2018.1934

34. Varadarajan AV, Poplin R, Blumer K, Angermueller C, Ledsam J, Chopra R, Keane PA, Corrado GS, Peng L, Webster DR. 2018. Deep Learning for Predicting Refractive Error From Retinal Fundus Images. *Investigative Ophthalmology & Visual Science.* 59(7):2861. doi:10.1167/iovs.18-23887

35. Poplin R, Varadarajan AV, Blumer K, Liu Y, McConnell MV, Corrado GS, Peng L, Webster DR. 2018. Prediction of Cardiovascular Risk Factors from Retinal Fundus Photographs via Deep Learning. *Nature Biomedical Engineering.* 2(3):158–164. doi:10.1038/s41551-018-0195-0

36. Lee CS, Tyring AJ, Deruyter NP, Wu Y, Rokem A, Lee AY. 2017. Deep-Learning based, Automated Segmentation of Macular Edema in Optical Coherence Tomography. *Biomedical Optics Express.* 8(7):3440. doi:10.1364/BOE.8.003440

37. Kermany D. 2018. Labeled Optical Coherence Tomography (OCT) and Chest X-Ray Images for Classification [Internet]. [accessed 2022 Mar 30]. doi:10.17632/RSCBJBR9SJ.2

38. De Fauw J, Ledsam JR, Romera-Paredes B, Nikolov S, Tomasev N, Blackwell S, Askham H, Glorot X, O'Donoghue B, Visentin D, et al. 2018. Clinically Applicable Deep Learning for Diagnosis and Referral in Retinal Disease. *Nature Medicine.* 24(9):1342–1350. doi:10.1038/s41591-018-0107-6

39. Sogancioglu E, Çallı E, van Ginneken B, van Leeuwen KG, Murphy K. 2021. Deep Learning for Chest X-ray Analysis: A Survey. *Medical Image Analysis.* 72:102125. doi:10.1016/j.media.2021.102125

40. Wang X, Peng Y, Lu L, Lu Z, Bagheri M, Summers RM. 2017. ChestX-ray8: Hospital-scale Chest X-ray Database and Benchmarks on Weakly-Supervised Classification and Localization of Common Thorax Diseases [Internet]. [accessed 2022 Mar 30]. doi:10.1109/CVPR.2017.369

41. Irvin J, Rajpurkar P, Ko M, Yu Y, Ciurea-Ilcus S, Chute C, Marklund H, Haghgoo B, Ball R, Shpanskaya K, et al. 2019. CheXpert: A Large Chest Radiograph Dataset with Uncertainty Labels and Expert Comparison. *AAAI.* 33:590–597. doi:10.1609/aaai.v33i01.3301590

42. Bustos A, Pertusa A, Salinas J-M, de la Iglesia-Vayá M. 2020. PadChest: A Large Chest x-ray Image Dataset with Multi-Label Annotated Reports. *Medical Image Analysis.* 66:101797. doi:10.1016/j.media.2020.101797

43. Zhu CS, Pinsky PF, Kramer BS, Prorok PC, Purdue MP, Berg CD, Gohagan JK. 2013. The Prostate, Lung, Colorectal, and Ovarian Cancer Screening Trial and Its Associated Research Resource. *JNCI Journal of the National Cancer Institute.* 105(22):1684–1693. doi:10.1093/jnci/djt281

44. Demner-Fushman D, Antani S, Simpson M, Thoma GR. 2012. Design and Development of a Multimodal Biomedical Information Retrieval System. *Journal of Computing Science and Engineering.* 6(2):168–177. doi:10.5626/JCSE.2012.6.2.168

45. Nguyen, Ha Quy, Pham, Hieu Huy, Tuan Linh, Le, Dao, Minh, Khanh, Lam. VinDr-CXR: An Open Dataset of Chest X-rays with Radiologist Annotations [Internet]. [accessed 2022 Apr 19].

46. Majkowska A, Mittal S, Steiner DF, Reicher JJ, McKinney SM, Duggan GE, Eswaran K, Cameron Chen P-H, Liu Y, Kalidindi SR, et al. 2020. Chest Radiograph Interpretation with Deep Learning Models: Assessment with Radiologist-adjudicated Reference Standards and Population-adjusted Evaluation. *Radiology.* 294(2):421–431. doi:10.1148/radiol.2019191293

47. SIIM ACR Pneumothorax Segmentation Data. [accessed 2022 Oct 5]. https://www.kaggle.com/datasets/jesperdramsch/siim-acr-pneumothorax-segmentation-data

48. Cohen JP, Morrison P, Dao L. 2020. COVID-19 Image Data Collection. arXiv:200311597 [cs, eess, q-bio] [Internet]. [accessed 2022 Apr 12]. http://arxiv.org/abs/2003.11597

49. Armato SG, McLennan G, Bidaut L, McNitt-Gray MF, Meyer CR, Reeves AP, Zhao B, Aberle DR, Henschke CI, Hoffman EA, et al. 2011. The Lung Image Database Consortium (LIDC) and Image Database Resource Initiative (IDRI): A Completed Reference Database of Lung Nodules on CT Scans. The LIDC/IDRI Thoracic CT Database of Lung Nodules. *Medical Physics.* 38(2):915–931. doi:10.1118/1.3528204

50. Grove O, Berglund AE, Schabath MB, Aerts HJWL, Dekker A, Wang H, Velazquez ER, Lambin P, Gu Y, Balagurunathan Y, et al. 2015. Quantitative Computed Tomographic Descriptors Associate Tumor Shape Complexity and Intratumor Heterogeneity with Prognosis in Lung Adenocarcinoma [Internet]. [accessed 2022 Oct 5]. doi:10.7937/K9/TCIA.2015.A6V7JIWX

51. Souid A, Sakli N, Sakli H. 2022. Toward an Efficient Deep Learning Model for Lung Pathologies Detection in X-ray Images. In: *International Wireless Communications and Mobile Computing (IWCMC)* [Internet]. Dubrovnik, Croatia: IEEE; [accessed 2022 Oct 5]; pp. 1028–1033.

52. Tang Y-X, Tang Y-B, Peng Y, Yan K, Bagheri M, Redd BA, Brandon CJ, Lu Z, Han M, Xiao J, Summers RM. 2020. Automated Abnormality Classification of Chest Radiographs Using Deep Convolutional Neural Networks. *NPJ Digital Medicine.* 3(1):70. doi:10.1038/s41746-020-0273-z

53. Chouhan V, Singh SK, Khamparia A, Gupta D, Tiwari P, Moreira C, Damaševičius R, de Albuquerque VHC. 2020. A Novel Transfer Learning Based Approach for Pneumonia Detection in Chest X-ray Images. *Applied Sciences.* 10(2):559. doi:10.3390/app10020559

54. Chhikara P, Singh P, Gupta P, Bhatia T. 2020. Deep Convolutional Neural Network with Transfer Learning for Detecting Pneumonia on Chest X-Rays. In: Jain LC, Virvou M, Piuri V, Balas VE, editors. *Advances in Bioinformatics, Multimedia, and Electronics Circuits and Signals* [Internet]. Vol. 1064. Singapore: Springer; [accessed 2022 Apr 12]; pp. 155–168.

55. Chen X, Chen Y, Liu H, Goldmacher G, Roberts CS, Maria DK, Ou W. 2019. PIN92 Pediatric Bacterial Pneumonia Classification Through Chest X-rays Using Transfer Learning. *Value in Health.* 22:S209–S210. doi:10.1016/j.jval.2019.04.962

56. Wu H, Xie P, Zhang H, Li D, Cheng M. 2020. Predict Pneumonia with Chest X-ray Images based on Convolutional Deep Neural Learning Networks. *IFS.* 39(3):2893–2907. doi:10.3233/JIFS-191438

57. RSNA Pneumonia Detection Challenge. [accessed 2022 Apr 12]. https://kaggle.com/competitions/rsna-pneumonia-detection-challenge

58. Two Public Chest X-ray Datasets for Computer-Aided Screening of Pulmonary Diseases - PMC. [accessed 2022 Apr 12]. https://www.ncbi.nlm.nih.gov/pmc/articles/PMC4256233/

59. Melendez J, van Ginneken B, Maduskar P, Philipsen RHHM, Reither K, Breuninger M, Adetifa IMO, Maane R, Ayles H, Sanchez CI. 2015. A Novel Multiple-Instance Learning-Based Approach to Computer-Aided Detection of Tuberculosis on Chest X-Rays. *IEEE Trans Med Imaging.* 34(1):179–192. doi:10.1109/TMI.2014.2350539

60. Chadaga K, Chakraborty C, Prabhu S, Umakanth S, Bhat V, Sampathila N. 2022. Clinical and Laboratory Approach to Diagnose COVID-19 Using Machine Learning. *Interdisciplinary Sciences: Computational Life Sciences* [Internet]. [accessed 2022 Apr 12]. doi:10.1007/s12539-021-00499-4

61. Stephen O, Sain M, Maduh UJ, Jeong D-U. 2019. An Efficient Deep Learning Approach to Pneumonia Classification in Healthcare. *Journal of Healthcare Engineering.* 2019:1–7. doi:10.1155/2019/4180949

62. Mittal A, Kumar D, Mittal M, Saba T, Abunadi I, Rehman A, Roy S. 2020. Detecting Pneumonia Using Convolutions and Dynamic Capsule Routing for Chest X-ray Images. *Sesors.* 20(4):1068. doi:10.3390/s20041068

63. Wang W, Feng H, Bu Q, Cui L, Xie Y, Zhang A, Feng J, Zhu Z, Chen Z. 2020. MDU-Net: A Convolutional Network for Clavicle and Rib Segmentation from a Chest Radiograph. *Journal of Healthcare Engineering.* 2020:1–9. doi:10.1155/2020/2785464

64. Rajaraman S, Thoma G, Antani S., Candemir S. 2019. Visualizing and Explaining Deep Learning Predictions for Pneumonia Detection in Pediatric Chest Radiographs. In: Hahn HK, Mori K, editors. *Medical Imaging 2019: Computer-Aided Diagnosis* [Internet]. San Diego, United States: SPIE; [accessed 2022 Oct 5]; p. 27.

65. Heo S-J, Kim Y, Yun S, Lim S-S, Kim J, Nam C-M, Park E-C, Jung I, Yoon J-H. 2019. Deep Learning Algorithms with Demographic Information Help to Detect Tuberculosis in Chest Radiographs in Annual Workers' Health Examination Data. *IJERPH*. 16(2):250. doi:10.3390/ijerph16020250

66. Sogancioglu E, Murphy K, Calli E, Scholten ET, Schalekamp S, Van Ginneken B. 2020. Cardiomegaly Detection on Chest Radiographs: Segmentation Versus Classification. *IEEE Access*. 8:94631–94642. doi:10.1109/ACCESS.2020.2995567

67. Li B, Kang G, Cheng K, Zhang N. 2019. Attention-Guided Convolutional Neural Network for Detecting Pneumonia on Chest X-Rays. In: *41st Annual International Conference of the IEEE Engineering in Medicine and Biology Society (EMBC)* [Internet]. Berlin, Germany: IEEE; [accessed 2022 Oct 5]; pp. 4851–4854.

68. Hurt B, Yen A, Kligerman S, Hsiao A. 2020. Augmenting Interpretation of Chest Radiographs With Deep Learning Probability Maps. *Journal of Thoracic Imaging*. 35(5):285–293. doi:10.1097/RTI.0000000000000505

69. Souid A, Sakli H. 2022. Xception-ResNet Autoencoder for Pneumothorax Segmentation. In: *IEEE 9th International Conference on Sciences of Electronics, Technologies of Information and Telecommunications (SETIT)* [Internet]. Hammamet, Tunisia: IEEE; [accessed 2022 Sep 21]; pp. 586–590.

70. Cardona Cardenas DA, Ferreira JR, Moreno RA, Rebelo MFS, Krieger JE, Gutierrez MA. 2021. Automated Radiographic Bone Suppression with Deep Convolutional Neural Networks. In: Gimi BS, Krol A, editors. *Medical Imaging 2021: Biomedical Applications in Molecular, Structural, and Functional Imaging* [Internet]. Online Only. USA: SPIE; [accessed 2022 Oct 5]; p. 46. doi:10.1117/12.2582210

71. Mortani Barbosa EJ, Gefter WB, Ghesu FC, Liu S, Mailhe B, Mansoor A, Grbic S, Vogt S. 2021. Automated Detection and Quantification of COVID-19 Airspace Disease on Chest Radiographs: A Novel Approach Achieving Expert Radiologist-Level Performance Using a Deep Convolutional Neural Network Trained on Digital Reconstructed Radiographs From Computed Tomography-Derived Ground Truth. *Investigative Radiology*. 56(8):471–479. doi:10.1097/RLI.0000000000000763

72. Larrazabal AJ, Martinez C, Glocker B, Ferrante E. 2020. Post-DAE: Anatomically Plausible Segmentation via Post-Processing With Denoising Autoencoders. *IEEE Transactions on Medical Imaging*. 39(12):3813–3820. doi:10.1109/TMI.2020.3005297

73. Xue C, Deng Q, Li X, Dou Q, Heng P-A. 2020. Cascaded Robust Learning at Imperfect Labels for Chest X-ray Segmentation. In: Martel AL, Abolmaesumi P, Stoyanov D, Mateus D, Zuluaga MA, Zhou SK, Racoceanu D, Joskowicz L, editors. *Medical Image Computing and Computer Assisted Intervention – MICCAI 2020* [Internet]. Vol. 12266. Cham: Springer International Publishing; [accessed 2022 Oct 5]; p. 579–588. doi:10.1007/978-3-030-59725-2_56

74. Gu Y, Lu X, Zhang B, Zhao Y, Yu D, Gao L, Cui G, Wu L, Zhou T. 2019. Automatic Lung Nodule Detection Using Multi-Scale Dot Nodule-Enhancement Filter and Weighted Support Vector Machines in Chest Computed Tomography. Wang Y, editor. *PLoS ONE*. 14(1):e0210551. doi:10.1371/journal.pone.0210551

75. Koulaouzidis G, Jadczyk T, Iakovidis DK, Koulaouzidis A, Bisnaire M, Charisopoulou D. 2022. Artificial Intelligence in Cardiology—A Narrative Review of Current Status. *JCM*. 11(13):3910. doi:10.3390/jcm11133910

76. Eng D, Chute C, Khandwala N, Rajpurkar P, Long J, Shleifer S, Khalaf MH, Sandhu AT, Rodriguez F, Maron DJ, et al. 2021. Automated Coronary Calcium Scoring Using Deep Learning with Multicenter External Validation. *NPJ Digital Medicine*. 4(1):88. doi:10.1038/s41746-021-00460-1

77. Pickhardt PJ, Graffy PM, Zea R, Lee SJ, Liu J, Sandfort V, Summers RM. 2020. Automated CT Biomarkers for Opportunistic Prediction of Future Cardiovascular Events and Mortality in an Asymptomatic Screening Population: A Retrospective Cohort Study. *The Lancet Digital Health.* 2(4):e192–e200. doi:10.1016/S2589-7500(20)30025-X

78. Zeleznik R, Foldyna B, Eslami P, Weiss J, Alexander I, Taron J, Parmar C, Alvi RM, Banerji D, Uno M, et al. 2021. Deep Convolutional Neural Networks to Predict Cardiovascular Risk from Computed Tomography. *Nature Communications.* 12(1):715. doi:10.1038/s41467-021-20966-2

79. Howard JP, Fisher L, Shun-Shin MJ, Keene D, Arnold AD, Ahmad Y, Cook CM, Moon JC, Manisty CH, Whinnett ZI, et al. 2019. Cardiac Rhythm Device Identification Using Neural Networks. *JACC: Clinical Electrophysiology.* 5(5):576–586. doi:10.1016/j.jacep.2019.02.003

80. Kim C, Lee G, Oh H, Jeong G, Kim SW, Chun EJ, Kim Y-H, Lee J-G, Yang DH. 2022. A Deep Learning–based Automatic Analysis of Cardiovascular Borders on Chest Radiographs of Valvular Heart Disease: Development/External Validation. *European Radiology.* 32(3):1558–1569. doi:10.1007/s00330-021-08296-9

81. Chakraborty C, Othman SB., Almalki FA, et al. 2023. FC-SEEDA: Fog Computing-based Secure and Energy Efficient Data Aggregation Scheme for Internet of Healthcare Things. *Neural Computing & Applications* doi: 10.1007/s00521-023-08270-0

82. Ben Othman S, Bahattab AA, Trad A and Youssef H. 2020. PEERP: A Priority-Based Energy-Efficient Routing Protocol for Reliable Data Transmission in Healthcare using the IoT. In *The 15th International Conference on Future Networks and Communications (FNC)*, Leuven, Belgium.

83. Ben Othman S, Almalki FA, Chakraborty C, Sakli H. 2022. Privacy-Preserving Aware Data Aggregation for IoT-based Healthcare with Green Computing Technologies, *Computers and Electrical Engineering*, 101, 108025. doi: 10.1016/j.compeleceng.2022.108025.

11 Deep Learning Methods for Brain Tumor Segmentation

Marwen Sakli, Chaker Essid, Bassem Ben Salah, and Hedi Sakli

11.1 INTRODUCTION

A brain tumor is a cellular growth in the brain that can be benign (noncancerous) or malignant (cancerous) in nature. It may originate in the brain, or it may have invaded the brain after growing in another part of the body (metastasis). The two main types of brain tumors are primary and secondary. The first type originates from intracranial cells or cells in structures adjacent to the brain. They can be benign or malignant. Whereas the second one is metastases. That is, they have developed in another part of the body and have spread to the brain. Thus, they are always malignant.

The most common primary tumors are gliomas (including astrocytomas, oligodendrogliomas, and glioblastomas), ependymomas, medulloblastomas, meningiomas, and acoustic neuromas. For example, gliomas represent 65% of all primary brain tumors. Brain metastases are much more common than primary tumors. Over 80% of people with brain metastases have more than one metastasis. Metastases from other parts of the body can spread to a single area of the brain or different parts of the brain. Many types of cancer can spread to the brain, such as breast cancer, lung, kidney, melanoma, thyroid, lymphoma, and leukemia. Brain lymphomas are increasingly frequent in people with weakened immune systems (such as AIDS patients), in the elderly, and, for unknown reasons, in people with normal immune systems.

The diagnosis of a brain tumor is first made by a clinical examination that identifies neurological symptoms that may indicate the presence of a brain tumor. When there is a suspicion of a tumor, brain magnetic resonance imaging (MRI) is essential to visualize the affected brain region and the size of the lesion. Thus, for the investigation, monitoring, and planning of brain tumor surgery, MRI is a crucial diagnostic tool.

To highlight various tissue features and regions of tumor dissemination, many complementary 3D MRI modalities are often obtained, including native T1, T1 with contrast agent (T1c), T2, and fluid-attenuated inversion recovery (FLAIR). T1 is effective in separating tumor cells from normal brain tissue. The tumor borders are

DOI: 10.1201/9781003366249-11

easier to see on T1ce. The fluid (edema) around the brain tumor may be seen in T2. Additionally, FLAIR may be used to distinguish an edema zone from cerebrospinal fluid [1]. Sagittal, axial, and coronal views of the MRI scans allow medical professionals to examine malignancies in three dimensions [2].

Due to the high complexity of the structure and appearance of the tumors, their borders are frequently hazy, and the tumors may spread into the nearby region of the brain. It is challenging to distinguish the affected tissue from the other healthy tissue in the surrounding area when segmenting brain tumors accurately from MRI images. As a result, manually delineating the border lines in the MRI scans takes time and is prone to inaccuracy. These issues would be resolved by automatic brain tumor segmentation utilizing MRI scans, which would enable a quick and accurate diagnosis by identifying the characteristics and precise location of the tumors. The patient may be cured if the treatment process started earlier.

Recently, researchers have tried to use deep learning (DL)-based algorithms [3] to segment and identify various tumors in medical scans, spurred on by the results reached. DL helps to exploit data more efficiently; its algorithms have developed rapidly worldwide [4]. It has been found that the use of a convolutional neural network (CNN) is capable of extracting relevant features from MRI images with the same level of performance as professionals. Especially, the U-Net architecture [5] is now having tremendous success, since the majority of winning contributions to recent medical picture segmentation competitions were entirely built around U-Net. It can capture fine and large segments of data from the encoder to the decoder via skip connections. Moreover, the totality of the extracted features is passed to the associated block of the upsampling convolution in the decoder thanks to these skip connections.

This work aims to automate MRI brain tumor segmentation. This task is based on the application of U-Net, which is one of the most common and efficient models employed in the field of medical imaging. The used dataset is BraTS 2020 challenge, which has 369 brain tumor MRI images with four modalities provided.

The rest of this investigation is structured as follows. Section 11.2 reviews similar papers found in the state of the art, whereas Section 11.3 details the proposed model for automated brain tumor MRI segmentation and simulation approaches. Section 11.4 contains a discussion and assessment of the proposed MRI segmentation model's findings. Lastly, Section 11.5 is a discussion of the conclusion and future initiatives.

11.2   RELATED WORKS

Traditional techniques and DL techniques are the two major types of developed models for automated brain tumor MRI segmentation. Traditional techniques rely on machine learning (ML) algorithms.

ML groups frequently face challenges in obtaining large-scale annotated medical imaging datasets for training and testing their algorithms. Consequently, some studies have relied on shorter proprietary datasets, making it difficult to show the full potential of their algorithms and even harder to compare their results to other published methods.

Medical image analysis challenges, by making large-scale, carefully labeled, multi-institution, real-world datasets publicly available for training, testing, and evaluating ML algorithms, play a critical role in developing ML applications for medical image analysis [6]. For over 10 years, the BraTS challenge has provided the community with a benchmarking platform to evaluate segmentation approaches, with the dataset size growing annually [6–10]. The dataset's availability, as well as the problem itself, have facilitated the building of numerous new efficient deep learning-based systems, such as DeepMedic [11] and nnU-Net [12].

Table 11.1 presents the BraTS challenges datasets' characteristics from 2012 to 2019 [6, 13].

Researchers also employed datasets provided by the Ischemic Stroke Lesion Segmentation (ISLES) challenges. The first one is ISLES 2015, which included 64 patients suffering from subacute stroke lesion segmentation (SISS). Sixty-six percent of its data is employed for training and the rest is reserved for testing the models [14]. The number of patients in ISLES 2017 increased to 75. The training dataset includes 43 subjects. The developed methods will be assessed using a testing set of 32 stroke subjects [15].

For brain tumor segmentation, various datasets were used. Figshare is a public Chinese contrast-enhanced MRI dataset from Tianjin Medical University and Nanfang Hospital. It includes 3,064 T1ce 512 × 512 pixels images from 233 patients. Three classes of brain tumors were found with the following distribution: 1,426 glioma, 708 meningioma, and 930 pituitary images [16].

The TCGA-GBM refers to the cancer genome atlas glioblastoma multiforme, which is another dataset that contains more than 500 various brain cancer samples. This dataset is available to researchers for academic purposes. It doesn't need ethical review because it examines a part of the body that doesn't require one. The most accurate images for brain tumor diagnosis were found when using T1-weighted post-contrast (T1-Gd) MRI sequences [17].

However, certain datasets are not available to the public. They are usually accessible on special request to specific researchers who created them to investigate the effectiveness of their method. For example, requesting access to the Combined Dataset requires agreeing to a licensing agreement. It contains over 15,300 MRI images collected from various sources [18]. Additionally, the BRAINIX dataset needs a special request when using the data [19].

Generally, all the images present in the datasets will be the subject of many segmentation techniques. The development of medicine has led to increased interest in image processing. Currently, new methods are being developed at an accelerated rate due to this growing field of study. Segmentation, or the creation of distinct areas in images, is one of many image-processing tasks performed by computers. This is accomplished by scanning an image and splitting it into segments that have similar pixel characteristics [20]. Image segmentation involves modifying how the image is displayed in a way that makes it easier to understand. It uses different techniques based on the features that help it segment images [7, 21]. The most common image segmentation methods are edge, threshold, region, and fuzzy theory-based segmentation.

TABLE 11.1

BraTS challenges datasets' characteristics from 2012 to 2019

BraTS Challenge	Total MRI images	Training set	Validation set	Test set	Tasks	Type of images
2012	50	35	—	15	Segmentation	Preoperative only
2013	60	35	—	25	Segmentation	Preoperative only
2014	238	200	—	38	Segmentation Disease progression	Longitudinal
2015	253	200	—	53	Segmentation Disease progression	Longitudinal
2016	391	200	—	191	Segmentation Disease progression	Longitudinal
2017	477	285	46	146	Segmentation Survival prediction	Preoperative only
2018	542	285	66	191	Segmentation Survival prediction	Preoperative only
2019	712	335	125	252	Segmentation Survival prediction	Preoperative only

Brain MRI image segmentation technics based on DL can be grouped into three major divisions: CNNs, fully convolutional networks (FCNs), and encoders and decoders (EAD).

The CNN belongs to the category of neural networks, and its weight distribution mechanism significantly reduces the complexity of the model. The CNN can directly use the image as input, automatically extract features, and have a high degree of invariance to changes such as image translation and scaling. In recent years, some network models based on CNNs [22], such as Network in Network [23], VGG [24], GoogLeNet [25], and ResNet [26], have been widely used in medical image segmentation. Among them, the VGG network has a strong feature extraction ability, which can ensure convergence with fewer training times. Although, because of the exploding and disappearing gradients due to the deepening of the network, when the depth of the network surpasses a particular threshold, the efficiency decrease. To address the problem of network degradation, He et al. [26] built a deep residual network (ResNet) that reached good performance on the segmentation challenge. Other teams of researchers [27, 28] grouped 3D convolutional densely connected neural networks to pretrain the model and then initialize it with the resulting weights. This method improves dice similarity coefficient (DSC) measurements in brain tumor MRI segmentation tasks. Havaei et al. [29] developed a cascaded two-path CNN that uses the feature output map of the first-stage CNN as additional input to the second-stage CNN. This method can effectively obtain rich background information and obtain better segmentation results. Lai et al. [30] first decreased the tail of the original image by 98%, modified the bias field using n4itk, then employed multiclass presegmentation through CNN, and finally got the last segmentation result using median filtering. This method vastly increases the segmentation DSC and PPV (positive predictive value). Salehi et al. [31] suggested employing 2D convolution to learn 3D visual information using a convolutional neural network technique based on autonomous context (Auto-Nets). To avoid complicated 3D convolution operations in segmentation, this approach leverages 2D convolution in axial, coronal, and sagittal MR images. Hussain and Anwar [32] added an induction structure to a correlation architecture consisting of parallel and linear CNN layers. This structure has shown promising results in brain tumor MR image segmentation, particularly in increasing the DSC measure to 90%. Kamnitsas et al. [11] used conditional random field postprocessing to provide smoother results on 3D brain tumor pictures. Saouli et al. [33] suggested a sequential CNN architecture and argued that an end-to-end incremental network may create and train CNN models at the same time. This approach yields an 88% average DSC measure. Hu and Deng [34] used a more hierarchical CNN (multi-cascaded CNN [MCCNN]) and fully connected conditional random fields (CRFs) in conjunction with the brain tumor segmentation approach. To accomplish the impact of batch segmentation and enhance accuracy, the brain tumor is first roughly segmented by a multiclassification CNN and then fine-segmented by a fully connected random field based on the rough segmentation findings. The segmentation technique based on CNN is capable of automatically extracting features and handling high-dimensional data, but it is prone to information loss during pooling and has poor interpretability. Image-level classification and regression tasks are more appropriate for applying the CNN structure than pixel-level classification since they both anticipate acquiring a likely value for image classification.

Image-level classification and regression tasks are more appropriate for applying the CNN structure than pixel-level classification since they both anticipate acquiring a likely value for image classification. FCN is more effective for semantic MRI segmentation. FCN has no restrictions on the size of the input, and there will be an upsampling procedure at the final convolution layer. This approach may accomplish the same outcome as the size of the input by estimating each pixel while keeping the spatial information in the input image to fulfill the pixel classification task. FCN is a technique for segmenting imaging at the pixel level. As a result, the semantic segmentation model based on FCN better meets the requirements of medical picture segmentation. Zhao et al. [35] presented an FCN–CRF combo for brain tumor segmentation. This approach employs a fusion mechanism to integrate segmented brain tumor samples after training two-dimensional slices in axial, coronal, and sagittal orientations. When compared to standard segmentation approaches, segmentation speed, and efficiency are increased. Xue and Hu [36] developed an FCN with feature integration and reuse modules (F2FCN). It reutilizes the features of various layers and employs the feature integration module to remove potential noise and improve layer fusion. This approach produces a high DSC and PPV. Zhou et al. [37] suggested a 3D atomic convolution feature pyramid to improve the model's discriminating capacity, which is utilized to segregate tumors of various sizes. The original foundation is then improved [38], a 3D dense connection architecture is provided, and a new feature pyramid module is constructed utilizing 3D convolution. This module is utilized to integrate multiscale contexts to increase segmentation accuracy. Liu [39] employed a ResNet-50–based dilated convolution refine (DCR) structure that is capable of successfully extracting local and global features and increasing to 92% the segmentation PPV measure. The FCN-based segmentation method can forecast the class of all pixels, transfer the image classification level to the semantic level, save the original image's location information, and provide a result size that is equal to the input image size. However, this technique has limited computation performance, consumes a lot of space in the memory, and has a tiny receptive field.

In general, the EAD structure consists of an encoder and a decoder. To obtain its characteristic map, the encoder trains and learns the input picture using a neural network. The decoder's role is to indicate the category of each pixel once the encoder has provided the feature map to pinpoint the segmentation effect. The structure of encoders in segmentation tasks based on the EAD structure is globally very close, largely drawn from the network structure of classification tasks, such as VGG. The goal of this is to determine the training weight parameters of the network by training a huge database. As a result, the difference in the decoder reflects the difference in the entire network to a significant extent, as well as the most important component influencing the segmentation effect. The SegNet model was developed by Badrinarayan and Kendall [40]. When compared to previous models, this model seems to have a deeper layer and performs better in semantic pixel segmentation. The model's encoder is a 13-layer VGG-16 network that can remember the position of the biggest pixel during the encoding phase. The segmentation outcomes are gathered by upsampling the bad resolution of the input features in the decoder. The FCN-based U-Net model is a popular brain tumor segmentation approach in which the network structure includes an encoder and a decoder, and a U-Net network skip connection will code paths, utilized to determine the characteristics of the image to the decoding path to the corresponding point, in the interest of finding the characteristics of the direct sampling under the coding stage into the decoding stage, so that it can learn more detailed features. Chen et al. [41] built a multilevel deep network that can collect multilevel image information by adding auxiliary classifiers to the Multi-Level DeepMedic and U-Net networks, allowing image segmentation. The DSC, PPV, and TPR scores were 83%, 73%, and 85%, respectively. Zhou and Siddiquee [42] presented several layered dense connection approaches to connect the EAD networks trying to eliminate the semantic gap between the feature mapping of EAD networks. Based on U-Net, Alom et al. [43] suggested a recursive neural network and a recursive residual convolutional neural network. Zhang and Lv [44] enhanced the segmentation performance of brain tumor MRI by including the residual network and attention mechanism into the classic U-Net network and proposing an attention residual U-Net. Fahsi et al. [45] employed a U-Net with a deletion layer as a brain MRI image segmentation model. Ladkat et al. [46] used a mathematical model with 3D attention U-Net. Spatial and channel attention enhances the quality of feature hierarchy encoding. As a result, by merging 3D trans and cross-feature interactions, 3D concentration units that enable 3D spatial and channel attention are built. Messaoudi et al. [47] presented an asymmetric U-Net including the EfficientNet network as an element of the encoding part. Because the input data is in 3D, the encoder's first layers are focused to reduce the third dimension trying to suit the EfficientNet network's input. Milletari et al. [48] presented the V-Net model as an extension of the 3D U-Net model, which used a 3D convolution check to expand the original U-Net model. Hua et al. [49] cascaded V-Net and employed the approach of segmenting the entire tumor first into subregions. The result was that the segmentation accuracy is superior to straightly used V-Net segmentation. The EAD segmentation technique can mix high-resolution and low-resolution information and detect characteristics at many scales, but there is only a short link between the encoding and decoding processes, which is not sufficient.

Other researchers segmented brain tumors in multimodal MR images using a high-resolution and non-local feature network (HNF-Net). The HNF-Net is built primarily on the parallel multiscale fusion (PMF) module that is capable to preserve high-resolution feature representation while also aggregating multiscale contextual information. The expectation–maximization attention (EMA) module is also included in the model to improve long-range dependent spatial contextual information while maintaining acceptable computational complexity. Chakraborty et al. [50] proposed a hybrid high and non-local feature network (H2NF-Net). In comparison to the original HNF-Net, the suggested H2NF-Net incorporates a two-stage cascaded HNF-Net to segment distinct subregions of the brain tumor.

Table 11.2 summarizes the benefits and limitations of the brain tumor MRI segmentation approaches based on DL. Table 11.3 details several mentioned methods to compare their results with the performances obtained from the proposed methods.

TABLE 11.2

Benefits and limitations of the brain tumor MRI segmentation approaches based on DL

DL segmentation technique	Benefits	Limitations
CNN [28, 29]	Common convolutional kernel. Characteristics extraction is automatic.	Minimal interpretability. Presence of local convergence. Easy information loss
FCN [37, 39]	Not required for image shape definition. All pixels are classified.	Real-time concept inefficiency. Inattention to detail. Spatial placement Inconsistency.
EAD [40, 41]	Multiscale characteristic detection. Low and high-resolution information is merged. Pixel location information is restored.	Inadequate contact between EAD. A huge number of variables. The computing speed is slow.

TABLE 11.3

Several mentioned methods to compare their results with the performances obtained from the proposed methods

Paper	Year	Model	Used dataset
Fahsi et al. [45]	2022	U-Net + Deletion Layer	BraTS 2020 BraTS 2018
Ladkat et al. [46]	2022	Mathematical model with 3 attention U-Net	BraTS 2020
Messaoudi et al. [47]	2021	Asymmetric U-Net incorporating EfficientNet	BraTS 2020
Jia et al. [37]	2020	H2NF-Net	BraTS 2020

11.3 METHODS

Figure 11.1 displays the proposed procedures that were applied in this investigation. The following sections will go through each stage of this workflow.

11.3.1 DATASET

In this work, the used dataset is BraTS 2020. It describes four different MRI modalities: (1) native (T1), (2) T1-Gd, (3) T2-weighted (T2), and (4) FLAIR volumes. They were obtained using varied clinical procedures and scanners from several (n = 19) organizations. These scans were manually segmented by one to four raters using

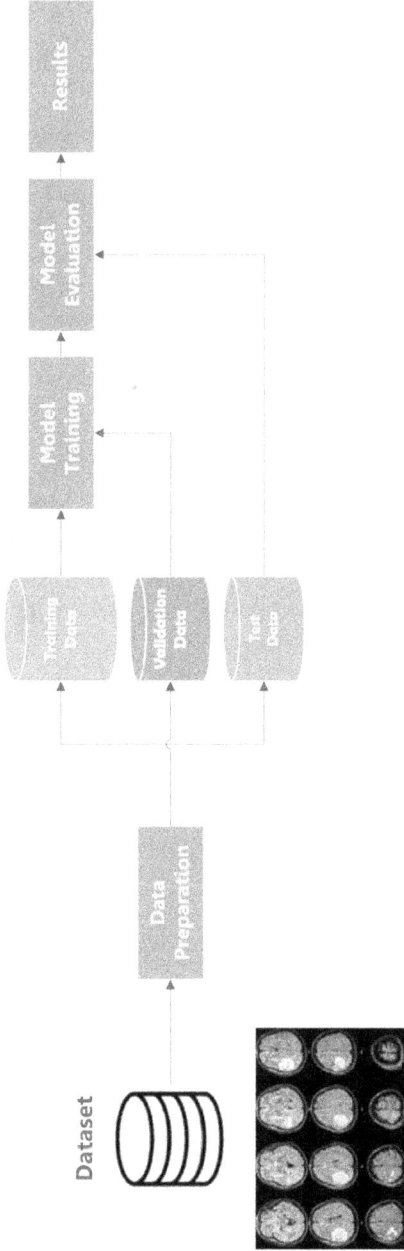

FIGURE 11.1   The proposed procedures.

the same annotation technique, and their annotations were approved by competent neuroradiologists. The necrotic non-enhancing tumor core (NCR/NET), the peritumoral edema (ED), and the GD-enhancing tumor (ET) are all annotated. After being coregistered to the same anatomical template, interpolated to the same resolution (1 mm^{-3}), and skull-stripped, the given data are disseminated [6–10]. Figure 11.2 illustrates the four modalities of the MRI and the annotation.

The BraTS 2020 challenge attempts to identify the clinical relevance of brain tumor multimodal MRI segmentation. It also focuses on (1) predicting patient overall survival from preoperative images (Task 1) and (2) differentiating real tumor recurrence from treatment-related effects on postoperative images (Task 3), using integrative studies of quantitative imaging phenomics characteristics and machine learning techniques [51].

BraTS 2020 includes training, validation, and testing datasets. This work focused on the training dataset, which contains 369 patients' brain MRIs, 293 from glioblastoma (GBM/HGG) and 76 from lower grade glioma (LGG) of patients with gliomas (both high and low grades), as well as their ground truth segmentations for evaluation [52]. The given data is provided as NIfTI files (*.nii.gz extension). Figure 11.3 presents the distribution of BraTS 2020 patients with gliomas.

11.3.2 DATA PREPARATION

The following paragraphs detail the rest of the data preparation steps of training, validation, and testing.

11.3.2.1 Data Preprocessing

The original size of the modality in the dataset is 240 × 240 × dep, i.e., the total number of images in each modality is dep = 155. Some of them refer to the starting or the ending of the modality and they don't contain any useful information. This seems useless for the segmentation task. Different values for dep were tried, and it was found that defining dep to 100 will enhance the model performance. In this work, the experiments show that optimal results are reached when using T1-Gd and FLAIR. In addition, all the chosen modality images were resized to 128 × 128. To resume, the output of this step is the generation of 73,800 slices with a size of 128 × 128.

11.3.2.2 Data Split

To train and test the model, a data split is needed. It starts by dividing the dataset into two sets with a ratio of 80:20, the training and validation set, and the test set, respectively. The first part is reserved for training the model and the second part is used for the evaluation of its performance. To optimize the model during the training, the validation data is obtained by splitting the training and validation data into two sets with an 85:15 ratio.

Figure 11.4 presents the partition of the dataset into training, validation, and test. In addition, Figure 11.5 illustrates the number of patient multimodal MRI images and the number of images in each set.

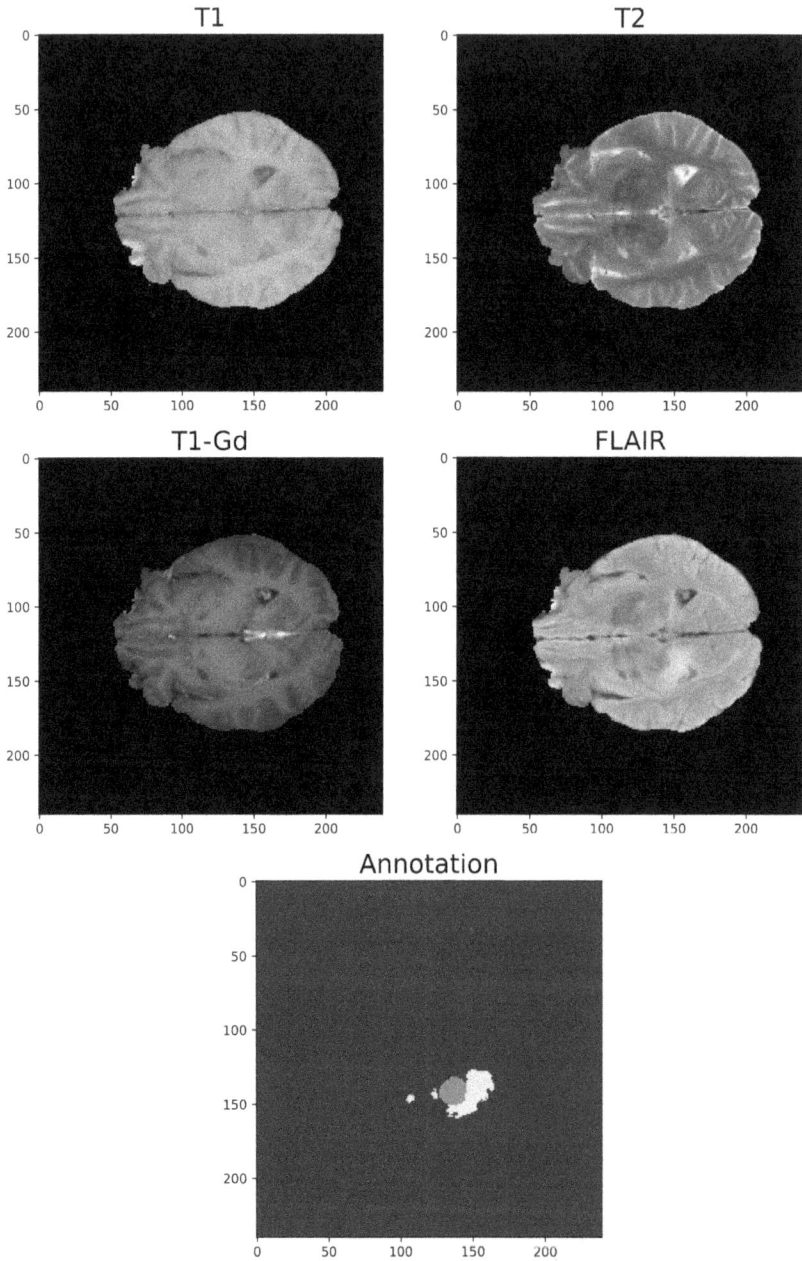

FIGURE 11.2 The four modalities of the MRI and the annotation.

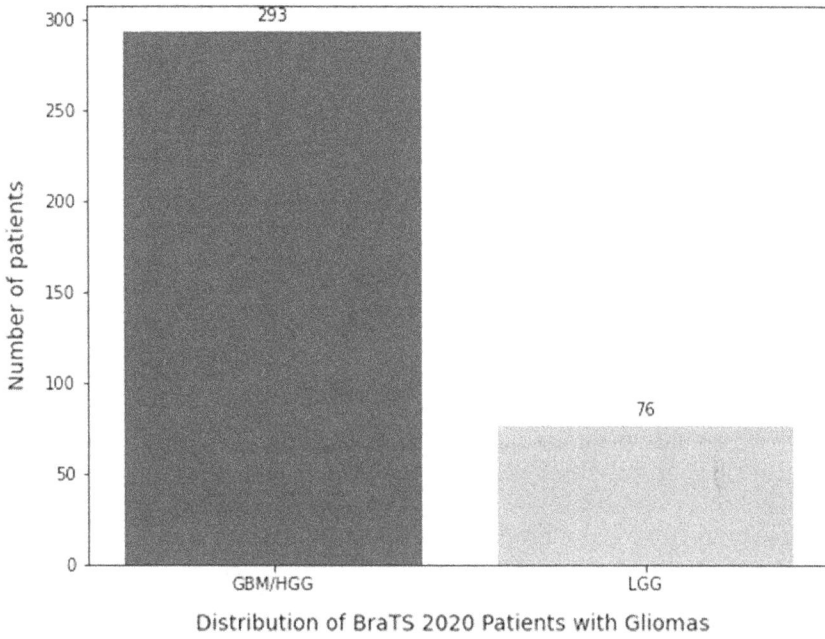

Distribution of BraTS 2020 Patients with Gliomas

FIGURE 11.3 The distribution of BraTS 2020 patients with gliomas.

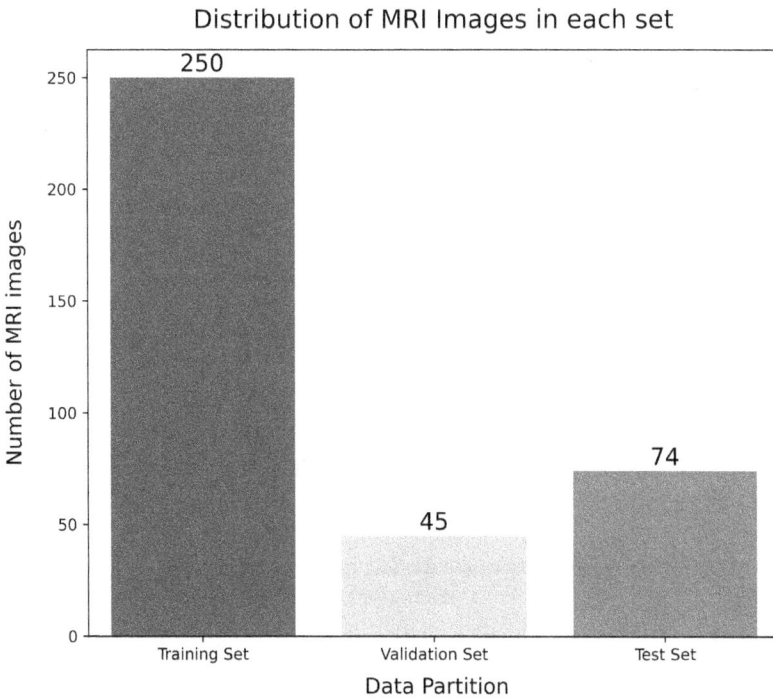

Distribution of MRI Images in each set

FIGURE 11.4 The partition of the dataset into training, validation, and test sets.

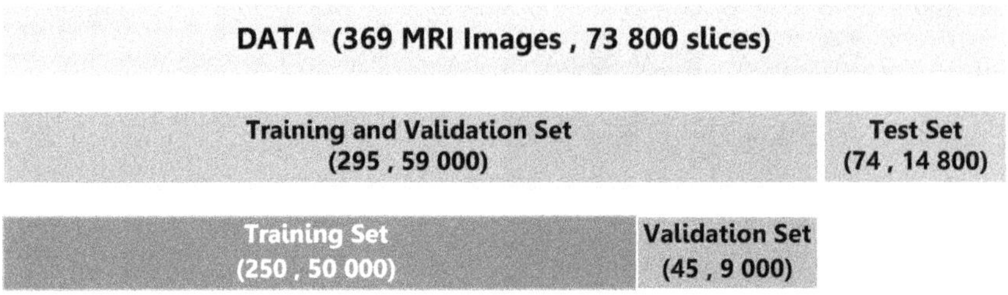

DATA (369 MRI Images , 73 800 slices)

Training and Validation Set (295 , 59 000)		Test Set (74 , 14 800)
Training Set (250 , 50 000)	Validation Set (45 , 9 000)	

FIGURE 11.5   The number of patient multimodal MRI images, and the number of slices in each set.

11.3.3 MODEL ARCHITECTURE

The U-NET architecture is composed of two "paths". The first one is the contraction path, also called the encoder. It is used to capture the context of an image. It is in fact an assembly of convolution layers and "max pooling" layers allowing the creation of a features map of the image and reducing its size in order to reduce the number of network parameters. The second path is the symmetric expansion path, also called the decoder. It also allows precise localization thanks to transposed convolution.

Figure 11.6 illustrates the architecture of the used U-Net.

11.3.4 TRAINING

The hyperparameters were determined through trial and error. Adam was used as the optimizer, with a learning rate of 0.001. In addition, the categorical cross-entropy is employed as a loss function.

The optimal hyperparameters for the neural network are 128×128 as the size of the input images and 2 as the number of channels that refer to the modalities used. Additionally, the batch size is limited to 1, and the number of epochs is fixed at 70 epochs. The learning rate (LR) schedule's purpose is to adjust the learning rate during the training. The optimized LR is ReduceLROnplateau.

11.3.5 METRICS

The segmentation resulting from a DL method can be either abnormal or normal, called positive class or negative class, respectively. The result of the prediction can also be true or false, which implies a correct or incorrect prediction, respectively. Thus, it can be summarized into four possible states:

- *True positive (TP)* – correct prediction of the positive class
- *True negative (TN)* – correct prediction of the negative class
- *False positive (FP)* – incorrect prediction of the positive class
- *False negative (FN)* – incorrect prediction of the negative class

In this work, the accuracy, precision, specificity, sensitivity, dice similarity coefficient, and intersection over union were provided to evaluate the model performance.

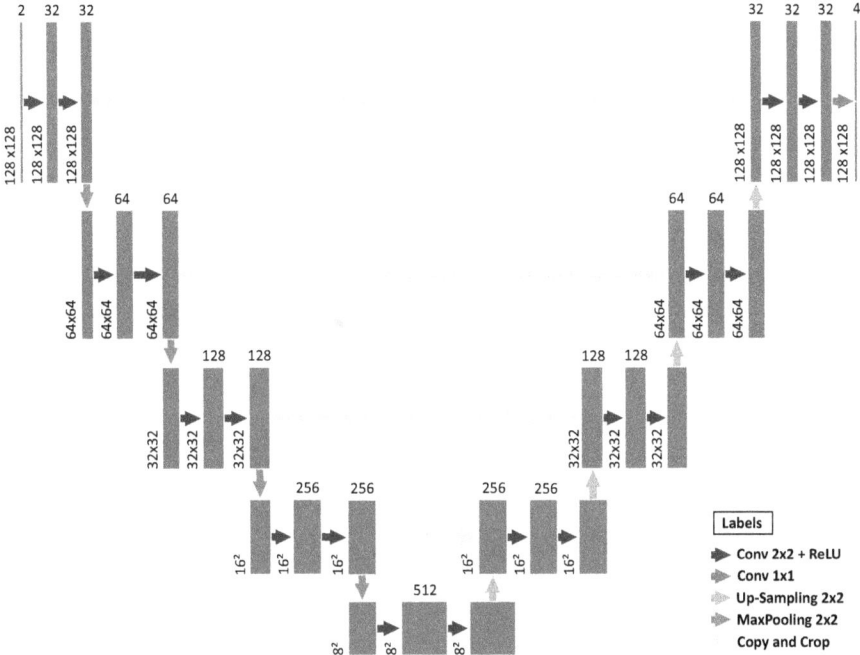

FIGURE 11.6   The architecture of the used U-Net.

11.3.5.1   Accuracy

Accuracy is defined as the fraction of brain tumor pixels that are correctly segmented as a tumor and normal tissue pixels that are truly predicted as normal.

$$Accuracy = \frac{TP + TN}{TP + TN + FP + FN} \tag{11.1}$$

11.3.5.2   Precision

Precision accurately depicts the purity of positive detections compared to the ground truth. In other words, it computes the ratio of real pixels with matching ground truth annotations to all predicted objects in a given image.

$$Precision = \frac{TP}{TP + FP} \tag{11.2}$$

11.3.5.3   Recall/Sensitivity (Se)

Sensitivity calculates the number of positive pixels in the ground truth that are also predicted as positive by the segmentation.

$$Se = \frac{TP}{TP + FN} \tag{11.3}$$

11.3.5.4 Specificity (Sp)

Specificity calculates the number of negative pixels in the ground truth that are also predicted as negative by the segmentation.

$$\mathrm{Sp} = \frac{TN}{TN + FP} \qquad (11.4)$$

11.3.5.5 Dice Similarity Coefficient (DSC)

A DSC is a segmentation performance metric that corresponds to the F1 score, which is the harmonic average of precision and recall. It estimates the overlap based on the intersection of X and Y, which refers to the segmented pixels and the ground truth.

$$\mathrm{DSC} = 2 \times \frac{|X \cap Y|}{|X| + |Y|} = 2 \times \frac{TP}{2TP + FN + FP} = 2 \times \frac{\mathrm{Pr}ecision \times \mathrm{Re}call}{\mathrm{Pr}ecision + \mathrm{Re}call} \qquad (11.5)$$

11.3.5.6 Intersection over Union (IoU)

IoU evaluates the area overlap between the actual and the predicted segmentation divided by the area of the union.

$$\mathrm{IoU} = \frac{Area\,of\,Overlap}{Area\,of\,Union} = \frac{TP}{TP + FN + FP} \qquad (11.6)$$

11.4 RESULTS AND DISCUSSION

11.4.1 Training and Validation Phase

11.4.1.1 Experiments

The training of the proposed models was done using Kaggle, which had the following characteristics:

- GPU: NVIDIA Tesla P100 16 Go
- CPU RAM: 13 GB

The total number of epochs used is 70. Each epoch takes 282 s. The training step duration is estimated at 5 h 29 min.

11.4.1.2 Accuracy

At the end of the training and validation of the proposed model, the accuracy obtained was 99.57% and 99.29%, respectively. Figure 11.7 represents the evolution of the accuracy during the training and validation.

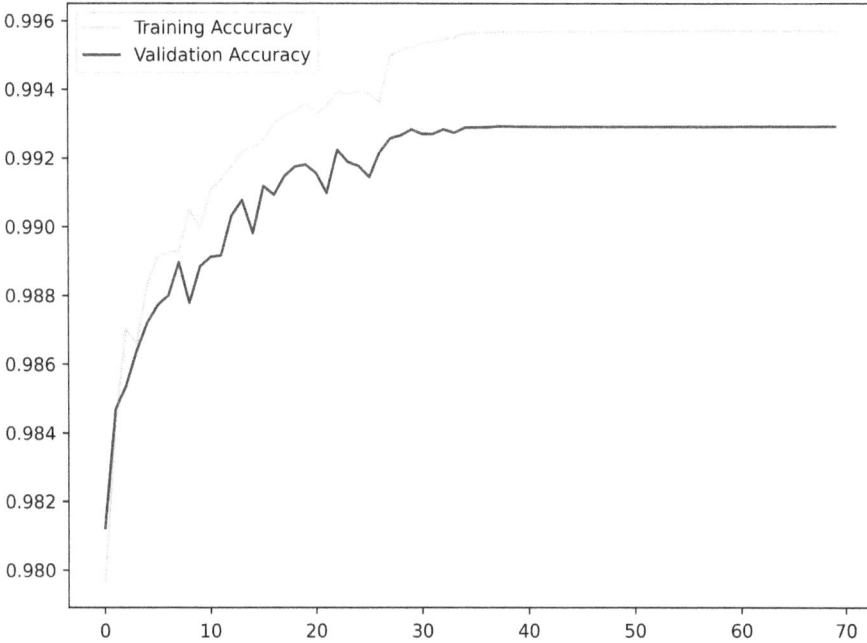

FIGURE 11.7   The evolution of the accuracy during the training and validation.

11.4.1.3   Precision

Concerning the precision, at the end of the training and validation, it reached 99.56% and 99.30%, respectively. Figure 11.8 shows the evolution of the precision metric for the proposed model.

11.4.1.4   Sensitivity

At the end of the training and validation of the proposed model, the sensitivity obtained was 99.57% and 99.29%, respectively. Figure 11.9 represents the evolution of the sensitivity during the training and validation.

11.4.1.5   Specificity

Regarding the specificity obtained by the end of the training and validation of the proposed model, it attained 99.85% and 99.76%, respectively. Figure 11.10 represents the evolution of the specificity during the training and validation.

11.4.1.6   IoU

Figure 11.11 illustrates the evolution of the IoU in the two steps. For the U-Net model, it reached 85.80% in the training and 86.06% in the validation.

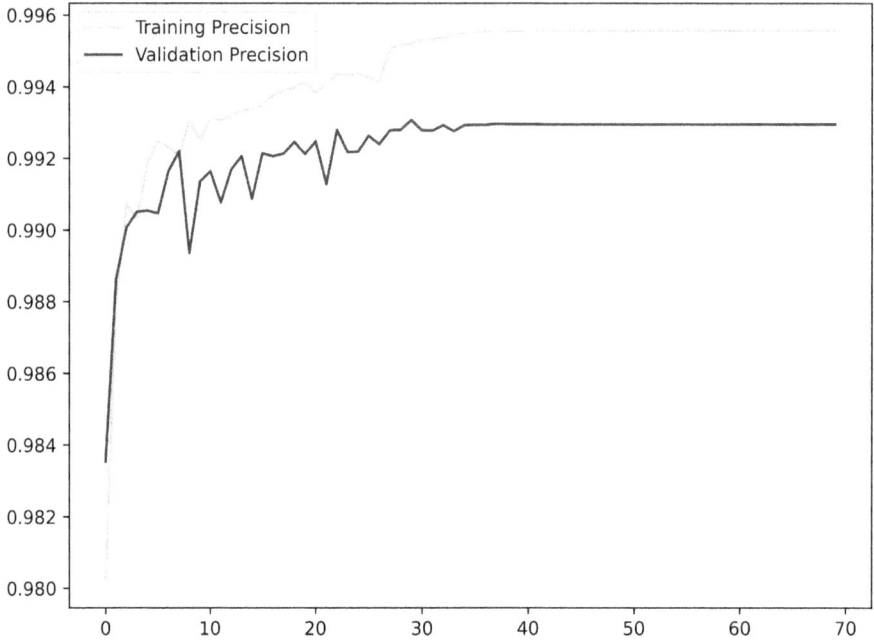

FIGURE 11.8　The evolution of the precision during the training and validation.

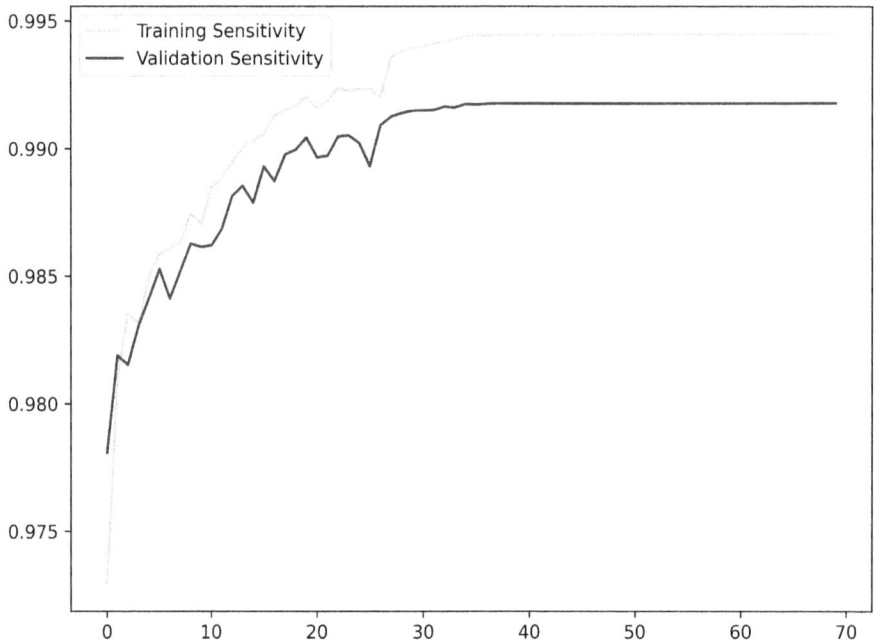

FIGURE 11.9　The evolution of the sensitivity during the training and validation.

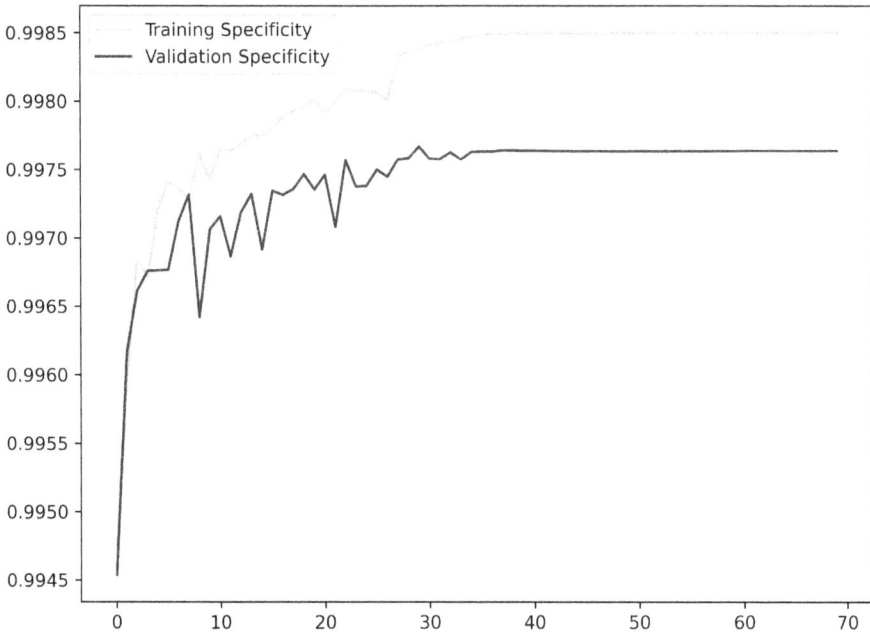

FIGURE 11.10 The evolution of the specificity during the training and validation.

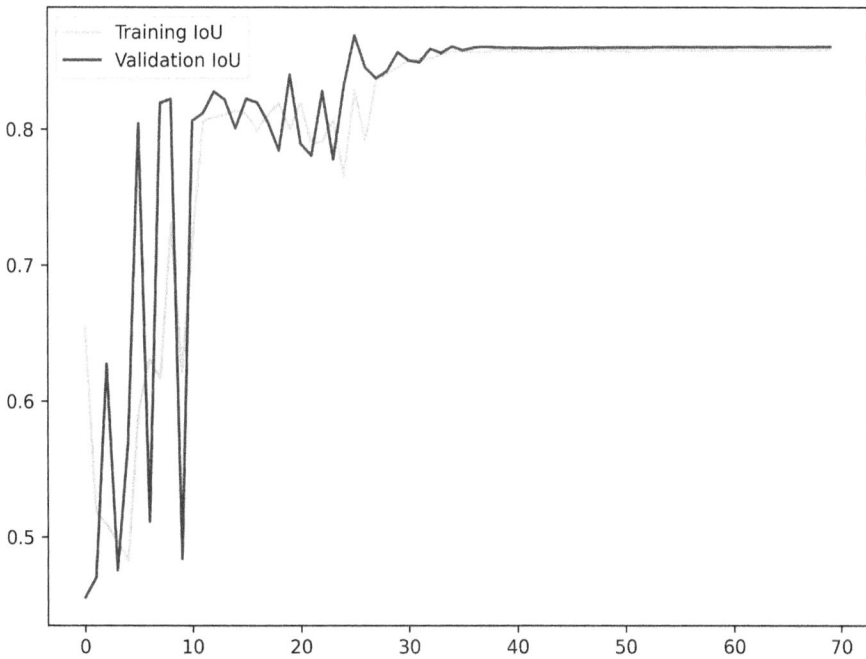

FIGURE 11.11 The evolution of the IoU during the training and validation.

11.4.1.7 DSC

Concerning the DSC, at the end of the training and validation, it reached 69.98% and 66.54%, respectively. Figure 11.12 shows the evolution of the DSC metric for the proposed model.

11.4.1.8 Loss

In terms of loss, the proposed model reached $1{,}18.10^{-02}$ and $2{,}15.10^{-02}$ in the two phases, respectively. Figure 11.13 presents the evolution of the loss function for the two models.

Globally, the saw teeth figured in these curves from to beginning of the training to epoch 35. Then, the proposed model converged from the 36th epoch for the totality of the metrics.

11.4.2 Test Phases

The total data reserved for testing the proposed model are 74 MRI images. Table 11.4 shows the metrics used to evaluate the performance of the proposed method.

Regarding accuracy, precision, sensitivity, and specificity, these metrics exceeded 99% when using the test set. The IoU reached 85.68%. However, the DSC attained 66.71%, which is not a competitive result, leading to 63.80%, 76.06%, and 71.90% for the DSC of the classes NCR/NET, ED, and ET, respectively.

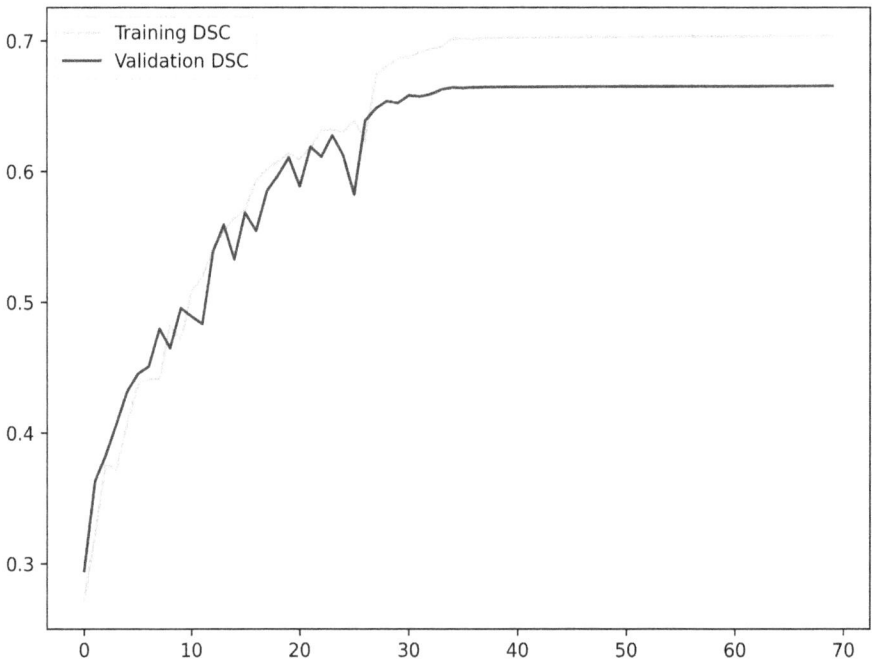

FIGURE 11.12   The evolution of the DSC during the training and validation.

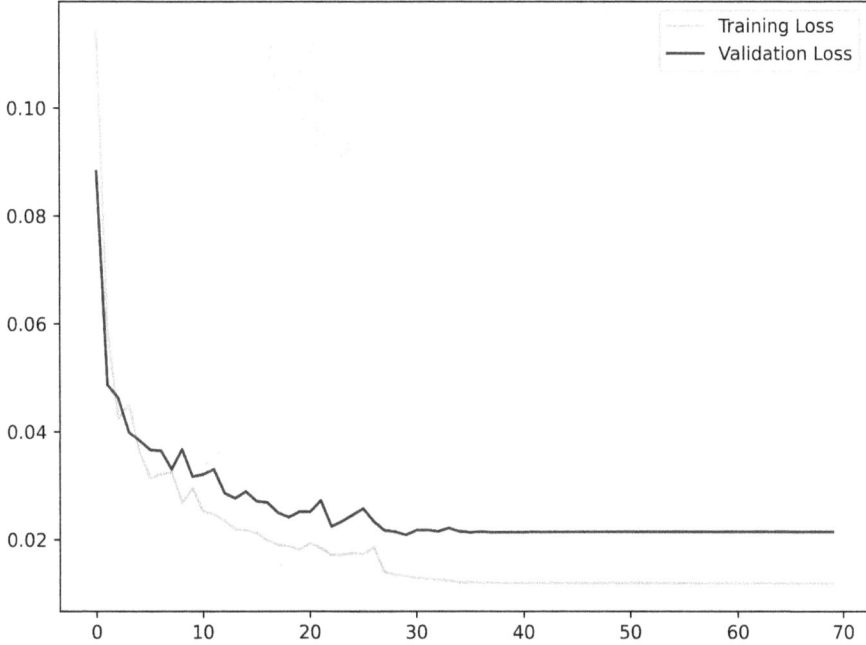

FIGURE 11.13 The evolution of the loss during the training and validation.

TABLE 11.4
Metrics used to evaluate the performance of the proposed method

Metrics	Values
Accuracy	0.9944
Precision	0.9945
Sensitivity	0.9934
Specificity	0.9981
Intersection over union	0.8569
Dice similarity coefficient	0.6671
Dice similarity coefficient (NCR/NET)	0.6381
Dice Similarity Coefficient (ED)	0.7606
Dice Similarity Coefficient (ET)	0.7190
Loss	0.0177

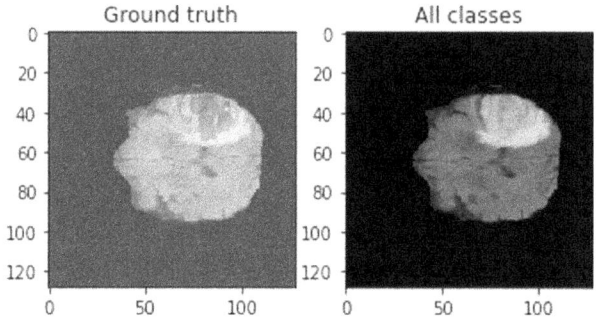

FIGURE 11.14 Test 1.

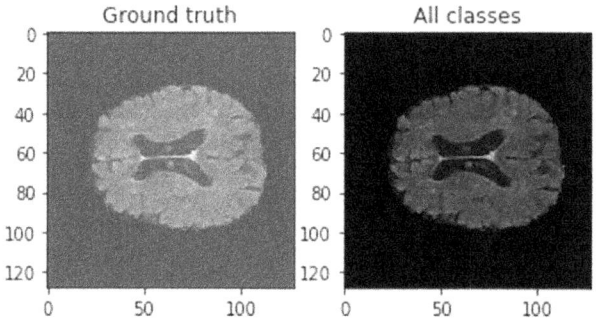

FIGURE 11.15 Test 2.

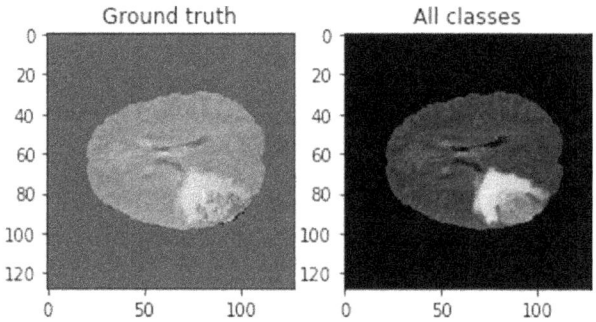

FIGURE 11.16 Test 3.

As examples, Figures 11.14, 11.15, and 11.16 represent three random brain tumor MRI slice segmentation tests 1, 2, and 3, respectively, predicted by the proposed method. So, for each test, the ground truth and all the class predictions are represented. In Figure 11.14, which shows a brain MRI slice without any tumor, the prediction of the suggested model does not include any segmented tumor.

TABLE 11.5

Comparison of the proposed models against various methods.

		Fahsi et al. [45]	Ladkat et al. [46]	Messaoudi et al. [47]	Jia et al. [37]	Proposed method
Accuracy		—	0.9890	—	—	**0.9944**
Precision		—	0.9900	—	—	**0.9945**
Sensitivity		—	0.9800	—	—	**0.9934**
DSC	NCR/NET	0.7613	0.7120	0.7520	**0.8537**	0.6381
	ED	0.5697	0.8230	0.868	**0.8879**	0.7606
	ET	0.7894	0.6030	0.6959	**0.8277**	0.7190

11.4.3 DISCUSSION

To evaluate this study with the results found in the state of the art, the metrics used are accuracy, precision, and sensitivity. In addition, the DSC of all the classes was utilized in this task.

Comparing the obtained results of the proposed method, accuracy, precision, and sensitivity outperformed all the mentioned methods. Considering the DSC, it is less performing, especially for the NCR/NET class. Globally, the ED class DSC, which refers to peritumoral edema, is the highest when compared to the other classes' DSC in all the mentioned investigations. The reached DSC of the class ED is higher than the result attained by Fahsi et al. [45]. Moreover, concerning the ET class DSC, it is higher than those of Ladkt et al. [46] and Messaoudi et al. [47]. Table 11.5 presents a detailed comparison of the proposed models against various methods.

11.5 CONCLUSION

This work demonstrates a powerful DL model for automated brain tumor MRI image segmentation based on U-Net. The used dataset counts 369 multimodal MRI images collected from 19 institutions. This work illustrates the efficiency of the DL approaches in the segmentation of medical images. The findings were also compared to and affirmed by values from recently published literature. Moreover, this study proves that the proposed methods can be easily adopted and perform well.

The suggested method has some disadvantages, including difficult computations and lack of interpretability due to the limitations in terms of resources. In the future, further tests should vary other parameters such as the number of neurons in the conventional layer and the drop-out. Modifying the architecture by introducing or altering layer(s), building U-Net with 3D conventional layers, and experimenting with different data preprocessing technics should also be undertaken. As a result of the upcoming research, the suggested approaches will be improved to be more suitable for a larger range of various medical imaging applications.

REFERENCES

1. S. Bauer, R. Wiest, L.-P. Nolte, and M. Reyes. (2013) "A survey of MRI-based medical image analysis for brain tumor studies." *Phys. Med. Biol.* 58(13): R97.
2. J. Juan-Albarracin, E. Fuster-Garcia, J. V. Manjon, M. Robles, F. Aparici, L. Martí-Bonmatí, and J. M. Garcia-Gomez. (2015) "Automated glioblastoma segmentation based on a multiparametric structured unsupervised classification." *PLoS One* 10(5): e0125143.
3. A. Souid, N. Sakli, and H. Sakli. (2021) "Classification and predictions of lung diseases from chest X-rays using MobileNet V2." *Appl. Sci.* 11(6): Art. no. 6. doi: 10.3390/app11062751.
4. N. Sakli, H. Ghabri, B. Othman Soufiene, F., Almalki, H., Sakli, O. Ali, and M. Najjari. (2022) "ResNet-50 for 12-lead electrocardiogram automated diagnosis." *Comput. Intell. Neurosci.* 2022: 1–16. doi: 10.1155/2022/7617551.
5. O. Ronneberger, P. Fischer, and T. Brox. (2015) "U-net: Convolutional networks for biomedical image segmentation." In *International Conference on Medical Image Computing and Computer-Assisted Intervention* 28: 234–241. doi: 10.1007/978-3-319-24574-4.
6. S. Bakas, M. Reyes, A. Jakab, S. Bauer, M. Rempfler, A. Crimi, and R. Takeshi Shinohara. (2018) "Identifying the best machine learning algorithms for brain tumor segmentation, progression assessment, and overall survival prediction in the BRATS challenge." *arXiv preprint arXiv:1811.02629.*
7. B. H. Menze, A. Jakab, S. Bauer, J. Kalpathy-Cramer, K. Farahani, J. Kirby, Y. Burren, N. Porz, J. Slotboom, R. Wiest, and L. Lanczi. (2015) "The multimodal brain tumor image segmentation benchmark (BRATS)." *IEEE Trans. Med. Imaging* 34(10): 1993–2024. doi: 10.1109/TMI.2014.2377694.
8. S. Bakas, H. Akbari, A. Sotiras, M. Bilello, M. Rozycki, J. S. Kirby, and C. Davatzikos. (2017) "Advancing the cancer genome atlas glioma MRI collections with expert segmentation labels and radiomic features." *Nat. Sci. Data* 4: 170117. doi: 10.1038/sdata.2017.117.
9. S. Bakas, H. Akbari, A. Sotiras, M. Bilello, M. Rozycki, J. Kirby, and C. Davatzikos. (2017) "Segmentation labels and radiomic features for the pre-operative scans of the TCGA-GBM collection." *Cancer Imaging Arch.* doi: 10.7937/K9/TCIA.2017.KLXWJJ1Q.
10. S. Bakas, H. Akbari, A. Sotiras, M. Bilello, M. Rozycki, J. Kirby, and C. Davatzikos. (2017) "Segmentation labels and radiomic features for the pre-operative scans of the TCGA-LGG collection." *Cancer Imaging Arch.* doi: 10.7937/K9/TCIA.2017.GJQ7R0EF.
11. Konstantinos Kamnitsas, Christian Ledig, Virginia FJ Newcombe, Joanna P Simpson, Andrew D Kane, David K Menon, Daniel Rueckert, and Ben Glocker. (2017) "Efficient multi-scale 3D CNN with fully connected CRF for accurate brain lesion segmentation." *Med. Image Anal.* 36: 61–78.
12. Fabian Isensee, Paul F. Jaeger, Simon A. A. Kohl, Jens Petersen, and Klaus H. Maier-Hein. (2021) "nnU-Net: A self-configuring method for deep learning-based biomedical image segmentation." *Nat. Methods* 18(2): 203–211.
13. L. Pei, L. Vidyaratne, M. M. Rahman, and K. M. Iftekharuddin. (2020) "Context aware deep learning for brain tumor segmentation, subtype classification, and survival prediction using radiology images." *Sci. Rep.* 10(1): 19726. doi: 10.1038/s41598-020-74419-9.
14. Ischemic stroke lesion segmentation|ISLES 2015. http://www.isles-challenge.org/ISLES2015/ (accessed on 10 December 2021).
15. Ischemic stroke lesion segmentation|ISLES 2017. http://www.isles-challenge.org/ISLES2017/ (accessed on 10 December 2021).
16. J. Cheng, W. Huang, S. Cao, R. Yang, W. Yang, and Q. Feng. (2015) "Correction: Enhanced performance of brain tumor classification via tumor region augmentation and partition." *PLoS One* 10(12): e0144479. doi: 10.1371/journal.pone.0144479.

17. L. Scarpace, L. Mikkelsen, T. Cha, S. Rao, S. Tekchandani, S. Gutman, and D. Pierce. (2016) "Radiology data from the cancer genome atlas glioblastoma multiforme [TCGA-GBM] collection." *Cancer Imaging Arch.* 11: 1.
18. A. Gumaei, M. M. Hassan, M. R. Hassan, A. Alelaiwi, and G. Fortino. (2019) "A hybrid feature extraction method with regularized extreme learning machine for brain tumor classification." *IEEE Access* 7: 36266–36273. doi: 10.1109/ACCESS.2019.2904145.
19. DICOM image library|Home. https://www.osirix-viewer.com/resources/dicom-image -library/brainix (accessed on 10 December 2021).
20. Z. Khan, N. Yahya, K. Alsaih, M. I. Al-Hiyali, and F. Meriaudeau. (2021) "Recent automatic segmentation algorithms of MRI prostate regions: A review." *IEEE Access* 9: 97878–97905. doi: 10.1109/ACCESS.2021.3090825.
21. N. Gordillo, E. Montseny, and P. Sobrevilla. (2013) "State of the art survey on MRI brain tumor segmentation." *Magn. Reson. Imaging* 31(8): 1426–1438. doi: 10.1016/j. mri.2013.05.002.
22. S. H. Chen, W. X. Liu, J. Qin, L. Chen, G. Bin, Y. Zhou, and B. Huang. (2017) "Research progress in computer-aided diagnosis of cancer based on deep learning and medical images." *J. Biomed. Eng.* 2: 160–165.
23. A. Krizhevsky, I. Sutskever, and G. E. Hinton. (2012) "ImageNet classification with deep convolutional neural networks." *Int. Conf. Neural Inf. Process. Syst.* 60: 1066.
24. K. Simonyan and A. Zisserman. (2014) "Very deep convolutional networks for large scale image recognition." *Comput. Sci.* 6: 1556.
25. C. Szegedy and Y. Liu. (2015) "Going deeper with convolutions." In *Proceedings of the IEEE Conference on Computer Vision and Pattern Recognition*, Boston, MA, USA, 7–12 June 2015, pp. 1–9.
26. K. W. He, X. Zhang, S. Ren, and J. Sun. (2016) "Deep residual learning for image recognition." In *Proceedings of the IEEE Conference on Computer Vision and Pattern Recognition (CVPR)*, Las Vegas, NV, USA, 27–30 June 2016, pp. 770–778.
27. T. Zhou, B. Q. Huo, and H. L. Lu. (2020) "Research on residual neural network and its application in medical image processing." *Chin. J. Electron.* 48: 1436–1447.
28. V. K. Anand and S. Grampurohit. (2021) "Brain tumor segmentation and survival prediction using automatic hard mining in 3D CNN architecture." *arXiv,* arXiv:2101.01546v1.
29. M. Havaei, A. Davy, F. D. Warde, A. Biard, A. Courville, Y. Bengio, C. Pal, P.-M. Jodoin, and H. Larochelle. (2017) "Brain tumor segmentation with deep neural networks." *Med. Image Anal.* 35: 18–31.
30. X. B. Lai, M. S. Xu, and X. M. Xu. (2019) "Multimodal MR image segmentation of glioblastoma based on multi-class CNN." *Chin. J. Electron.* 47: 140–149.
31. S. Salehi, D. Erdogmus, and A. Gholipour. (2017) "Auto-context convolutional neural network(auto-net) for brain extraction in magnetic resonance imaging." *IEEE Trans. Med. Imaging* 36: 2319–2330.
32. S. Hussain and S. M. Anwar. (2018) "Segmentation of glioma tumors in brain using deep convolutional neural network." *Neuro Comput.* 282: 248–261.
33. R. Saouli, M. Akil, and R. Kachouri. (2018) "Fully automatic brain tumor segmentation using end-to-end incremental deep neural networks in MRI images." *Comput. Methods Programs Biomed.* 166: 39–49.
34. K. Hu and S. H. Deng. (2019) "Brain tumor segmentation using multi-cascaded convolutional neural networks and conditional random field." *IEEE Access* 7: 2615–2629.
35. X. Zhao, Y. Wu, G. Song, Z. Li, Y. Zhang, and Y. Fan. (2017) "A deep learning model integrating FCNNs and CRFs for brain tumor segmentation." *Med. Image Anal.* 43: 98–111.
36. J. Xue and J. Y. Hu. (2020) "Hypergraph membrane system based F^2 fully convolutional neural network for brain tumor segmentation." *Appl. Soft Comput. J.* 94: 106454.

37. Z. X. Zhou, Z. S. He, and Y. Y. Jia. (2020) "AFP-Net: A 3D fully convolutional neural network with atrous-convolution feature pyramid for brain tumor segmentation via MRI images." *Neuro Comput.* 402: 03097.

38. Z. X. Zhou, Z. S. He, M. F. Shi, J. L. Du, and D. D. Chen. (2020) "3D dense connectivity network with atrous convolutional feature pyramid for brain tumor segmentation in magnetic resonance imaging of human head." *Comput. Biol. Med.* 121: 103766.

39. D. Liu, H. Zhang, M. Zhao, X. Yu, S. Yao, and W. Zhou. (2018) "Brain tumor segmentation based on dilated convolution refine networks." In *Proceedings of the 16th IEEE International Conference on Software Engineering Research, Management and Application*, Kunming, China, 13–15 June 2018, pp. 113–120.

40. V. Badrinarayan and A. Kendall. (2017) "SegNet: A deep convolutional encoder-decoder architecture for image segmentation." *IEEE Trans. Pattern Anal. Mach. Intell.* 39: 2481–2495.

41. S. C. Chen, C. X. Ding, and M. F. Liu. (2019) "Dual-force convolutional neural networks for accurate brain tumor segmentation." *Pattern Recog.* 88: 90–100.

42. Z. W. Zhou and M. R. Siddiquee. (2018) "U-Net++: A nested U-net architecture for medical image segmentation." In *International Workshop on Deep Learning in Medical Image Analysis Deep Learning in Medical Image Analysis and Multimodal Learning for Clinical Decision Support.* Cham, Switzerland; Berlin/Heidelberg, Germany: Springer, pp. 3–11.

43. M. Z. Alom, M. Hasan, C. Yakopcic, T. M. Taha, and K. Asari. (2018) "Recurrent residual convolutional neural network based on U-net (R2U-Net) for medical image segmentation." *Comput. Vis. Pattern Recogn.* 5: 06955.

44. J. Zhang and X. Lv. (2020) "Ares U-Net: Attention residual U-net for brain tumor segmentation." *Symmetry* 12: 721.

45. M. Fahsi, C. Mouilah, and N. Mahammed. (2022) "An hyperparameter optimization study of brain tumor medical image segmentation using U-net." *Turk. J. Comput. Math. Educ.* 13(2): Art. n° 2.

46. A. S. Ladkat, Sunil L. Bangare, Vishal Jagota, Sumaya Sanober, Shehab Mohamed Beram, Kantilal Rane, and Bhupesh Kumar Singh. (2022) "Deep neural network-based novel mathematical model for 3D brain tumor segmentation." *Comput. Intell. Neurosci.* 2022: e4271711. doi: 10.1155/2022/4271711.

47. H. Messaoudi, A. Belaid, M. L. Allaoui, A. Zetout, M. S. Allili, S. Tliba, D. B. Salem, and P.-H. Conze. (2021) "Efficient embedding network for 3D brain tumor segmentation." In *Brainlesion: Glioma, Multiple Sclerosis, Stroke and Traumatic Brain Injuries.* Cham, pp. 252–262. doi: 10.1007/978-3-030-72084-1_23.

48. F. Milletari, N. Navab, and S. A. Ahmadi. (2016) "V-Net: Fully convolutional neural networks for volumetric medical image segmentation." In *Proceedings of the International Conference on 3D Vision*, Stanford, CA, USA, 25–28 October 2016, pp. 565–571.

49. R. Hua, Q. Huo, Y. Gao, H. Sui, B. Zhang, Y. Sun, S. Mo, and F. Shi. (2020) "Segmenting brain tumor using cascaded V-nets in multimodal MR images." *Front. Comput. Neurosci.* 14: 9.

50. C. Chakraborty, S. B. Othman, F. A. Almalki, and H. Sakli. (2023) "FC-SEEDA: Fog computing-based secure and energy efficient data aggregation scheme for internet of healthcare things." *Neural Comput. Appl.* doi: 10.1007/s00521-023-08270-0.

51. S. Ben Othman, A. A. Bahattab, A. Trad, and H. Youssef. (2020) "PEERP: A priority-based energy-efficient routing protocol for reliable data transmission in healthcare using the IoT." In *The 15th International Conference on Future Networks and Communications (FNC)*, Leuven, Belgium, 9–12 August 2020.

52. S. Ben Othman, F. A. Almalki, C. Chakraborty, and H. Sakli. (2022) "Privacy-preserving aware data aggregation for IoT-based healthcare with green computing technologies." *Comput. Electr. Eng.* 101: 108025. doi: 10.1016/j.compeleceng.2022.108025.

12 Face Mask Detection and Temperature Scanning for the COVID-19 Surveillance System Based on Deep Learning Models

Nagarjuna Telagam, D Ajitha, Nehru Kandasamy, and Ben Othman Soufiene

12.1 INTRODUCTION

The premise of this chapter is that in a pandemic crisis, a face mask is an essential item that everyone should wear to prevent the spread of disease. This project uses an MLX90614 contactless temperature sensor to monitor body temperature and a Raspberry Pi camera to determine whether someone is wearing a mask. We offer the COVID-19 internal safety system, which is economical and practical. The Raspberry Pi CPU connects all of the modules and sensors.

An efficient mask detector model was created using a deep learning model that can work in Raspberry Pi with low latency and high performance. The deep learning models were developed and compared using various algorithms' precision, accuracy, and validation losses. Deep learning is a machine learning subclass that uses three or more layers of neural networks. These neural networks try to mimic human brain function by allowing them to "learn" from enormous volumes of data, yet they fall short. Whereas a single-layer neural network can only make estimates, adding hidden layers improves and optimizes the network's accuracy. Artificial intelligence services utilize the deep learning approach for automation applications such as television, digital assistants, and fraud detection. The machine learning algorithms are well structured for labeled data. Machine learning methods depend on structured and labeled data to make predictions. The input data are specified in groups of tables. Deep learning methods reduce the preprocessing of data in machine learning. These algorithms analyze different data, such as text, photographs, and feature extraction.

DOI: 10.1201/9781003366249-12

The deep learning features can identify the ears and noses of various animals, such as cats, dogs, and hamsters.

A deep learning technique is utilized to detect a mask on a face in the system's face mask detection architecture. The model was trained using labeled picture data, with the pictures being faces with and without masks. The suggested approach correctly recognizes a face mask with 98.7% accuracy. Because it almost looks like the individual is wearing a mask, the developed system has trouble classifying faces covered by hands. When a person without a face mask travels in a vehicle, the system cannot find that person effectively. It isn't easy to differentiate each person's face in a densely populated region. In this case, identifying people without a face mask would be highly challenging for this proposed method [1].

Convolutional neural networks (CNNs) and VGG16-based deep learning models have developed a face mask recognition system to identify people who aren't wearing masks in a crowd. Data augmentation, dropout, normalization, and transfer learning are all concepts used in the proposed study. For training, validation, and testing, the model obtained 96.35%, 96.35%, and 97.42% accuracy, respectively, using CNN; and 99.47%, 98.59%, and 98.97% accuracy, respectively, using VGG16. A smaller number of datasets are used in this model: almost 1,315 images and applied masks on images [2].

Machine learning technologies such as TensorFlow, Keras, OpenCV, and SciKit-Learn are utilized for face detection. This proposed method identifies the face that is covered by a mask. The other advantage is it can also identify the moving face in a mask. This proposed approach has an accuracy of 95.77%. However, this method also suffers from critical drawbacks such as variable angles and lack of clarity [3]. The authors proposed a CNN model for training face mask detection using TensorFlow and Keras. The approach is to work with real-time videos to detect the face mask, the model is trained on various datasets [4, 6]. The authors developed machine learning models based on security cameras to detect people who are not wearing a face mask and thus prevent COVID-19 transmission. This approach yields fewer convolution layers and lower accuracy [5]. The method of artificial intelligence in the healthcare environment is cost-effective and highly reliable. The combination of deep learning and machine learning methods, called hybrid models, is used for mask detection. The dataset is taken for different people, such as with-mask and without-mask scenarios. The Raspberry Pi detects real-time data with a webcam. Infrared thermography sensors are used to detect body temperatures. A door controller is used to help security guards in various applications [7]. The screening of people in malls, especially via body temperature, was used to identify COVID-19. Manual temperature systems have many drawbacks, such as human error. The authors implemented an automated temperature scanner system that takes live images of people and detects their temperature. The system is connected to Raspberry Pi [8]. The Arduino Uno is used to detect temperature, and it depends on the infrared detecting component and influences PC vision methods to perform a social separating check square measure. The authors implemented a programmed scanning system including a locator, temperature scanner, and monitor [9]. Table 12.1 reviews the related works of mask detection methods and scanning systems.

TABLE 12.1

Related works of mask detection methods and scanning systems

Reference	Dataset used	Method used	Performance metrics
Echtioui et al. 2020 [10]	CXR Images	CNN method	Accuracy of 91.4%
Ozturk et al. 2020 [11]	CXR Images	DarkCovidNet	For multiclass cases, the accuracy is 87.02%
Wang et al. 2021 [12]	CXR Images	Deep CNN model	Accuracy of 93.3%
Shah et al. 2021 [13]	CT scan images	Distinct deep learning techniques	Accuracy of 82.1%
Sedik et al. 2021 [14]	Radiography dataset	CNN and ConvLSTM	Accuracy of the first model was 95%; 88% for the second model
Loey et al. 2020 [15]	Medical face mask images	ResNET-50	Adam optimizer (0.81) is better than the AP of SGDM (0.61)
Nieto-Rodríguez et al. 2015 [16]	Medical face mask images	Gentle AdaBoost	True positive ratio is throughout 95%; the false positives are under 40
Loey et al. 2021 [17]	Medical face mask images of three datasets: RMFD, SMFD, and LFW	DT, SVM, and ensemble algorithm	SVM classifier is better than the DT classifier; highest validation accuracy achieved by the DT classifier in DS3 was 98.

12.2   PROPOSED SYSTEM

Figure 12.1 is divided into two sections: the first is for face mask detection training, and the second is to apply face mask detection. The first section has three significant scenarios, and the dataset is loaded using PyTorch in the Google Colab platform. Later, the number of images is adjusted to train the model, and these face mask images are prepared using TensorFlow or Keras. The serialization of the face mask classified to the disk is done at the end of the first section. The second section is for classifying the face mask images from the disk. After classification, the faces are detected from the real-time video stream. The image processing libraries are imported into the platform to perform the image segmentation, augmentation, and resizing tasks. After the face detection, the model will evaluate the data and determine whether there is a mask or no mask in the image. After the block diagram analysis, this chapter presents a deep learning model that automatically monitors whether people wear masks or not in public. In Figure 12.1, the drawn architecture shows how the proposed technology prevents COVID-19 from spreading.

The TensorFlow and Keras algorithms and a CNN model are used in our system to assess whether someone is wearing a face mask. We'll start by training the system with the Kaggle Dataset, Keras, and TensorFlow, then load the face mask classifier

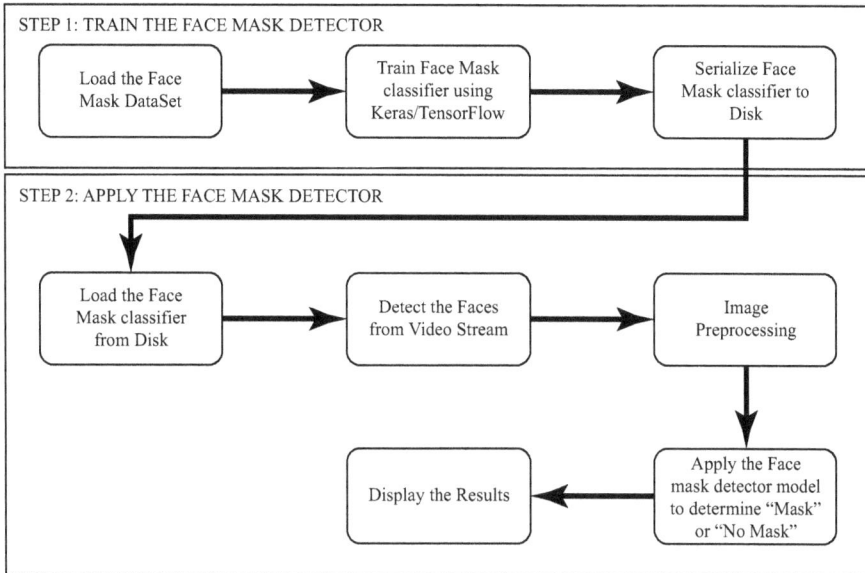

FIGURE 12.1 Architecture for face mask detection.

from the disc, recognizing faces in real-time video. In addition, MobileNet is utilized for training many images and categorizing high-quality photos in this operation. Keras is used to load the image dataset, and the photographs are then turned into an array. The input picture is preprocessed and appended to the data list using MobileNet. Personal face identification and face mask detection are the key contributions of the proposed system. MobileNet and OpenCV are used to do both of these tasks in real time. A square box with red and green is displayed on each individual's face, with red indicating the absence of a mask and green indicating the presence of a mask.

We offer an automated temperature scanner and face mask-detecting entrance provider system. In this system, a contactless temperature scanner and a mask monitor are employed. Without a temperature and mask scan, a person will be denied access. Only those who meet both criteria are permitted to enter. The system utilizes a temperature sensor and a camera connected to a Raspberry Pi system that controls everything. If the system identifies a person as having a high temperature or not wearing a mask, it sounds a buzzer and prevents them from entering. Figure 12.2 shows the architecture of the Raspberry automation system. Figure 12.2 shows the hardware used in the automated system. The components include the camera, power supply, battery, motor, and different sensors. In this system, Camera Module 3 with 12 megapixels is used; the temperature sensors DHT22 and BME280 are used in the system for accurate readings. This hardware kit works in the −45 degrees to +85 degrees temperature range, so the external power supply is between 0 and 15 volts maximum. The face detection codes are dumped into the Raspberry Pi integrated

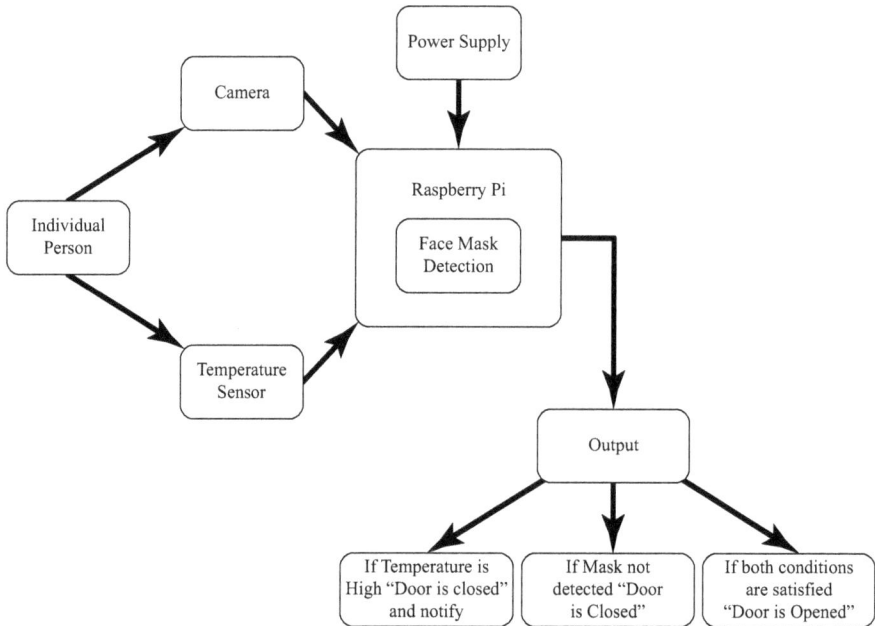

FIGURE 12.2   The architecture of the Raspberry automation system.

circuit, so the kit generates the output after the image analysis. The scenario is classified into three parts. The first part depends on temperature sensor values. If the value of DHT22 is very high, the automated system door is closed and authorities are notified.

Similarly, if a mask is undetected, the door is automatically closed and won't allow the user to enter the premises. In the third condition, if the temperature sensor DHT22 value is within the limits and a mask is detected, the door is opened for the person to enter the premises. The sequence of steps is shown in Figure 12.2.

12.3 METHODOLOGY

12.3.1 DATASET

Masks play a crucial role in protecting the health of individuals against respiratory diseases, and masks were one of the few precautions available for COVID-19 in the absence of immunization. With this dataset, it is possible to create a model to detect people wearing masks, not wearing masks, or wearing masks improperly. We used the dataset comprised of two folders – with and without face mask images – from Prajna Bhandary's GitHub account [18]. The face images were comprised of diverse skin colors, various angles, different occlusions, etc. Figure 12.3 and Figure 12.4 show the sample images in the two folders in the dataset. The size of the dataset is 2.0 GB, and the folder consists of 3,584 images out of which 1,792 images are from

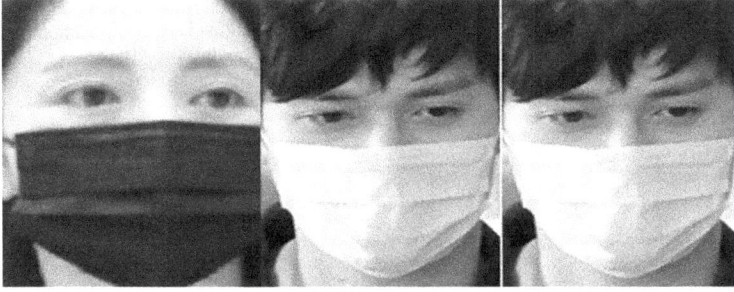

FIGURE 12.3 Images in the with mask folder.

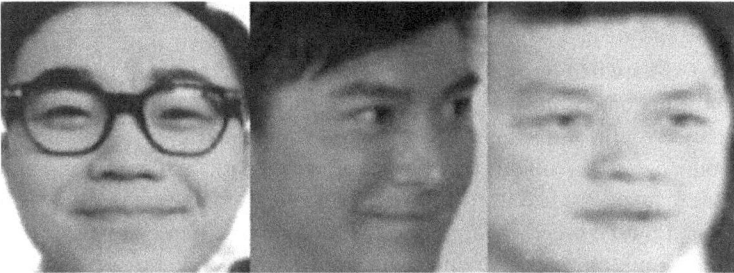

FIGURE 12.4 Images in the without mask folder.

the with mask folder and the remaining 1,792 images are from the without mask folder.

12.3.2 CONVOLUTIONAL NEURAL NETWORK

A CNN is an artificial neural network commonly used for image recognition, computer vision, and natural language processing tasks. In a CNN, the input is typically an image, and the network uses convolutional layers to extract features from the image. Convolutional layers consist of a set of learnable filters that slide over the input image to detect patterns in local regions. The outputs of these filters are then passed through activation functions and pooling layers, which reduce the spatial dimensions of the feature maps. The resulting feature maps are then passed through one or more fully connected layers, which perform classification or regression tasks based on the extracted features. In the case of image classification, the final layer usually outputs a probability distribution over the different classes of objects that the network has been trained to recognize. CNNs are highly effective at image recognition tasks because they can learn hierarchical representations of visual features, which can capture complex patterns in images. They have been used in various applications, including medical image analysis and natural language processing. Figure 12.5 shows the architecture of a CNN.

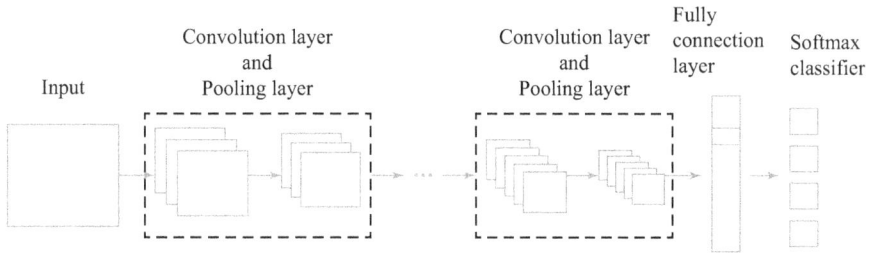

FIGURE 12.5   The architecture of CNN.

In this model, each input image will undergo a series of convolutional layers with filters, pooling, and contour steps involved in the CNN model. The convolutional layer extracts the features from the input image. It operates on an image matrix and filter, which results in feature gaps. In the pooling layer, the parameters are reduced. The matrix is flattened into a vector and sent to a fully connected layer as input. An activation function categorizes the images. The deep learning method uses matrix multiplication for the implementation of neural networks. Here CNN uses a convolution operator, which combines two functions in the mathematical formula to generate the other function. The third function expresses how the shape of one function is redesigned by the other. In simple words, two images that can be represented as matrices are multiplied to give an output used to extract features from the image. A CNN belongs to artificial neurons dependent on mathematical function and is composed of multiple layers. The activation map uses the transitory image method through a convolutional layer. The image recognition software is also called a CNN. There are two main parts in a CNN architecture:

- A convolution tool that identifies and separates the various types of features in the image to analyze the process is called feature extraction.
- A fully connected layer that utilizes the convolution process's output predicts the image's class based on the features eliminated in previous stages.

The most crucial advantage of a CNN compared to its previous versions of deep learning is that it automatically detects significant features without any human administration. The main drawback of a CNN is the inability to be spatially invariant to the input data.

12.3.2.1 MobileNetV2 Model

MobileNetV2 is a CNN architecture designed for mobile and embedded devices. It was introduced in 2018 by researchers at Google in their paper "MobileNetV2: Inverted Residuals and Linear Bottlenecks." MobileNetV2 improves upon the original MobileNet architecture by introducing two new key features: inverted residuals and linear bottlenecks. Inverted residuals are residual connections with a twist: instead of adding the input to the output, the input is first expanded to a higher-dimensional space using a 1×1 convolutional layer, then processed by a depthwise convolutional layer, and finally projected back down to a lower-dimensional space using another 1×1 convolutional layer. This design allows for more efficient use of computation resources by reducing the number of parameters while increasing the expressivity of the network. Overall, MobileNetV2 achieves state-of-the-art accuracy on several image classification benchmarks while maintaining a small model size and low computational requirements, making it well-suited for deployment on mobile and embedded devices, as shown in Figure 12.6.

12.3.2.2 Xception Model

Xception is a CNN architecture developed by Google researchers in 2016. It is a variation of the Inception architecture, which was introduced earlier. The name "Xception" stands for "extreme Inception," and it was designed to improve upon the Inception architecture by using depthwise separable convolutions, which are more computationally efficient than the standard convolutions used in previous architectures. Depthwise separable convolutions are composed of two steps: a depthwise convolution that filters each input channel separately, and a pointwise convolution that combines the filtered outputs from the depthwise convolution. This approach significantly reduces the number of parameters needed to train the model, while maintaining its accuracy. The Xception architecture consists of 36 convolutional layers and several skip connections. It has been used for various computer vision tasks, such as image classification, object detection, and semantic segmentation, and has achieved state-of-the-art results on several benchmarks. Overall, Xception is an effective and efficient neural network architecture that has been widely adopted in the computer vision community, as shown in Figure 12.7.

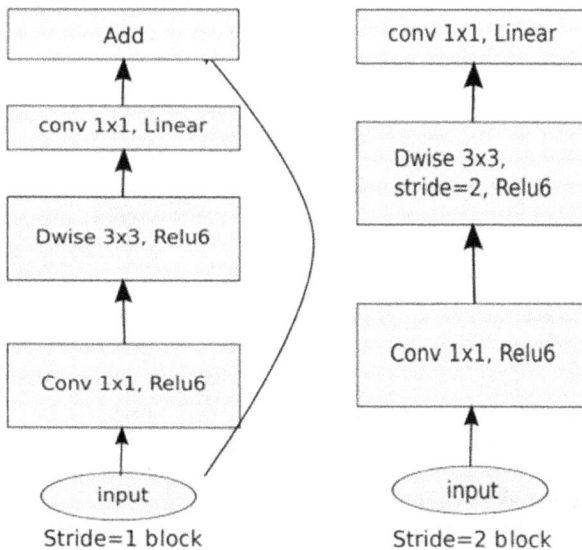

FIGURE 12.6 MobileNetV2 architecture.

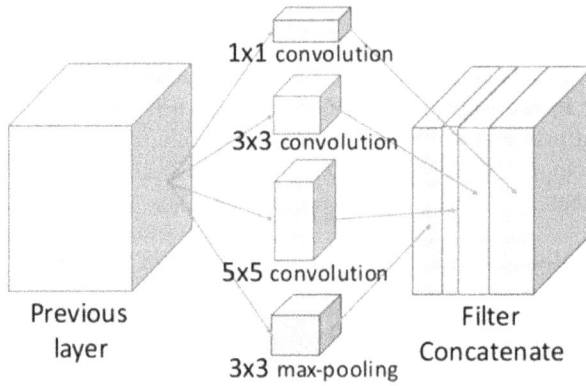

FIGURE 12.7   Xception architecture.

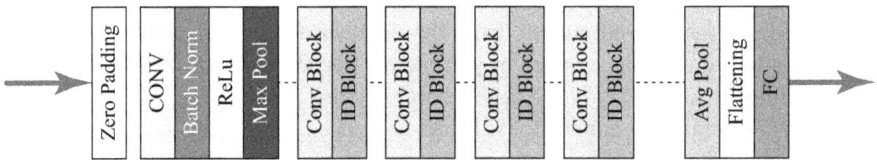

FIGURE 12.8   ResNet50 architecture.

12.3.2.3   ResNet50 Model

ResNet50 is a deep neural network model that belongs to a family of models called ResNets (residual networks). It was developed by Microsoft Research Asia and is used for image classification and object detection tasks. ResNet50 consists of 50 layers of neural networks, including convolutional layers, batch normalization layers, activation layers, and fully connected layers. The key innovation in ResNet50 is the use of residual connections, which allows the model to bypass some layers and directly connect the input to the output of the later layers. This helps in preventing the vanishing gradient problem, where the gradients become too small to update the weights in the earlier layers. The architecture of ResNet50 has several blocks, each containing convolutional layers followed by batch normalization, activation, and residual connections. The output of each block is then passed on to the next block, and the network's final output is passed through a softmax layer to generate predictions. ResNet50 has achieved state-of-the-art performance on several image classification benchmarks, including the ImageNet dataset, and is widely used in various computer vision applications, as shown in Figure 12.8.

12.3.2.4   InceptionV3 Model

InceptionV3 is a deep CNN architecture that was introduced by Google in 2015. It is one of the models in the Inception family of models, which are designed to be efficient in terms of computational resources while maintaining high accuracy

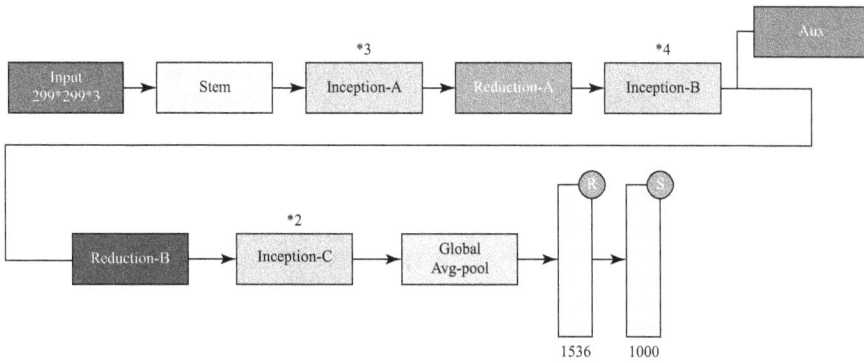

FIGURE 12.9   InceptionV3 architecture.

on large-scale image classification tasks. The InceptionV3 model consists of multiple layers of convolutional, pooling, and activation functions, followed by fully connected layers for classification. One of the key features of InceptionV3 is the use of "Inception modules", which are designed to perform parallel convolutions at different scales and combine the results computationally efficiently. In addition to image classification, InceptionV3 can be used for other computer vision tasks, such as object detection and image segmentation. It has been trained in large-scale image datasets such as ImageNet and has achieved high accuracy on these datasets. Overall, InceptionV3 is a powerful deep learning model that has been widely used in various computer vision applications, as shown in Figure 12.9.

12.3.2.5   VGG16 Model

VGG16 is a CNN architecture proposed by the Visual Geometry Group (VGG) at the University of Oxford in 2014. The VGG16 model is composed of 16 layers, including 13 convolutional layers and 3 fully connected layers. The architecture of VGG16 is characterized by using small convolutional filters (3×3) with a stride of 1 pixel and a max-pooling layer with a stride of 2 pixels. This simple design enables the VGG16 model to learn very deep representations of images. The VGG16 model was trained on the ImageNet dataset, containing over 1.2 million labeled images from 1,000 object categories. The VGG16 model achieved state-of-the-art performance on the ImageNet classification task, achieving a top-5 error rate of 7.32%. The VGG16 model is widely used in computer vision applications, such as object recognition, object detection, and image segmentation. The model is also frequently used as a starting point for transfer learning, where the pretrained VGG16 weights are used to initialize the weights of a new model trained on a different dataset, as shown in Figure 12.10.

12.4   RESULTS

In this section, the performance analysis of the proposed architecture is done based on the applied variables; the accuracy of CNN, InceptionV3, MobileNetV2,

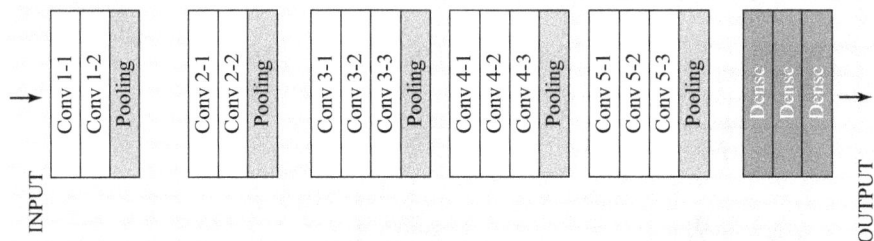

FIGURE 12.10 VGG16 architecture.

```
Epoch 15/20
89/89 [==============================] - 36s 406ms/step - loss: 0.0281 - accuracy: 0.9908 - val_loss: 0.0325 - val_accuracy: 0.9888
Epoch 16/20
89/89 [==============================] - 36s 401ms/step - loss: 0.0381 - accuracy: 0.9884 - val_loss: 0.0321 - val_accuracy: 0.9874
Epoch 17/20
89/89 [==============================] - 36s 403ms/step - loss: 0.0335 - accuracy: 0.9884 - val_loss: 0.0310 - val_accuracy: 0.9888
Epoch 18/20
89/89 [==============================] - 36s 403ms/step - loss: 0.0286 - accuracy: 0.9908 - val_loss: 0.0384 - val_accuracy: 0.9833
Epoch 19/20
89/89 [==============================] - 36s 405ms/step - loss: 0.0259 - accuracy: 0.9933 - val_loss: 0.0300 - val_accuracy: 0.9916
Epoch 20/20
89/89 [==============================] - 36s 405ms/step - loss: 0.0253 - accuracy: 0.9929 - val_loss: 0.0271 - val_accuracy: 0.9888
[INFO] evaluating network...
              precision    recall  f1-score   support

   with_mask       0.99      0.99      0.99       358
without_mask       0.99      0.99      0.99       359

    accuracy                           0.99       717
   macro avg       0.99      0.99      0.99       717
weighted avg       0.99      0.99      0.99       717
```

FIGURE 12.11 MobileNetV2 model accuracy and loss results.

ResNet50, Xception, and VGG16 are done in the algorithms. These values are compared with the other algorithms as well. For the close investigation of the results, the sensitivity, accuracy, and specificity were obtained for each method. Other terms that describe these parameters are true positive, true negative, false positive, and false negative. The total number of subjects with positive tests, subjects with negative tests, and subjects of the study were used to compute the confusion matrix and accuracy of different approaches.

12.4.1 MobileNetV2 Model

MobileNetV1 is comprised of two layers. The first layer is depthwise convolution; it uses lightweight filtering with a single convolutional filter per input channel. The second layer is pointwise convolution; it's responsible for building new features using a linear combination of input channels. The activation function ReLU6 is used in MobileNetV1. MobileNetV2 consists of two blocks. The first block is the residual block with a stride of 1, and the second residual block is for downsizing with a stride of 2. This algorithm has three layers for both types of blocks. The first layer is 1×1 convolution, the second layer is depthwise convolution, and the third layer is another 1×1 convolution without any linearity in it. Figure 12.11 shows the iterations in the

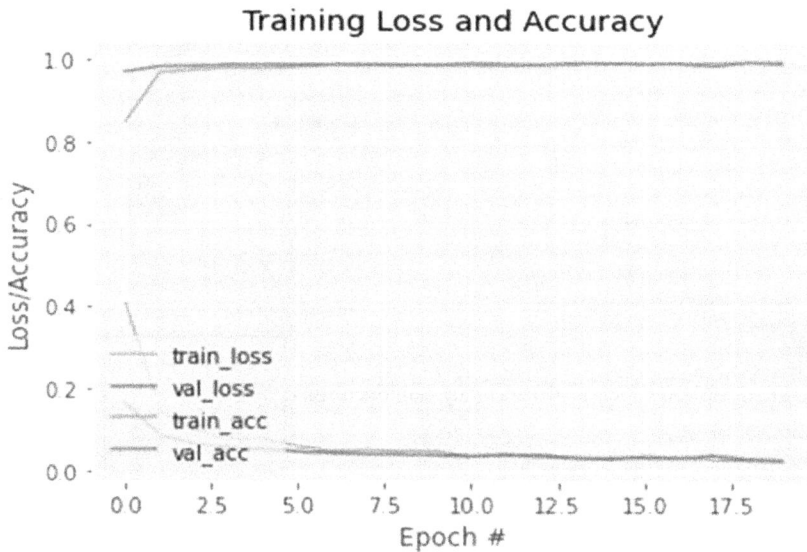

FIGURE 12.12 Plot for training loss and accuracy for MobileNetV2.

evaluating network based on the number of epochs. The training accuracy and testing accuracy are calculated, based on the confusion matrix values. The datasets of images with a mask and without a mask are calculated. The precision values are 0.99, the recall value is 0.99, the F1 score is 0.99, the support is 358 for with mask, and 717 for accuracy.

Figure 12.11 shows the Python code screenshot with metric performance evaluation, and Figure 12.12 shows the plot between the loss/accuracy and epochs. The number of epochs is shown in the x-axis between 0 to 20, on a scale of 2.5. MobileNetV2 outperforms MobileNetV1 and ShuffleNet (1.5) with comparable model sizes and computational costs. With a width multiplier of 1.4, MobileNetV2 (1.4) outperforms ShuffleNet (×2) and NASNet with faster inference time.

12.4.2 XCEPTION MODEL

The Xception model performance metrics are evaluated based on epochs, depthwise separable convolution, and shortcuts between convolution blocks as in ResNet, and this architecture has efficient architecture. Figure 12.13 shows the Python code screenshot with metric performance evaluation, and12.14 Figure 12.14 shows the plot between epoch and loss/accuracy for the Xception model. The accuracy lies between 90% and 97% based on the epoch's values.

12.4.3 VGG16 MODEL

The convolutional neural network, also called ConvNet, is a form of an artificial neural network (ANN). This network has input, output, and hidden layers. VGG16 is also a

```
Epoch 15/20
89/89 [==============================] - 50s 563ms/step - loss: 0.0238 - accuracy: 0.9922 - val_loss: 0.0286 - val_accuracy: 0.9874
Epoch 16/20
89/89 [==============================] - 50s 563ms/step - loss: 0.0243 - accuracy: 0.9933 - val_loss: 0.0295 - val_accuracy: 0.9888
Epoch 17/20
89/89 [==============================] - 50s 564ms/step - loss: 0.0214 - accuracy: 0.9933 - val_loss: 0.0278 - val_accuracy: 0.9874
Epoch 18/20
89/89 [==============================] - 50s 563ms/step - loss: 0.0251 - accuracy: 0.9926 - val_loss: 0.0269 - val_accuracy: 0.9874
Epoch 19/20
89/89 [==============================] - 50s 561ms/step - loss: 0.0211 - accuracy: 0.9944 - val_loss: 0.0241 - val_accuracy: 0.9902
Epoch 20/20
89/89 [==============================] - 50s 562ms/step - loss: 0.0222 - accuracy: 0.9951 - val_loss: 0.0241 - val_accuracy: 0.9902
[INFO] evaluating network...
              precision    recall  f1-score   support

  with_mask        0.99      0.99      0.99       358
without_mask        0.99      0.99      0.99       359

    accuracy                           0.99       717
   macro avg        0.99      0.99      0.99       717
weighted avg        0.99      0.99      0.99       717
```

FIGURE 12.13   Xception model accuracy and loss results.

```
Epoch 15/20
89/89 [==============================] - 47s 526ms/step - loss: 0.1688 - accuracy: 0.9538 - val_loss: 0.1162 - val_accuracy: 0.9721
Epoch 16/20
89/89 [==============================] - 47s 528ms/step - loss: 0.1644 - accuracy: 0.9570 - val_loss: 0.1169 - val_accuracy: 0.9679
Epoch 17/20
89/89 [==============================] - 48s 539ms/step - loss: 0.1573 - accuracy: 0.9556 - val_loss: 0.1076 - val_accuracy: 0.9721
Epoch 18/20
89/89 [==============================] - 47s 532ms/step - loss: 0.1531 - accuracy: 0.9531 - val_loss: 0.1032 - val_accuracy: 0.9735
Epoch 19/20
89/89 [==============================] - 49s 545ms/step - loss: 0.1461 - accuracy: 0.9559 - val_loss: 0.0996 - val_accuracy: 0.9749
Epoch 20/20
89/89 [==============================] - 47s 527ms/step - loss: 0.1358 - accuracy: 0.9637 - val_loss: 0.0961 - val_accuracy: 0.9749
[INFO] evaluating network...
              precision    recall  f1-score   support

  with_mask        0.98      0.97      0.97       358
without_mask        0.97      0.98      0.97       359

    accuracy                           0.97       717
   macro avg        0.97      0.97      0.97       717
weighted avg        0.97      0.97      0.97       717
```

FIGURE 12.14   Screenshot of training loss and accuracy for the Xception model.

family of CNNs mostly used for computer vision models. Researchers from Oxford University evaluated the network based on depth with 3×3 convolution filters. They pushed the depth to 19 weight layers, making it approximately 138 trainable parameters. Figure 12.15 shows the Python code along with screenshots that show that the number of epochs plays a major role in accuracy calculation. Figure 12.16 shows the response for training loss and testing accuracy in VGG16. The number of epochs is changed in the interval of 2.5 times. The training loss decreases when the number of epochs increases. The validation loss also decreases at the same time. The training accuracy increases when the number of epochs increases. At 2.5 epochs, the accuracy is 60%. Similarly, the accuracy remains at saturation when the number of epochs reaches above 20. The original VGG model was trained for two to three weeks.

12.4.4   INCEPTIONV3 MODEL

The multiple deep layers of convolution operations are used in InceptionV3 models. The model suffers from overfitting of the data. Inception V1 uses multiple filters

```
Epoch 15/20
89/89 [==============================] - 47s 526ms/step - loss: 0.1688 - accuracy: 0.9538 - val_loss: 0.1162 - val_accuracy: 0.9721
Epoch 16/20
89/89 [==============================] - 47s 528ms/step - loss: 0.1644 - accuracy: 0.9570 - val_loss: 0.1169 - val_accuracy: 0.9679
Epoch 17/20
89/89 [==============================] - 48s 539ms/step - loss: 0.1573 - accuracy: 0.9556 - val_loss: 0.1076 - val_accuracy: 0.9721
Epoch 18/20
89/89 [==============================] - 47s 532ms/step - loss: 0.1531 - accuracy: 0.9531 - val_loss: 0.1032 - val_accuracy: 0.9735
Epoch 19/20
89/89 [==============================] - 49s 545ms/step - loss: 0.1461 - accuracy: 0.9559 - val_loss: 0.0996 - val_accuracy: 0.9749
Epoch 20/20
89/89 [==============================] - 47s 527ms/step - loss: 0.1358 - accuracy: 0.9637 - val_loss: 0.0961 - val_accuracy: 0.9749
[INFO] evaluating network...
              precision   recall  f1-score   support

   with_mask       0.98     0.97      0.97       358
without_mask       0.97     0.98      0.97       359

    accuracy                          0.97       717
   macro avg       0.97     0.97      0.97       717
weighted avg       0.97     0.97      0.97       717
```

FIGURE 12.15   VGG16 model accuracy and loss results.

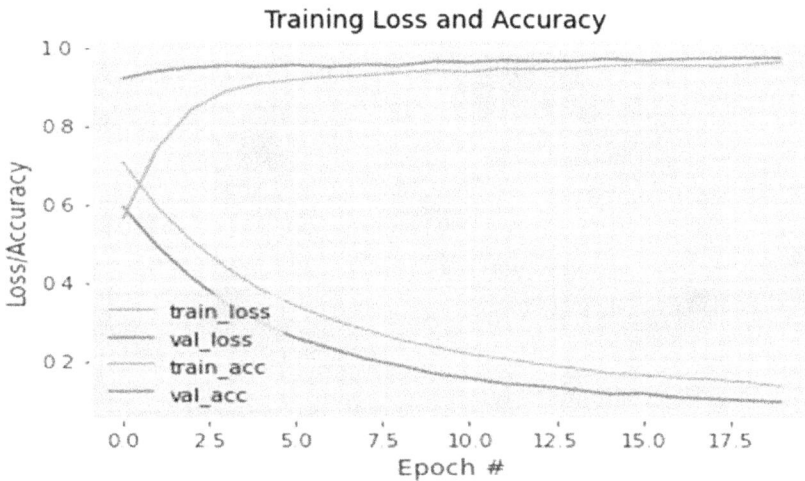

FIGURE 12.16   Plot for training loss and accuracy for VGG16.

of various sizes on the same level. Instead of deep layers, parallel layers are used in this model to make it deeper. InceptionV3 is the most advanced version of the InceptionV1 model. It uses several methods for optimizing the network for better adaption, has higher efficiency, has a deeper network compared to the InceptionV1 and V2 models, is less expensive, and uses auxiliary classifiers [19].

Figure 12.17 shows the Python code along with screenshots that show that the number of epochs plays a major role in accuracy calculation. The training loss and accuracy are shown in Figure 12.18. This model provides accuracy near 95% for 5-plus epochs. Even after increasing the number of epochs from 5 to 20, the accuracy remains constant.

```
Epoch 15/20
89/89 [==============================] - 38s 427ms/step - loss: 0.0369 - accuracy: 0.9905 - val_loss: 0.0125 - val_accuracy: 0.9958
Epoch 16/20
89/89 [==============================] - 38s 427ms/step - loss: 0.0313 - accuracy: 0.9898 - val_loss: 0.0062 - val_accuracy: 0.9972
Epoch 17/20
89/89 [==============================] - 38s 425ms/step - loss: 0.0280 - accuracy: 0.9905 - val_loss: 0.0096 - val_accuracy: 0.9958
Epoch 18/20
89/89 [==============================] - 38s 427ms/step - loss: 0.0215 - accuracy: 0.9940 - val_loss: 0.0161 - val_accuracy: 0.9944
Epoch 19/20
89/89 [==============================] - 39s 443ms/step - loss: 0.0304 - accuracy: 0.9894 - val_loss: 0.0159 - val_accuracy: 0.9930
Epoch 20/20
89/89 [==============================] - 38s 427ms/step - loss: 0.0254 - accuracy: 0.9908 - val_loss: 0.0071 - val_accuracy: 0.9958
[INFO] evaluating network...
              precision    recall  f1-score   support

   with_mask       1.00      0.99      1.00       358
without_mask       0.99      1.00      1.00       359

    accuracy                           1.00       717
   macro avg       1.00      1.00      1.00       717
weighted avg       1.00      1.00      1.00       717
```

FIGURE 12.17   InceptionV3 model accuracy and loss results.

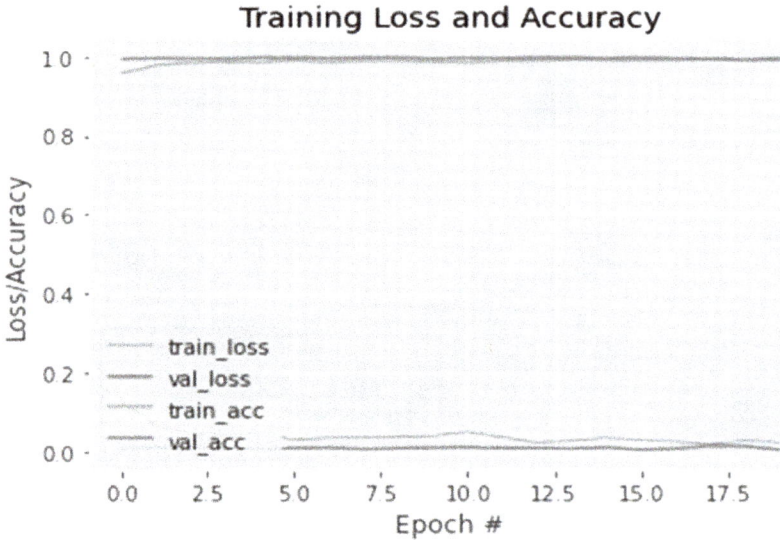

FIGURE 12.18   Plot for training loss and accuracy for InceptionV3.

12.4.5   RESNET50 MODEL

ResNet50 is a CNN that is 50 layers deep. The pretrained version of the network is trained on the database. The network learns rich feature representations of the wide range of mask images. Figure 12.19 shows the ResNet50 accuracy and loss results based on the number of epochs. Figure 12.20 shows the loss and accuracy between epochs. The training loss decreases based on the number of epochs, and the accuracy increases slightly based on the number of epochs.

```
Epoch 15/20
89/89 [==============================] - 47s 532ms/step - loss: 0.5399 - accuracy: 0.7584 - val_loss: 0.4706 - val_accuracy: 0.8312
Epoch 16/20
89/89 [==============================] - 48s 534ms/step - loss: 0.5220 - accuracy: 0.7757 - val_loss: 0.4600 - val_accuracy: 0.8424
Epoch 17/20
89/89 [==============================] - 47s 532ms/step - loss: 0.5264 - accuracy: 0.7658 - val_loss: 0.4564 - val_accuracy: 0.8480
Epoch 18/20
89/89 [==============================] - 46s 512ms/step - loss: 0.5193 - accuracy: 0.7675 - val_loss: 0.4478 - val_accuracy: 0.8410
Epoch 19/20
89/89 [==============================] - 45s 507ms/step - loss: 0.5165 - accuracy: 0.7728 - val_loss: 0.4453 - val_accuracy: 0.8312
Epoch 20/20
89/89 [==============================] - 45s 507ms/step - loss: 0.5144 - accuracy: 0.7665 - val_loss: 0.4373 - val_accuracy: 0.8842
[INFO] evaluating network...
              precision    recall  f1-score   support

   with_mask       0.87      0.90      0.89       358
without_mask       0.90      0.87      0.88       359

    accuracy                           0.88       717
   macro avg       0.88      0.88      0.88       717
weighted avg       0.88      0.88      0.88       717
```

FIGURE 12.19 ResNet50 model accuracy and loss results.

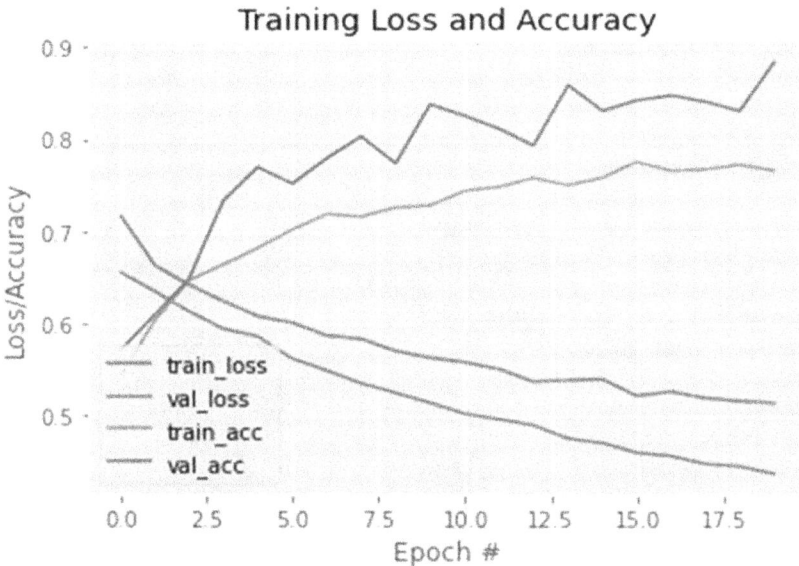

FIGURE 12.20 Plot for training loss and accuracy for ResNet50 model.

Table 12.2 shows the comparison results of various deep learning methods. The comparison is based on a facial mask conducted on Raspberry Pi hardware components. Based on the confusion matrix and average accuracies, InceptionV3 has better accuracy than MobileNetV2. Based on 20 epochs, the InceptionV3 model has an accuracy of 98%, and MobileNet has an accuracy of 96% in 100 epochs. Still, as the training performance of InceptionV3 increases, it can be improved further if we run the training for more epochs. Table 12.3 shows the comparative result analysis of

TABLE 12.2
Accuracy results obtained for various algorithms

Model	Accuracy	Precision	Recall	F1 score
InceptionV3	98.29%	0.98	0.99	0.99
MobileNetV2	97.08%	0.96	0.96	0.98
ResNet50	88.78%	0.87	0.90	0.89
Xception	95.51%	0.98	0.97	0.97
VGG16	95.37%	0.97	0.97	0.98

TABLE 12.3
Comparative analysis with the conventional systems

Reference	Dataset	Algorithm	Accuracy (%)	Comparison
Rahman et al. 2020 [20]	Kaggle 1,539 images	CNN architecture	98.7%	Difficulties in classifying faces covered by hands since it almost looks like the person wearing a mask
Das et al. 2020 [21]	Kaggle 8,538 images	CNN architecture	94.58%	Indistinct moving faces in the video stream make it more difficult
Sakshi et al. 2021 [22]	Kaggle and random images	MobileNetV2	98.9%	Difficulty in identifying mask if there are multiple faces
Suresh et al. 2021 [23]	Kaggle 3,918 images	MobileNetV2	98%	Uses a custom dataset with applied mask images
Adusumalli et al. 2021 [24]	Kaggle 3,835 images	MobileNetV2	98%	Difficulty in identifying mask if there are multiple faces
Islam et al. 2020 [25]	1,300 images	CNN architecture	97%	Used fewer datasets and only CNN is used
Sanjaya et al. 2020 [26]	Kaggle and RMFD 3,846 Images	MobileNetV2	96.85%	Fewer convolution layers and less accuracy
Negi et al. 2021 [27]	Kaggle 1,315 images	VGG16	98.59%	Used fewer datasets and applied masks on images
Proposed system	**Kaggle dataset from GitHub repository of 3,584 images**	**InceptionV3, MobilNetV2**	**98.29%, 97.08%**	**No difficulty in identifying the face even if multiple masks are present; higher number of images for training and testing; high convolution less with maximum accuracy**

the various articles published in the past three years. The proposed model has more advantages than the conventional methods, as explained in Table 12.3.

12.4.6 Mask Detection Results

Figure 12.21 shows the components connected using Raspberry Pi. An LCD board is connected to the corresponding PIN configuration. The infrared sensor and temperature sensor are also connected to the PIN configuration. The camera, motor, and other components are connected to the microcontroller circuit with the PIN configuration. The figure shows the hardware used in the automated system. This system uses Camera Module 3 with 12 megapixels. The DHT22 and BME280 temperature sensors are used in the system for accurate readings. This hardware kit works in the −45 degrees to +85 degrees temperature range, so the external power supply is between 0 and 15 volts maximum. The face detection codes are dumped into the Raspberry Pi IC, so the kit generates the output after the image analysis. The scenario is classified into three parts. The first part depends on temperature sensor values. If the value of DHT22 is very high, the automated system door is closed and the authorities are notified. Similarly, if a mask is undetected, the door is automatically closed and won't allow the person to enter the premises. In the third condition, if the temperature sensor DHT22 value is within limits and if a mask is properly detected, then the door is opened for the person to enter the premises.

Figure 12.22 is divided into three parts. Figure 12.22a is the deep learning method classification based on the camera. The user is wearing the mask properly. The InceptionV3 method runs the problem and generates the mask detection output. Figure 12.22b shows the user is wearing a mask, but is not wearing it properly. The algorithm detects that a mask is not present. Figure 12.22c shows the user not wearing a mask at all, so the algorithm detects no mask.

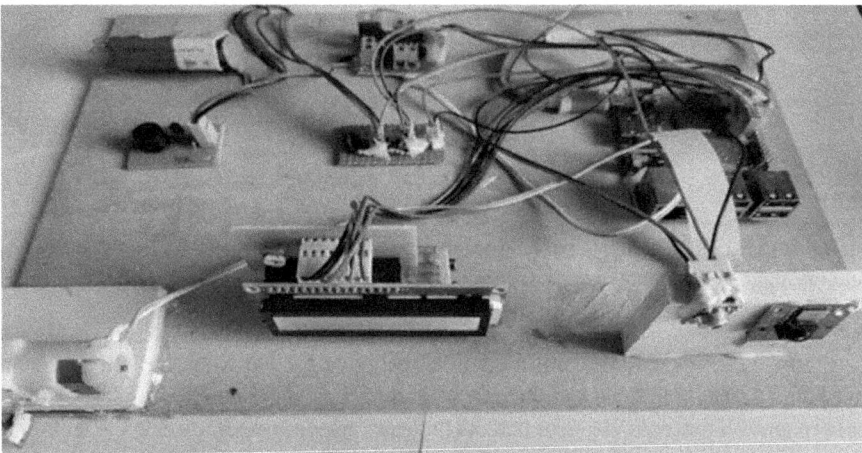

FIGURE 12.21 Project front view of hardware components.

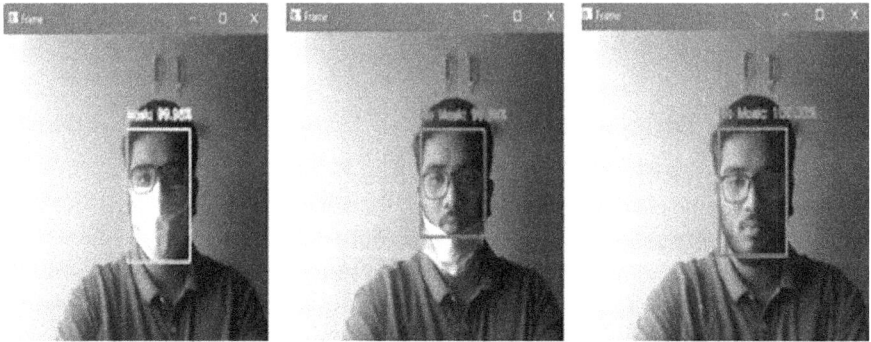

FIGURE 12.22   (a) Result obtained on camera for mask detection. (b) Result obtained on camera when the mask is not adequately worn. (c) Result obtained on camera when there is no mask.

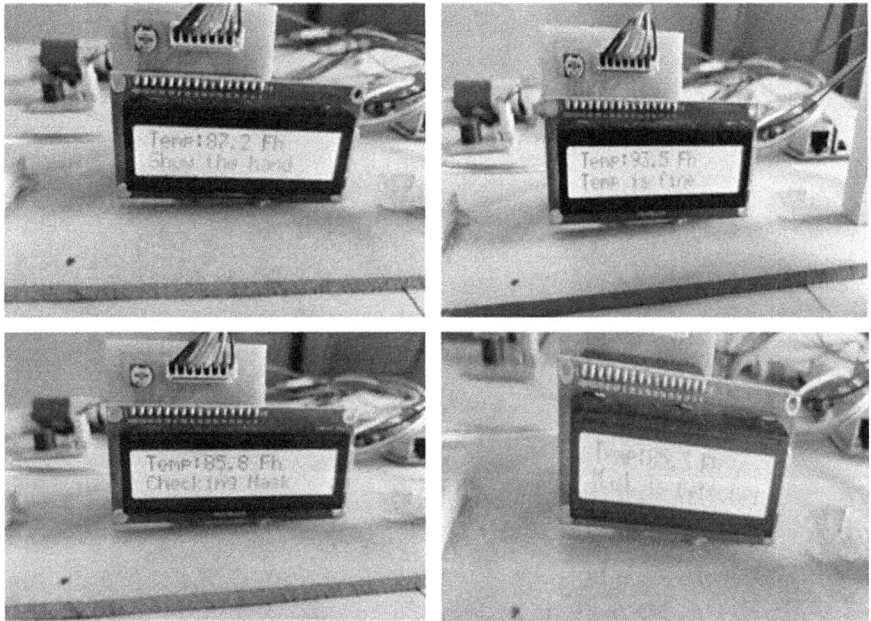

FIGURE 12.23   (a) Detecting the temperature by asking to show the hand. (b) If the temperature is in the normal human body range. (c) Checking for a mask. (d) If a mask is detected.

Figure 12.23 shows the scenario that happened in the hardware circuit. The scan mask entry system first checks the user's hands to check the temperature. The medical sensor or temperature sensor detects the entry user's temperature. If the temperature is below 93°F, the gate is not opened; if the temperature is above 93°F, then the camera checks for a mask. The algorithm checks the user's face and identifies the

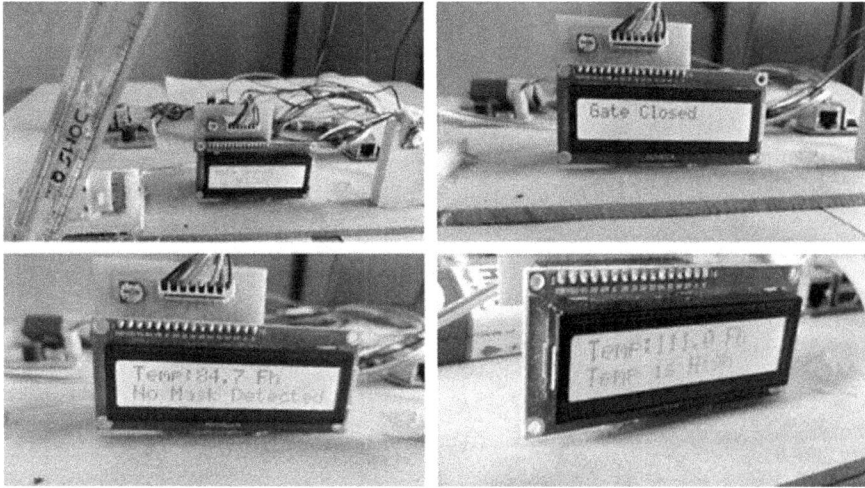

FIGURE 12.24 (a) When a mask is detected, the gate will open. (b) After some time, the gate will close. (c) When no mask is detected. (d) When a high temperature is detected.

facial mask. The InceptionV3 model identifies the mask and generates the accuracy. The corresponding scenarios are shown in Figure 12.23.

The entry system is connected to the motor, where the generated results are programmed to the motor section in Raspberry Pi. The gate closes or opens based on the case. The gate is closed when the temperature is too high, the same way as if the temperature is low. If a mask is detected, the gate opens. The corresponding scenarios are shown in Figure 12.24.

The visual studio is used in this project for execution and debugging unit tests in the hardware components. This includes the project templates and frameworks with multiple platforms to work with. The unit testing runs all the units in the background and shows the code coverage live, as shown in Figure 12.25. It uses a single window to organize the run, debug the tests, and configure the data after every build.

The Proteus Design Suite is the proprietary software tool suite used primarily for electronic design automation. It's one of the Windows applications for schematic capture and printed circuit board. In this project, the hardware is designed by selecting the hats or breakout boards from the gallery. Control of the program can be done using Python script. The entire project is simulated in Proteus with debugging tools. Figure 12.26 shows the simulated result with a mask detected with high accuracy, and Figure 12.27 shows the simulated result with no mask detected.

12.5 CONCLUSION AND FUTURE SCOPE

In this research, we designed a deep learning model using the MobileNetV2 algorithm, which gave us an accuracy of 98.29%, which is better than other results and efficiently works for detecting masks. We have chosen MobileNetV2 and

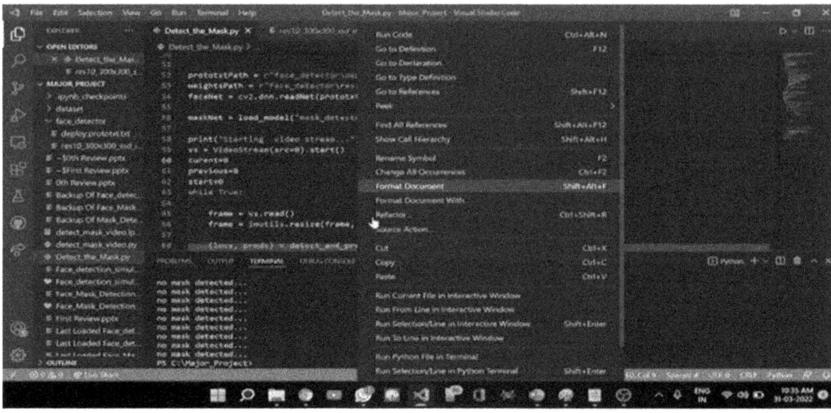

FIGURE 12.25   Visual studio output for the automated system project.

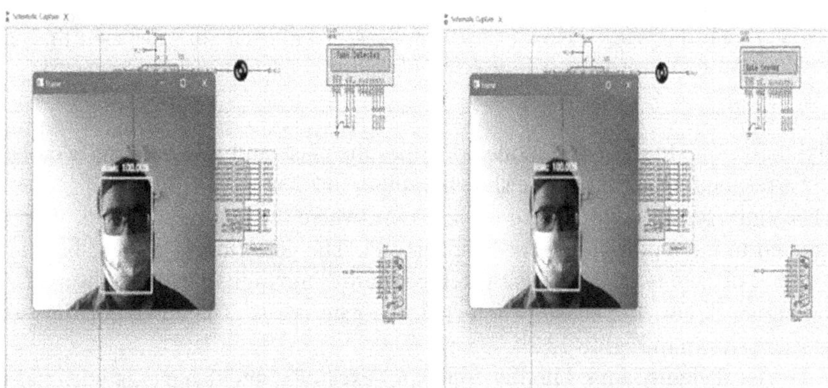

FIGURE 12.26   Proteus Design Suite simulated output for mask detection.

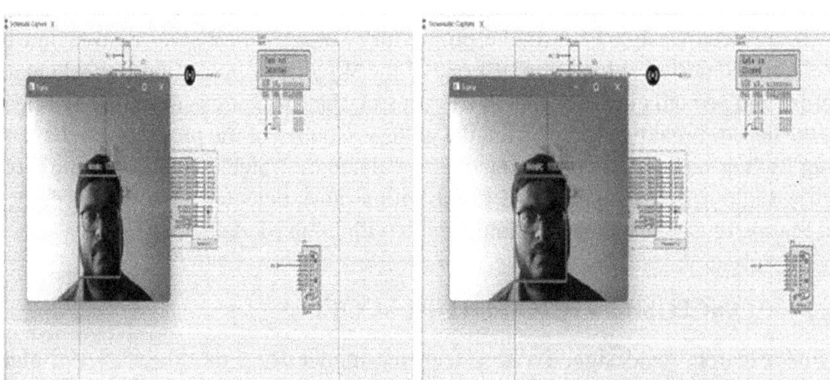

FIGURE 12.27   Proteus Design Suite simulated output for without mask detection.

InceptionV3 other than Xception, which have better accuracy because InceptionV3 and MobileNetV2 perform well in embedded systems and have low latency results. It is necessary to check body temperature and whether a person is wearing a mask to avoid the spread of COVID-19. So, to achieve this, we have designed this automation system. We dumped the code into the Raspberry Pi, which efficiently detects a mask. Continuous temperature and mask scan monitoring is done using the temperature sensor. The entry system will open if the person is wearing a mask and has a normal body temperature.

REFERENCES

1. M. M. Rahman, M. M. H. Manik, M. M. Islam, S. Mahmud, and J.-H. Kim, "An Automated System to Limit COVID-19 Using Facial Mask Detection in Smart City Network," in *IEEE International IOT, Electronics and Mechatronics Conference (IEMTRONICS)*, 2020, pp. 1–5, doi: 10.1109/IEMTRONICS51293.2020.9216386.
2. A. Das, M. Wasif Ansari and R. Basak, "Covid-19 Face Mask Detection Using TensorFlow, Keras and OpenCV," in *IEEE 17th India Council International Conference (INDICON)*, 2020, pp. 1–5, doi: 10.1109/INDICON49873.2020.9342585.
3. S. Sakshi, A. K. Gupta, S. Singh Yadav, and U. Kumar, "Face Mask Detection System using CNN," in *International Conference on Advance Computing and Innovative Technologies in Engineering (ICACITE)*, 2021, pp. 212–216, doi: 10.1109/ICACITE51222.2021.9404731.
4. K. Suresh, M. Palangappa, and S. Bhuvan, "Face Mask Detection by using Optimistic Convolutional Neural Network," in *6th International Conference on Inventive Computation Technologies (ICICT)*, 2021, pp. 1084–1089, doi: 10.1109/ICICT50816.2021.9358653.
5. Adusumalli, H., Kalyani, D., Sri, R. K., Pratapteja, M., Rao, P. V. R. D. P. "Face Mask Detection Using OpenCV," in *Proceedings of the International Conference on Intelligence Communication Technologies and Virtual Mobile Networks* (ICICV), 1304–1309, 2021.
6. C. Szegedy, V. Vanhoucke, S. Ioffe, J. Shlens, and Z. Wojna, "Rethinking the Inception Architecture for Computer Vision," in *Proceedings of the IEEE Conference on Computer Vision and Pattern Recognition (CVPR)*, June 2016, pp. 2818–2826.
7. A. D. Mahalle, "Artificial Intelligence Based Mask Detection with Thermal Scanning and Hand Sanitization Based Entry System," *Turkish Journal of Computer and Mathematics Education (TURCOMAT)*, 12(13), 2021, pp. 299–304.
8. H. Mani, D. R. Arumugam, A. Karuppasamy, G. Soundiran, and S. Mani, "IoT Temperature and Mask Scan Entry for Covid Prevention," in *AIP Conference Proceedings* (Vol. 2408, No. 1, p. 030002). AIP Publishing LLC, 2021.
9. Priyanka Sawale and Dhiraj Vyawahare, "Temperature and Mask Scan Entry System using IoT," *Recent Trends in Computer Graphics and Multimedia Technology*, 3(2), 2021.
10. A. Echtioui, W. Zouch, M. Ghorbel, C. Mhiri, and H. Hamam, "Detection Methods of COVID-19," *SLAS TECHNOLOGY: Translating Life Sciences Innovation*, 25(6), 2020, pp. 566–572.
11. T. Ozturk, M. Talo, E. A. Yildirim, U. B. Baloglu, O. Yildirim, and U. Rajendra Acharya, "Automated Detection of COVID-19 Cases Using Deep Neural Networks with X-Ray Images," *Computers in Biology and Medicine*, vol. 121, 2020, Article ID 103792.

12. L. Wang, Z. Q. Lin, and A. Wong, "Covid-net: A Tailored Deep Convolutional Neural Network Design for Detection of Covid-19 Cases from Chest X-Ray Images," *Scientific Reports*, 10(1), 2020, pp. 1–12.

13. V. Shah, R. Keniya, A. Shridharani, M. Punjabi, J. Shah, and N. Mehendale, "Diagnosis of COVID-19 Using CT Scan Images and Deep Learning Techniques," *Emergency Radiology*, 49, 2021, pp. 1–9.

14. A. Sedik, M. Hammad, F. E. Abd El-Samie, B. B. Gupta, and A. A. Abd El-Latif, "Efficient Deep Learning Approach for Augmented Detection of Coronavirus Disease," *Neural Computing & Applications*, 18, 2021, pp. 1–18.

15. M. Loey, G. Manogaran, M. H. N. Taha, and N. E. M. Khalifa, "Fighting Against COVID-19: A Novel Deep Learning Model based on YOLO-v2 with ResNet-50 for Medical Face Mask Detection," *Sustainable Cities and Society*, 65, 2021, Article ID 102600.

16. A. Nieto-Rodríguez, M. Mucientes, and V. M. Brea, "System for Medical Mask Detection in the Operating Room Through Facial Attributes," in *Proceedings of the Iberian Conference on Pattern Recognition and Image Analysis*. Springer, Santiago de Compostela, Spain, June 2015, pp. 138–145.

17. M. Loey, G. Manogaran, M. H. N. Taha, and N. E. M. Khalifa, "A Hybrid Deep Transfer Learning Model with Machine Learning Methods for Face Mask Detection in the Era of the COVID-19 Pandemic," *Measurement*, vol. 167, 2021, Article ID 108288.

18. https://github.com/prajnasb/observations

19. W. You, C. Shen, X. Guo, X. Jiang, J. Shi, and Z. Zhu, "A Hybrid Technique based on Convolutional Neural Network and Support Vector Regression for Intelligent Diagnosis of Rotating Machinery," *Advances in Mechanical Engineering*, 9(6), 2017, 1687814017704146.

20. M. M. Rahman, M. M. H. Manik, M. M. Islam, S. Mahmud, and J. H. Kim, "An Automated System to Limit COVID-19 Using Facial Mask Detection in Smart City Network," in *IEEE International IOT, Electronics and Mechatronics Conference (IEMTRONICS)*, IEEE, 2020, pp. 1–5.

21. A. Das, M. W. Ansari, and R. Basak, "Covid-19 Face Mask Detection Using TensorFlow, Keras and OpenCV," in *IEEE 17th India Council International Conference (INDICON)*, IEEE, 2020, pp. 1–5.

22. S. Sakshi, A. K. Gupta, S. S. Yadav, and U. Kumar, "Face Mask Detection System Using CNN," in *International Conference on Advance Computing and Innovative Technologies in Engineering (ICACITE)*, IEEE, 2021, pp. 212–216.

23. Suresh, K., Palangappa, M. B., and Bhuvan, S. "Face Mask Detection by Using Optimistic Convolutional Neural Network," in *6th International Conference on Inventive Computation Technologies (ICICT)*, IEEE, 2021, pp. 1084–1089.

24. H. Adusumalli, D. Kalyani, R. K. Sri, M. Pratapteja, and P. P. Rao, "Face Mask Detection Using Opencv," in *Third International Conference on Intelligent Communication Technologies and Virtual Mobile Networks (ICICV)*, IEEE, 2021, pp. 1304–1309.

25. Chakraborty, C., Othman, S.B., Almalki, F.A., et al. "FC-SEEDA: Fog Computing-based Secure and Energy Efficient Data Aggregation Scheme for Internet of Healthcare Things," *Neural Comput & Applic*, 2023. https://doi.org/10.1007/s00521-023-08270-0

26. Soufiene Ben Othman, Abdullah Ali Bahattab, Abdelbasset Trad and Habib Youssef, "PEERP: A Priority-Based Energy-Efficient Routing Protocol for Reliable Data Transmission in Healthcare Using the IoT," in *The 15th International Conference on Future Networks and Communications (FNC)*, Leuven, Belgium, 2020.

27. Soufiene Ben Othman, Faris A. Almalki, Chinmay Chakraborty, and Hedi Sakli, "Privacy-Preserving Aware Data Aggregation for IoT-Based Healthcare with Green Computing Technologies," *Computers and Electrical Engineering*, 101, 2022, 108025, doi: 10.1016/j.compeleceng.2022.108025.

13 Diabetic Disease Prediction Using Machine Learning Models and Algorithms for Early Classification and Diagnosis Assessment

AAA Aayush, Jawahar Sundaram, S Devaraju,
Sujith Jayaprakash, Harishchander Anandaram,
and C Manivasagan

13.1 INTRODUCTION

According to a 2021 World Health Organization estimate, there were 422 million cases of diabetes in 2014, up from 108 million in 1980. Compared to high-income countries, the prevalence has increased more quickly in low- and middle-income nations. The body's ineffective use of insulin results in type 2 diabetes, also known as non-insulin-dependent or adult-onset diabetes. More than 95% of people with diabetes have type 2 diabetes. The primary causes of this kind of diabetes are obesity and inactivity. The link between type 2 diabetes and elevated heart disease and stroke risk has long been understood. More recent research has demonstrated that having diabetes raises your risk of developing dementia. Studies reveal a strong correlation between type 2 diabetes and Alzheimer's. In this study, big data analytics and machine learning (ML) algorithms are employed to develop a model that will forecast the disease and issue early warnings. Researchers' interest in creating ML models to predict conditions has significantly increased. Breast cancer prediction, therapeutic discovery in psychiatry, prediction of heart diseases, monkeypox prediction, and COVID-19 prediction are some of the significant research work focused on by researchers across the globe. As medical data is growing substantially, the

DOI: 10.1201/9781003366249-13

intervention of big data analytics and ML algorithms has paved the way for several research works and has given enough solutions to emerging problems in the medical industry. Prolific researchers worldwide have concentrated on several important research projects, including the prediction of breast cancer, therapeutic discoveries in psychiatry, heart disease predictions, monkeypox predictions, and COVID-19 predictions [5, 6, 7]. Healthcare produces an almost unimaginable amount of data every second. The intervention of big data analytics and ML algorithms has led the way for numerous studies and provided enough solutions to the rising difficulties in the medical field due to the significant growth of medical data. With knowledge derived from large dataset analysis, a skill that has recently arisen, clinical and healthcare providers, suppliers, policymakers, and patients are having encouraging experiences. Because of its ability to predict outcomes, machine learning has significantly contributed to medicine. A considerable amount of the cost of healthcare worldwide is caused by chronic diseases.

13.2   MATERIALS AND METHODS

This section includes the predictive proposed model for type 1 diabetes. Google Colaboratory and Python, RStudio, and Weka were used for the disease prediction implementation. The packages NumPy, Matplotlib, Pandas, and Scikit-Learn were used for analyzing the data [10].

13.2.1   Data Collection

The dataset used is from the National Institute of Diabetes and Digestive and Kidney Diseases. The dataset for disease prediction includes females at least 21 years old of Pima Indian heritage. The number of instances is 768, and there are nine attributes [4]. Table 13.1 is a description of the dataset. All these features affect people with diabetes. All these attributes are not null and tell the data type of the attribute.

TABLE 13.1
Dataset description

Attribute name	Attribute description
Pregnancies (P)	Number of times pregnant
Glucose (G)	2-hour plasma glucose + oral glucose tolerance test
Blood Pressure (BP)	Diastolic blood pressure (DBP)
Skin Thickness (ST)	Skin fold thickness (SFT)
Insulin (I)	Serum insulin (SI)
BMI	Body mass index
Diabetes Pedigree Function (DPF)	Diabetes pedigree function
Age (A)	Age
Outcome (O)	Class variable (0 or 1) / (T/F)

13.2.2   DATA PREPROCESSING

For data preprocessing, we will be using Excel. The motive is that the data must be free from errors and can be interpreted by machine algorithms. So, the data will be converted into a more functional and efficient format. There are various steps, including data cleaning, data transformation, and data reduction for the preprocessing dataset.

13.2.3   DATA CLEANING

A median will fill in missing values in the attribute. The median will be a better approach for missing values as the dataset is positively skewed. Now checking outliers, we will use the boxplot diagram or the interquartile range formula that finds the Q1 and Q3 and their interquartile difference range. After that, we will be seeing the upper bound (Q3 + [1.5 × (Q3 – Q1)]) and lower bound (Q1 – [1.5 × (Q3 – Q1)]) and using the formula = if(cell > upper bound, cell < lower bound). If it returns true, it means it is an outlier and if false then it is not an outlier.

Figure 13.1 is the boxplot of all nine attributes. The dots represent the outliers, and the box represents the upper, lower, and middle quartiles. We can see that there are many outliers for Diabetes Pedigree Function. For removing outliers, we will use Weka and Excel.

Table 13.2 represents the outliers for Pregnancies, Glucose, Blood Pressure, Skin Thickness, Insulin, BMI, Diabetes Pedigree Function, Age, and Outcome, which we found using the Excel interquartile range formula. Two attributes do not have outliers. The remaining attributes have outliers, which can badly affect our algorithm, as outliers can mislead our training process resulting in lesser accurate models and, ultimately, poor overall results.

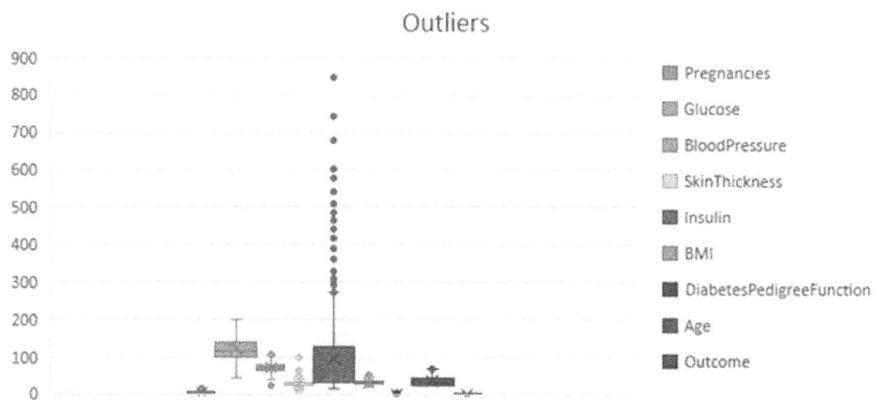

FIGURE 13.1   Attribute representation.

TABLE 13.2
Outlier count for attributes

Attribute	Outlier count
Pregnancies	4
Glucose	6
Blood Pressure (BP)	0
Skin Thickness (ST)	44
Insulin (I)	9
BMI	29
Diabetes Pedigree Function (DPF)	9
Age (A)	0

13.2.4 DATA VISUALIZATION

Data visualization is the process of displaying data using common images like infographics, charts, and even animations. These informational visual representations make it easy to understand complex data relationships and data-driven conclusions.

Figure 13.2 represents the *histogram* matrix for Pregnancies, Glucose, Blood Pressure, Skin Thickness, Insulin, BMI, Diabetes Pedigree Function, Age, and Outcome. There is a total of nine attributes, so nine charts represent each attribute's histogram. From this chart, the skewness of the dataset can be identified. This histogram matrix was obtained with the help of scatter_matrix from pandas. There are ten bins for each of the charts except Outcome, as Outcome only had two variables, 0 and 1.

Figure 13.3 represents the *scatterplot* matrix for Pregnancies, Glucose, Blood Pressure, Skin Thickness, Insulin, BMI, Diabetes Pedigree Function, Age, and Outcome. From the figure, we can see the relation between two features when one is dependent on the other, and we can conclude that the scatteredness is huge so variables are not dependent on each other. With nine features we get 81 outcomes, so we have 81 charts and each diagonal represents a histogram as both independent and dependent variables are the same.

Figure 13.4 represents the *pair plot* of Pregnancies, Glucose, Blood Pressure, Skin Thickness, Insulin, BMI, Diabetes Pedigree Function, Age, and Outcome. From the figure, we can understand the relationship explained by two sets of variables. This helps in many classification models such as the best-fit line in regression. We can also see the scatter of variables.

Figure 13.5 represents the *correlation* matrix of the attributes Pregnancies, Glucose, Blood Pressure, Skin Thickness, Insulin, BMI, Diabetes Pedigree Function, Age, and Outcome. We can see there is no correlation between the attributes, but only some attributes have moderate correlation as they are correlated with each other but in the remaining cases there is a positive correlation but poor correlation. The diagonal shows the correlation of the attribute with itself.

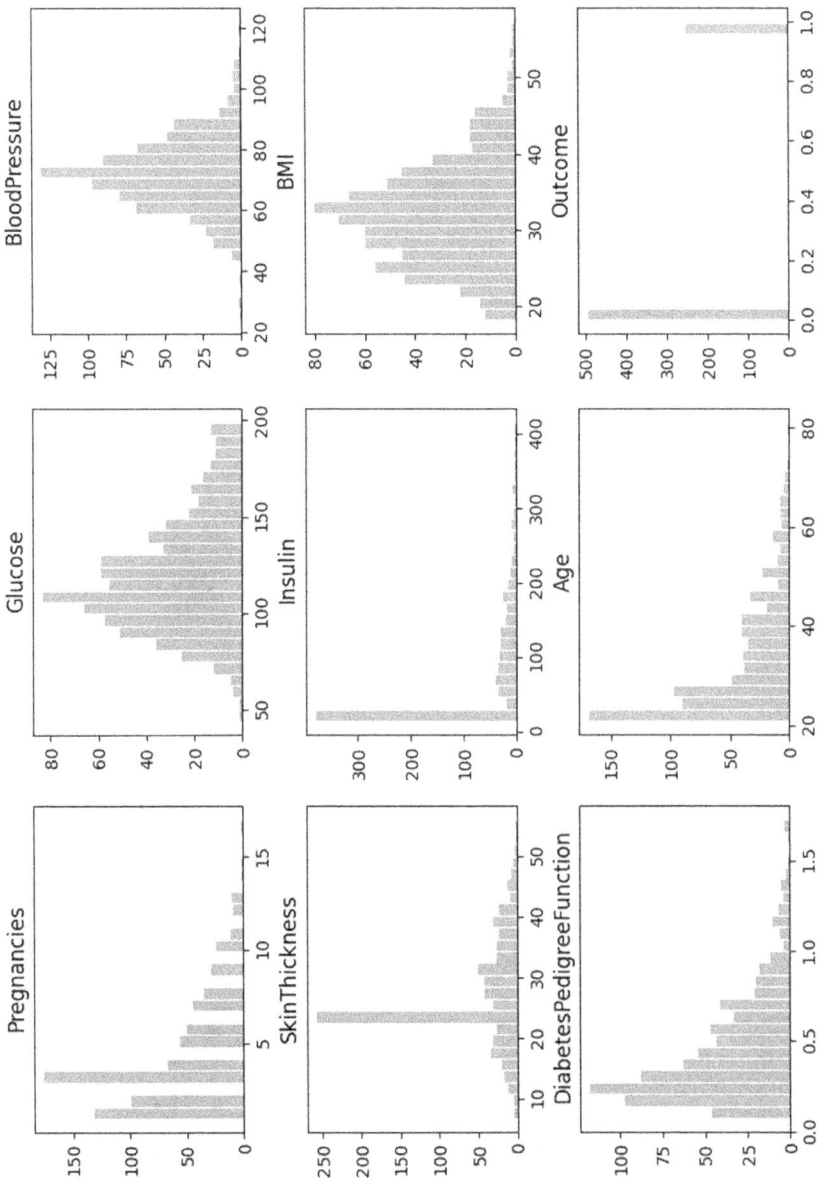

FIGURE 13.2 Histogram matrix.

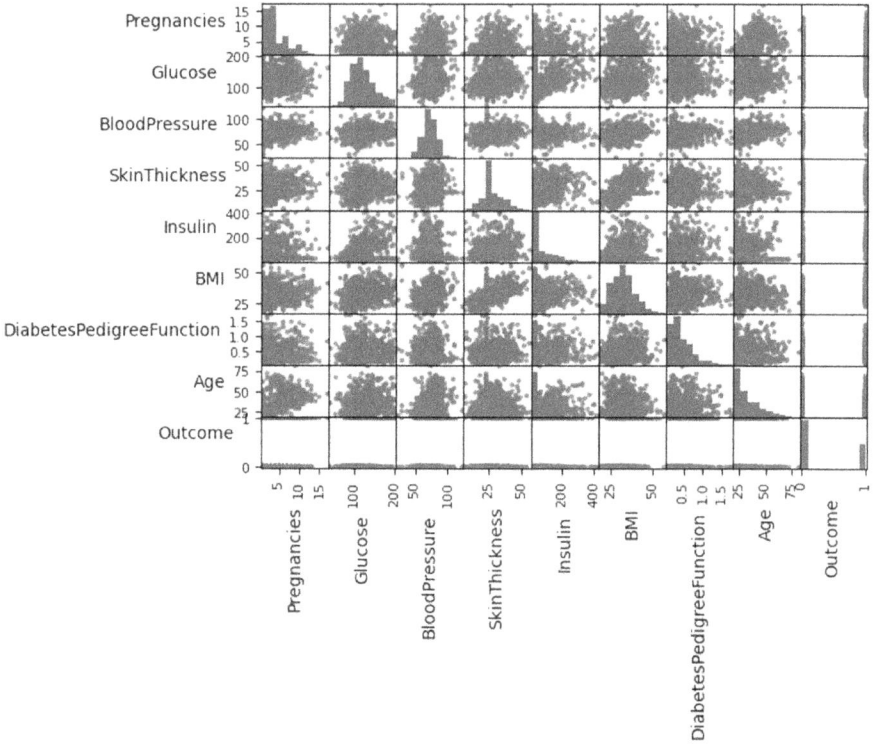

FIGURE 13.3   Scatterplot matrix.

We can use the MinMaxScaler to transform data, as high values may affect the model so scaling is necessary. MinMaxScaler transforms data into the range of 0 to 1, as we don't have any negative values in this dataset. This will help in maintaining the original shape of the dataset. We will also use StandardScaler to compare the accuracy of both scalers. StandardScaler transforms the data into standard normal distribution.

13.2.5   DATA ANALYSIS

With the help of the visualizations, we can see the relationships among the attributes. With the help of correlation, we can see that Age and Pregnancy have a good moderate relationship of 0.55, i.e., with the increase in age, there is an increase in pregnancies. BMI and Skin Thickness also have a reasonable correlation, which is good as skin layers become progressively thicker with increasing BMI. Diabetes occurs when the blood sugar is too high. But there is no relationship between Insulin and Skin Thickness, so the correlation is negative and weak. Type 2 diabetes depends on various attributes, and we can see all relations between them. Note that this data is based on the female samples collected.

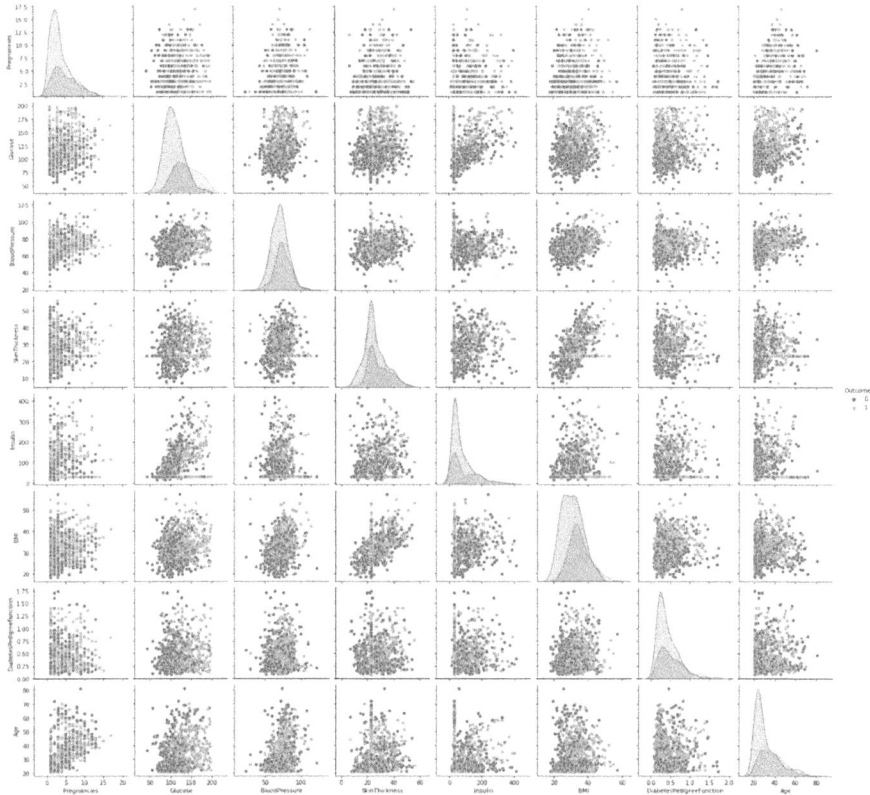

FIGURE 13.4　Pair plot matrix.

We can see the descriptive statistics of all the diabetic and non-diabetic patients with all dataset attributes and the descriptive statistics of the dataset.

Table 13.3 tells the meaning of all the dataset's attributes classified into diabetic (1) and non-diabetic (0). There are a total of 492 non-diabetic and 251 diabetic patients.

Table 13.4 shows the descriptive statistics of dataset attributes. This table reveals the mean, count, std, min value, max value, and lowest, middle, and highest quartiles. These values were obtained after removing the outliers and extreme values and before scaling the data.

From the descriptive statistics of Table 13.4, we can tell many things. Normal blood pressure (BP) is 80/120, and the average is 72, so BP is low in females and sometimes diabetes may lower the BP level. And the average BMI is also greater than 25, so the women are in the obesity range. The glucose level is 120; the normal range is 70–100 mg/dl, so the glucose level is also high.

The average of all the attributes is either low or high after removing outliers and extreme values. More than 25% of values are not normal so the person might have diabetes, and many may have prediabetes.

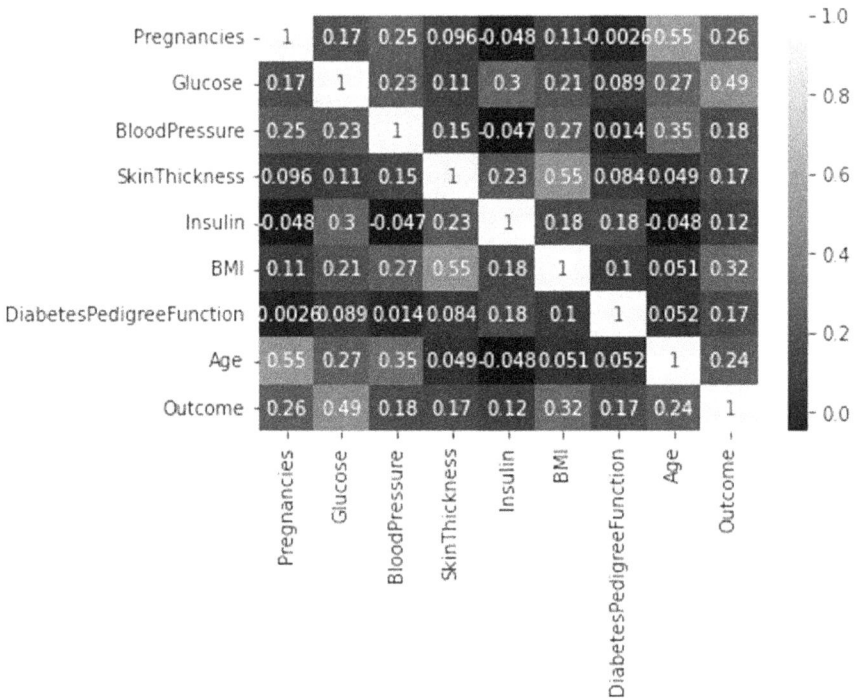

FIGURE 13.5   Correlation matrix.

TABLE 13.3
Mean value for dataset attributes

	P	G	BP	ST	I	BMI	DPF	A
O								
0	3.75	110.01	70.78	25.83	77.39	30.70	0.42	31.21
1	5.39	140.43	75.33	28.98	96.49	35.13	0.52	37.06

In Figure 13.6 the proposed model for diabetic disease is illustrated with the pre-processing method, train and test data, ML diabetes diseases prediction, and different parameters for evaluating the proposed model.

13.3   MACHINE LEARNING MODEL

The *Naïve* Bayes (NB) algorithm is an easy and effective method for classification using the Naïve Bayes classifier. The base of the Naïve Bayes classification uses the Bayes theorem with a robust feature independence assumption. We get good results

TABLE 13.4
Descriptive statistics for attributes

	P	G	BP	ST	I	BMI	DPF	A	O
count	743	743	743	743	743	743	743	743	743
mean	4.30	120.29	72.32	26.89	83.84	32.19	0.45	33.19	0.33
std	3.04	29.67	12.01	8.57	78.06	6.65	0.29	11.70	0.47
min	1	44	24	7	14	18.2	0.07	21	0
25%	2	99	64	23	30.5	27.4	0.24	24	0
50%	3	116	72	23	30.5	32	0.36	29	0
75%	6	138	80	32	120	36.25	0.61	40.5	1
max	17	199	122	56	414	57.3	1.73	81	1

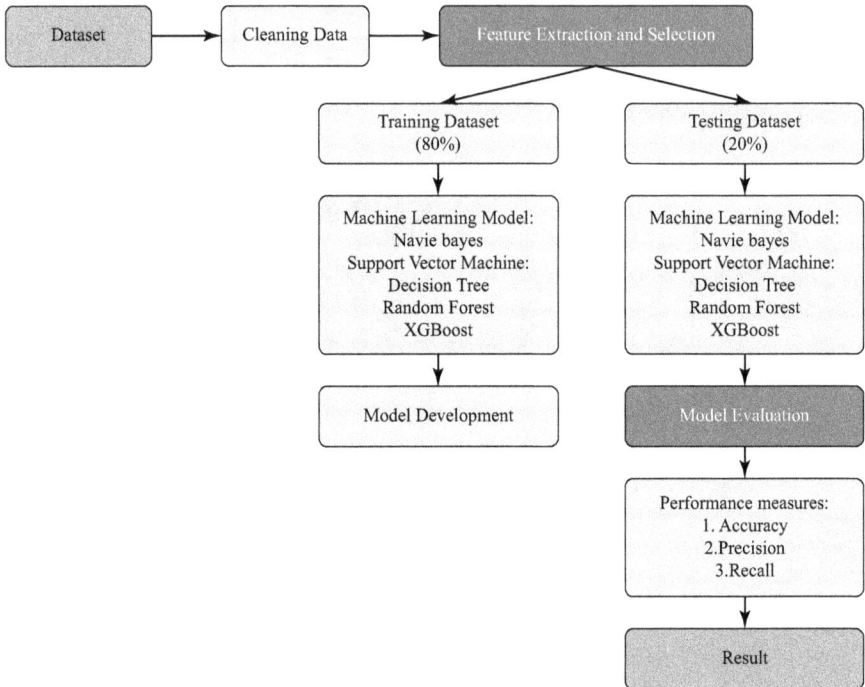

FIGURE 13.6   Predictive model for diabetes.

when we apply the Naïve Bayes classifier to studying textual data. But when we have numerical values, we can use Gaussian Naïve Bayes. When an attribute has continuous values, we presumptively assume that each class's values are distributed along a Gaussian or normal distribution.

The *support vector machine* (SVM) algorithm is based on the supervised ML model [1]. It represents the dataset with few outliers in n-dimensional space; "n" is the number that represents features or attributes. The goal of SVM is to create a hyperplane that divides the preprocessed data into several sorts, and the hyperplane should be as far away from the different kinds as possible. And then, using the predict function and trained SVM classifier, we will create a model that can predict diabetes.

In the *decision tree* (DT) approach [2], a predetermined goal variable is built into a tree or graph-based structure based on parameters. One must move from root to leaf and traverse until the conditions are met before making a decision.

Random forest (RF) [3] is a dimensionality reduction technique, a classifier consisting of a few decision trees. For words like classification, regression, and others, it is one of the ensemble approaches. The ranking of the variables' relevance may be done using it.

Extreme Gradient Boosting (*XGBoost*) is a distributed, scalable gradient-boosted decision tree (GBDT) machine learning framework. The top machine learning library for regression, classification, and ranking issues, it offers parallel tree boosting.

One of the supervised learning methods for machine learning is *k-nearest neighbor* (KNN) [9]. KNN is a no-parametric and supervised learning classifier. KNN categorizes items based on their distance from other objects in the training set, also known as their nearest measure.

13.4   RESULTS AND DISCUSSIONS

This section includes the results of the disease prediction method and how reliable the technique is. We will be considering accuracy (A), precision (P), recall (R), F1 score (F1), and confusion matrix (CM). We will also see how close a measurement is to its actual value. We will also do a Fisher hypothesis test on the confusion matrix to check the dependence.

Accuracy is how frequently the algorithm correctly identifies a data point may be determined by its accuracy.

$$\frac{TP + TN}{TP + FP + TN + FN} \tag{13.1}$$

Table 13.5 discusses the accuracy of the different algorithms: support vector machine, XGBoost, random forest, decision tree, Naïve Bayes, and k-nearest neighbor with MinMaxScaler and StandardScaler. The graphical representation is shown in Figure 13.7. We can conclude that random forest gives the highest accuracy with StandardScaler, followed by random forest and support vector machine with MinMaxScaler.

Precision (also called positive predictive value) is the fraction of relevant instances among the retrieved instances. Written as a formula:

$$\frac{TP}{(TP + FP)} \tag{13.2}$$

Table 13.6 shows the algorithm's precision with the MinMaxScaler and StandardScaler, as well as the non-diabetic (0) accuracy. Figure 13.8 shows the

---

TABLE 13.5
Accuracy of the algorithms

Algorithm	Accuracy (A)	
	MinMaxScaler	StandardScaler
Support vector machine (SVM)	0.77	0.76
Decision tree (DT)	0.70	0.70
Random forest (RF)	0.77	0.79
XGBoost (XGB)	0.75	0.75
Naïve Bayes (NB)	0.70	0.70
K-nearest neighbor (KNN)	0.72	0.72

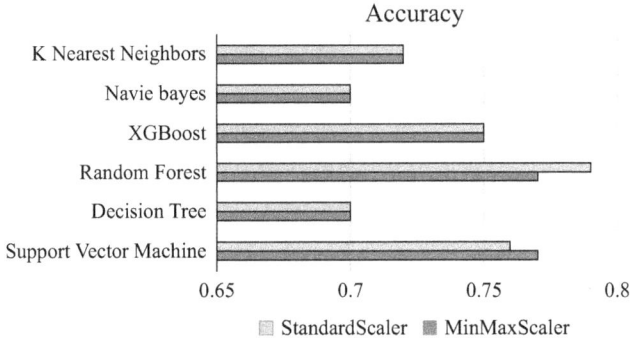

FIGURE 13.7 Accuracy representation.

TABLE 13.6
Precision of the algorithms

Algorithm	Precision (in points for non-diabetic)	
	MinMaxScaler	StandardScaler
Support vector machine (SVM)	0.78	0.77
Decision tree (DT)	0.77	0.76
Random forest (RF)	0.82	0.82
XGBoost (XGB)	0.80	0.80
Naïve Bayes (NB)	0.77	0.77
K-nearest Neighbor (KNN)	0.75	0.75

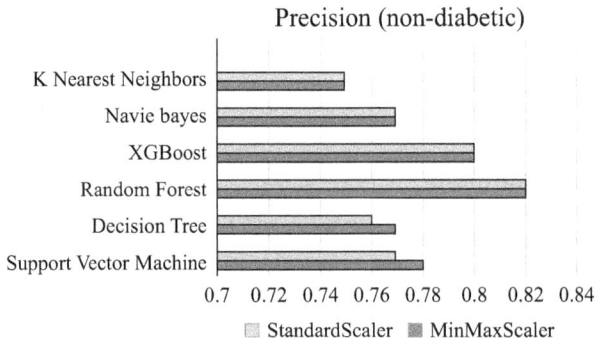

FIGURE 13.8 Precision representation.

graphical representation of Table 13.6. We can conclude that the random forest gives the highest precision with both scalers, followed by XGBoost. So, we can say that in accuracy, the scalers are equal.

Recall (also known as sensitivity) is the fraction of relevant instances that were retrieved. Written as a formula:

$$\frac{TP}{(TP + FN)} \tag{13.3}$$

So, from Table 13.7, we can see the recall of the algorithm with MinMaxScaler and StandardScaler and shows the recall for non-diabetic (0). Figure 13.9 is the graphical representation of Table 13.7. From the results, we can conclude that SVM gives the highest recall, followed by random forest with both scalers. So, we can say that in the recall, the scalers are close to each other.

The mean value of recall and accuracy is the *F1 score*. This score accounts for both false negatives and false positives.

TABLE 13.7
Recall of the algorithms

	Recall (in points for non-diabetic)	
Algorithm	MinMaxScaler	StandardScaler
Support vector machine (SVM)	0.91	0.90
Decision tree (DT)	0.79	0.81
Random forest (RF)	0.85	0.88
XGBoost (XGB)	0.84	0.84
Naïve Bayes (NB)	0.80	0.80
K-nearest neighbor (KNN)	0.88	0.88

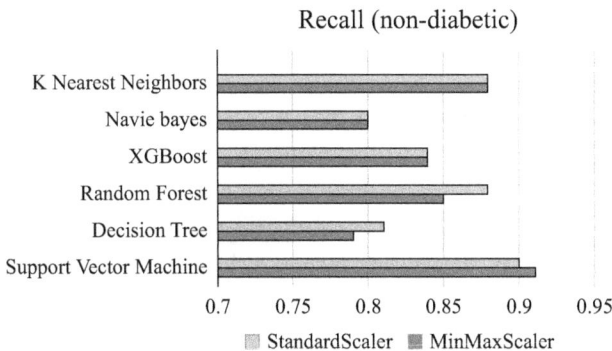

FIGURE 13.9 Recall representation.

$$\frac{2 \times \textbf{\textit{Precision}} \times \textbf{\textit{Recall}}}{\textbf{\textit{precision}} + \textbf{\textit{Recall}}} \tag{13.4}$$

From Table 13.8, we can see the F1 score of the algorithm with the MinMaxScaler and StandardScaler, and the F1 score for non-diabetic (0). Figure 13.10 shows the graphical representation of Table 13.8. The table represents that the random forest gives the highest precision with both scalers, followed by the support vector machine.

The *accuracy rate can be improved* with the implementation of soft voting and hard voting. We need to import the voting classifier in terms of different parameters. So, from Table 13.9, we can see the improved accuracy with the help of the voting classifier on all five algorithms with the MinMaxScaler and StandardScaler. Figure 13.11

TABLE 13.8
F1   score of the algorithms

Algorithm	F1 score (in points for non-diabetic)	
	MinMaxScaler	StandardScaler
Support vector machine (SVM)	0.84	0.83
Decision tree (DT)	0.78	0.78
Random forest (RF)	0.83	0.85
XGBoost (XGB)	0.82	0.82
Naïve Bayes (NB)	0.78	0.78
K-nearest neighbor (KNN)	0,81	0.81

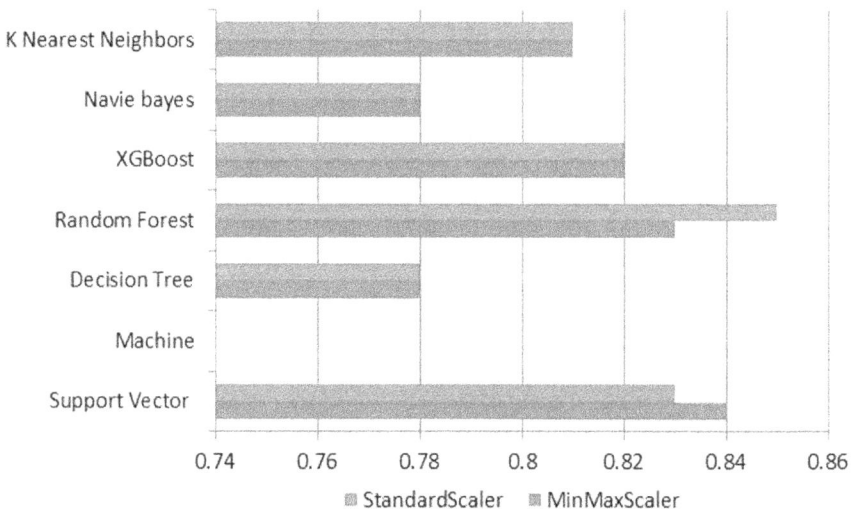

FIGURE 13.10   F1 score representation.

TABLE 13.9

Improved accuracy of the algorithms

	Improved accuracy using voting classifier	
Algorithm	MinMaxScaler	StandardScaler
Support vector machine (SVM)	0.78	0.77
Decision tree (DT)	0.74	0.73
Random forest (RF)	0.78	0.78
XGBoost (XGB)	0.76	0.76
Naïve Bayes (NB)	0.76	0.76
K-nearest Neighbor (KNN)	0.77	0.76

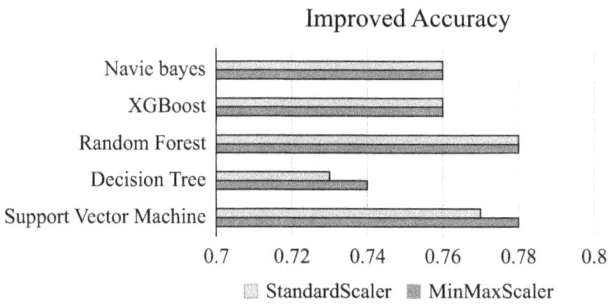

FIGURE 13.11 Improved accuracy representation.

shows the graphical representation of Table 13.9. We can conclude that random forest gives the highest precision with both scalers followed by the support vector machine.

A *confusion matrix* (CM) is used in machine learning to evaluate the effectiveness of the classification method. In the CM, columns indicate the predicted class, and rows represent the actual class.

Table 13.10 represents the structure of the confusion matrix that is as follows:

- Actual class (AC): The Actual Class for classifier before building.
- Predicted class (PC): The Predicted Class for classifier after building.
- True positive (TP): Number of predicted instances positive (diabetic) and are positive (diabetic).
- False positive (FP): Number of predicted instances positive (diabetic) but are actually negative (non-diabetic).
- True negative (TN): Number of instances predicted negative (non-diabetic) and are negative (non-diabetic).
- False negative (FN): Number of instances predicted negative (non-diabetic) but are actually positive (diabetic).

TABLE 13.10

Confusion matrix

		Predicted		
		FALSE (99)	TRUE (50)	
	Confusion matrix	Tested non-diabetic	Tested diabetic	Total
Actual	FALSE (99) Tested non-diabetic	TN	FP	99
	TRUE (50) Tested diabetic	FN	TP	50
Total		99	50	149

TABLE 13.11

Confusion matrix for support vector machine

Support vector machine (SVM)								
MinMaxScaler		Predicted (P)		StandardScaler			Predicted (P)	
		FALSE	TRUE				FALSE	TRUE
Confusion Matrix (CM)				Confusion matrix (CM)				
Actual (A)	FALSE	90	9		Actual	FALSE	89	10
	TRUE	26	24			TRUE	26	24

TABLE 13.12

Confusion matrix for decision tree

Decision tree (DT)							
MinMaxScaler				StandardScaler			
Confusion matrix (CM)		Predicted (P)		Confusion matrix (CM)		Predicted (P)	
		FALSE	TRUE			FALSE	TRUE
Actual (A)	FALSE	78	21	Actual	FALSE	80	19
	TRUE	23	27		TRUE	25	25

Table 13.11 represents the confusion matrix of the support vector machine on both the MinMaxScaler and StandardScaler. The MinMaxScaler gives better output in this case.

Table 13.12 represents the confusion matrix of the decision tree on both the MinMaxScaler and StandardScaler. StandardScaler gives better output in this case.

Table 13.13 represents the confusion matrix of random forest on the MinMaxScaler and StandardScaler. StandardScaler gives better output in this case.

TABLE 13.13
Confusion matrix for random forest

Random forest (RF)							
MinMaxScaler				StandardScaler			
Confusion matrix (CM)		Predicted (P)		Confusion matrix (CM)		Predicted (P)	
		FALSE	TRUE			FALSE	TRUE
Actual (A)	FALSE	84	15	Actual	FALSE	87	12
	TRUE	19	31		TRUE	19	31

TABLE 13.14
Confusion matrix for XGB

XGBoost (XGB)							
MinMaxScaler				StandardScaler			
Confusion matrix (CM)		Predicted (P)		Confusion matrix (CM)		Predicted (P)	
Actual (A)		FALSE	TRUE	Actual		FALSE	TRUE
	FALSE	83	16		FALSE	83	16
	TRUE	21	29		TRUE	21	29

TABLE 13.15
Confusion matrix for Naïve Bayes

Naïve Bayes (NB)							
MinMaxScaler				StandardScaler			
Confusion matrix (CM)		Predicted (P)		Confusion matrix (CM)		Predicted (P)	
		FALSE	TRUE			FALSE	TRUE
Actual (A)	FALSE	79	20	Actual	FALSE	79	20
	TRUE	24	26		TRUE	24	26

Table 13.14 represents the confusion matrix of XGBoost on both the MinMaxScaler and StandardScaler. Both scalers give equal output.

Table 13.15 represents the confusion matrix of Naïve Bayes on both the MinMaxScaler and the StandardScaler. Both scalers give equal output.

Table 13.16 represents the confusion matrix of k-nearest neighbor on both the MinMaxScaler and StandardScaler. Both scalers give equal output in this case.

So, Tables 13.11, 13.12, 13.13, 13.14, 13.15, and 13.16 represent the confusion matrix of the support vector machine, decision tree, random forest, XGBoost, Naïve Bayes, and KNN, respectively, on both the MinMaxScaler and StandardScaler. From

TABLE 13.16

Confusion matrix for KNN

K-nearest Neighbor (KNN)

MinMaxScaler			StandardScaler		
Confusion matrix (CM)	Predicted (P)		Confusion matrix (CM)	Predicted (P)	
	FALSE	TRUE		FALSE	TRUE
Actual (A) FALSE	87	12	Actual FALSE	87	12
TRUE	29	21	TRUE	29	21

TABLE 13.16

Confusion matrix with hypothesis contingency

Confusion matrix (CM)		Predicted (P)	
		Fail to reject	Reject
Actual (A)	H_0 is true	TN Correct decision Confidence level (Prob $1 - \alpha$)	FP Type I error Significance level (Prob α)
	H_0 is false	FN Type II error Fail to reject (Prob β)	TP Correct decision: power (Prob $1 - \beta$)

this, we can see that Naïve Bayes and XGBoost give equal output on both scalers. These tables represent the values for diabetic patients. With the help of the Fisher test, we can say that there is a dependency between variables. Knowing one value can help us to know the value of the other.

$$H_0 = the \ variables \ are \ independent$$

$$H_1 = the \ variables \ are \ dependent$$

As the value of p is less than 0.05 in all the tables, we may reject and say there is significant dependence between variables. There is a relationship between diabetic and non-diabetic prediction.

We can also relate the confusion matrix with the hypothesis contingency table for better inferences.

For Table 13.16:

$$H_0 = the \text{ person is non} - diabetic$$

$$H_1 = the \text{ person is diabetic}$$

The type I prediction is represented as 'α' and the type II prediction is represented as 'β' errors.

A type I error occurs when a researcher rejects a null hypothesis that is confirmed by the population (false positive). Type II errors occur when a researcher fails to reject an incorrect null hypothesis in the population (false negative). The researcher can lessen the danger of type I and type II errors even though they cannot be totally avoided [8].

As we have more type I and type II errors to reduce, we can increase the amount of the dataset, as currently, the amount of the testing dataset is 149. As we increase size, there is a decrease in error, and power is improved. But still, there is a minor effect between the MinMaxScaler and StandardScaler. Usually, the type I error is fixed at 0.05, resulting in a fixed error, and the type II error is then fixed at 0.10. Then the investigator is willing to accept a 10% chance of missing an association between the diabetic and non-diabetic. Thus (*Prob 1 − β*) results in 90%. There is a 90% chance of association between them. So, they should be as small as possible. And we fix the value of the type I error as low as possible, which could increase the value of the type II error, so the sample size should be increased, and the value should be taken so low that the other value should also be kept low. Ideally, $\alpha = 0.05$ is fixed, so $\beta = 0.10$ or 0.20, resulting in a good 90% or 80% power.

Table 13.17 represents the *combined confusion matrix* of all algorithms, by which we can draw a chart (Figure 13.12) to compare the TP, TN, FP, and FN. So, both TP and TN are good, and FP and FN should be reduced.

In machine learning, a *classification report* (CR) is a performance evaluation measurement.

Table 13.18 represents the classification report for the support vector machine with both the MinMaxScaler and StandardScaler. This table shows the accuracy and precision, recall, F1 score, support for diabetic and non-diabetic, macro average, and weighted average for these column variables.

Table 13.19 represents the classification report for the decision tree with both the MinMaxScaler and StandardScaler. This table shows the accuracy and precision, recall, F1 score, support for diabetic and non-diabetic, macro average, and weighted average for these column variables.

Table 13.20 represents the classification report for random forest with both the MinMaxScaler and StandardScaler. This table shows the classification report.

Table 13.21 represents the classification report for Naïve Bayes with both the MinMaxScaler and StandardScaler. This table shows the classification report.

TABLE 13.17
Combined confusion matrix

Algorithm	TP		TN		FP		FN	
	MinMaxScaler	StandardScaler	MinMaxScaler	StandardScaler	MinMaxScaler	StandardScaler	MinMaxScaler	StandardScaler
Support vector machine (SVM)	24	24	90	89	9	10	26	26
Decision tree (DT)	26	26	79	79	20	20	24	24
Random forest (RF)	27	25	78	80	21	19	23	25
XGBoost (XGB)	31	31	84	87	15	12	19	19
Naïve Bayes (NB)	29	29	83	83	16	16	21	21
K-nearest neighbor (KNN)	29	29	87	87	12	12	21	21

Combined Confusion Matrix

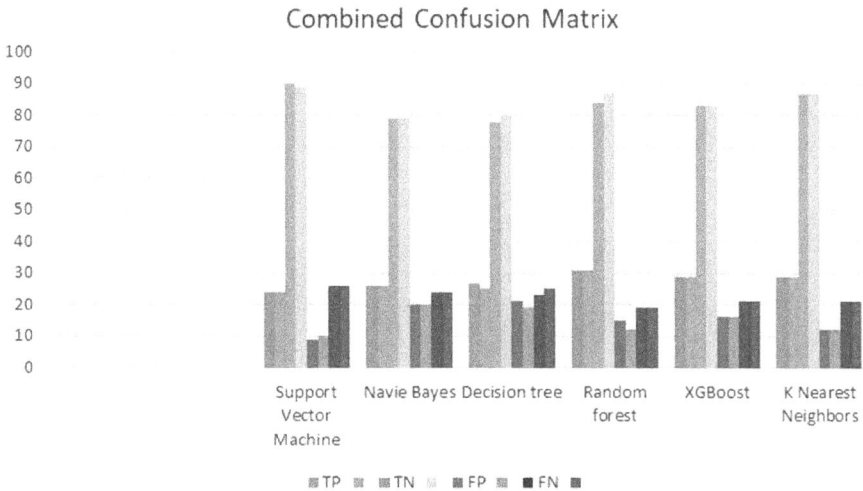

FIGURE 13.12   Predictive comparison of the algorithms' confusion matrices.

Table 13.22 represents the classification report for XGBoost with both the MinMaxScaler and Standard Scaler. This table shows the classification report.

Table 13.23 represents the classification report for k-nearest neighbor with both the MinMaxScaler and StandardScaler. This table shows the classification report. This table also shows the accuracy and precision, recall, F1 score, support for diabetic and non-diabetic, macro average, and weighted average for these column variables.

13.5   CONCLUSION AND FUTURE ENHANCEMENT

Predictive analytics is very significant in the healthcare industry. So, a model was created for predicting diabetics. We used six popular machine learning algorithms (support vector machine, decision tree, random forest, XGBoost, Naïve Bayes, and KNN) with two scalers (MinMaxScaler and StandardScaler). From this model, we got the highest accuracy for random forest using standard scaling, 79%, followed by support vector machine at 77%. After using a voting classifier, our accuracy remained the same in the random forest case. Still, our accuracy in the support vector machine increased by 78%. Other performance measures, including precision, recall, F1 score, and confusion matrix, were also calculated. From the Fisher test, we can also see that the predicted and actual diabetic and non-diabetic depend on each other. So, if the actual dataset is improved, the predicted result will also be improved.

So, for future reference, the result can be improved if the size of the dataset is increased, as we only had 768 subjects. If the size increases, we might get better results with proper data cleaning techniques like removing missing outliers and extreme values. Feature selection can also be used to increase performance. Other attributes can also be considered, such as physical activity, diet, family history, or suffering from any other disease.

TABLE 13.18

Classification report for the support vector machine

Support vector machine (SVM)

	MinMaxScaler					StandardScaler			
	Precision (P)	Recall (R)	F1 score (F1)	Support (S)		Precision (P)	Recall (R)	F1 score (F1)	Support (S)
0	0.78	0.91	0.84	99	0	0.77	0.90	0.83	99
1	0.73	0.48	0.58	50	1	0.71	0.48	0.57	50
Accuracy (A)			0.77	149	Accuracy (A)			0.76	149
Macro Avg (MA)	0.75	0.69	0.71	149	Macro Avg (MA)	0.74	0.69	0.70	149
Weighted Avg (WA)	0.76	0.77	0.75	149	Weighted Avg (WA)	0.75	0.76	0.74	149

TABLE 13.19

Classification report for the decision tree

	Decision tree (DT)							
	MinMaxScaler				StandardScaler			
	Precision (P)	Recall (R)	F1 score (F1)	Support (S)		Precision (P)	Recall (R)	F1 score (F1)	Support (S)
0	0.77	0.79	0.78	99	0	0.76	0.81	0.78	99
1	0.56	0.54	0.55	50	1	0.57	0.50	0.53	50
Accuracy (A)			0.70	149	Accuracy (A)			0.70	149
Macro Avg (MA)	0.66	0.66	0.67	149	Macro Avg (MA)	0.67	0.65	0.66	149
Weighted Avg (WA)	0.66	0.70	0.70	149	Weighted Avg (WA)	0.70	0.70	0.70	149

TABLE 13.20

Classification report for random forest

Random forest (RF)

	MinMaxScaler					StandardScaler			
	Precision (P)	Recall (R)	F1 score (F1)	Support (S)		Precision (P)	Recall (R)	F1 score (F1)	Support (S)
0	0.82	0.85	0.83	99	0	0.82	0.88	0.85	99
1	0.67	0.62	0.65	50	1	0.72	0.62	0.67	50
Accuracy (A)			0.77	149	Accuracy (A)			0.79	149
Macro Avg (MA)	0.74	0.73	0.74	149	Macro Avg (MA)	0.77	0.75	0.76	149
Weighted Avg (WA)	0.77	0.77	0.77	149	Weighted Avg (WA)	0.79	0.79	0.79	149

TABLE 13.21

Classification report for Naïve Bayes

Naïve Bayes (NB)

	MinMaxScaler					StandardScaler			
	Precision (P)	Recall (R)	F1 score (F1)	Support (S)		Precision (P)	Recall (R)	F1 score (F1)	Support (S)
0	0.77	0.80	0.78	99	0	0.77	0.80	0.78	99
1	0.57	0.52	0.54	50	1	0.57	0.52	0.54	50
Accuracy (A)			0.70	149	Accuracy (A)			0.70	149
Macro Avg (MA)	0.67	0.66	0.66	149	Macro Avg (MA)	0.67	0.66	0.66	149
Weighted Avg (WA)	0.70	0.70	0.70	149	Weighted Avg (WA)	0.70	0.70	0.70	149

TABLE 13.22

Classification report for XGBoost (XGB)

XGBoost (XGB)

MinMaxScaler

	Precision (P)	Recall (R)	F1 score (F1)	Support (S)
0	0.80	0.84	0.82	99
1	0.64	0.58	0.61	50
Accuracy (A)			0.75	149
Macro Avg (MA)	0.72	0.71	0.71	149
Weighted Avg (WA)	0.75	0.75	0.75	149

StandardScaler

	Precision (P)	Recall (R)	F1 score (F1)	Support (S)
0	0.80	0.84	0.82	99
1	0.64	0.58	0.61	50
Accuracy (A)			0.75	149
Macro Avg (MA)	0.72	0.71	0.71	149
Weighted Avg (WA)	0.75	0.75	0.75	149

TABLE 13.23

Classification report for K-nearest neighbor

K-nearest neighbor (KNN)

MinMaxScaler

	Precision (P)	Recall (R)	F1 score (F1)	Support (S)
0	0.75	0.88	99	99
1	0.64	0.42	0.51	50
Accuracy (A)			0.72	149
Macro Avg (MA)	0.69	0.65	0.66	149
Weighted Avg (WA)	0.71	0.72	0.71	149

StandardScaler

	Precision (P)	Recall (R)	F1 score (F1)	Support (S)
0	0.75	0.88	99	99
1	0.64	0.42	0.51	50
Accuracy (A)			0.72	149
Macro Avg (MA)	0.69	0.65	0.66	149
Weighted Avg (WA)	0.71	0.72	0.71	149

REFERENCES

1. V. Roy, P. K. Shukla, A. K. Gupta, V. Goel, P. K. Shukla, and S. Shukla, Taxonomy on EEG artifacts removal methods, issues, and healthcare applications. *Journal of Organizational and End User Computing*, 33(1), 19–46, 2021.
2. P. Argentiero, R. Chin, and P. Beaudet. An automated approach to the design of decision tree classifiers. *IEEE Transactions on Pattern Analysis and Machine Intelligence*, 1, 51–57, 1982.
3. L. Breiman. Random forests. *Machine Learning*, 45(1), 5–32, 2001.
4. https://www.kaggle.com/datasets/mathchi/diabetes-data-set [dataset link, Kaggle diabetes]
5. A. E. Budson. What's the relationship between diabetes and dementia? (2022) [Blog]. Retrieved from https://www.health.harvard.edu/blog/whats-the-relationship-between -diabetes-and-dementia-202107122546
6. P. Galetsi, K. Katsaliaki, and S. Kumar. Big data analytics in health sector: Theoretical framework, techniques and prospects. *International Journal of Information Management*, 50, 206–216, 2020. doi: 10.1016/j.ijinfomgt.2019.05.003
7. G. Battineni, G. Sagaro, N. Chinatalapudi, and F. Amenta. Applications of machine learning predictive models in the chronic disease diagnosis. *Journal of Personalized Medicine*, 10(2), 21, 2020. doi: 10.3390/jpm10020021
8. Soufiene Ben Othman, Faris A. Almalki, Chinmay Chakraborty, and Hedi Sakli. Privacy-preserving aware data aggregation for IoT-based healthcare with green computing technologies. *Computers and Electrical Engineering*, 101, 2022, 108025. doi: 10.1016/j.compeleceng.2022.108025.
9. Soufiene Ben Othman, Abdullah Ali Bahattab, Abdelbasset Trad and Habib, Youssef. PEERP: A priority-based energy-efficient routing protocol for reliable data transmission in healthcare using the IoT. The 15th International Conference on Future Networks and Communications (FNC), August 9–12, 2020, Leuven, Belgium.
10. C. Chakraborty, S.B. Othman, F.A. Almalki, et al. FC-SEEDA: Fog computing-based secure and energy efficient data aggregation scheme for Internet of healthcare things. *Neural Computing & Applications*, 2023. doi: 10.1007/s00521-023-08270-0

14 Defeating Alzheimer's: AI Perspective from Diagnostics to Prognostics
Literature Summary

*Iheb Elghaieb, Abdelbaki Souid,
Ahmed Zouinkhi, and Hedi Sakli*

14.1 INTRODUCTION

Alzheimer's disease is a common type of dementia that causes cognitive decline and memory loss. In North America and Europe, Alzheimer's disease and other related dementias have become a major public health concern. In 2019, it was estimated that over 5.6 million people in North America and Europe who were 65 or older had Alzheimer's disease, representing 10% of the population in those regions. This number is expected to rise as the population continues to age, and the number of people with Alzheimer's disease is likely to increase significantly. The majority of the care needed by people with Alzheimer's disease is provided by family members, friends, and other unpaid caregivers. In 2018, American caregivers of people with Alzheimer's disease and related dementias provided 18.5 billion hours of unpaid care, valued at $233.9 billion. This represents a significant financial and emotional burden on caregivers, who often have to balance their caregiving responsibilities with their own work, family, and personal obligations [1]. The tissue loss associated with Alzheimer's disease primarily affects the brain's gray matter, which is responsible for processing information from the senses and controlling muscle movement. As the disease progresses, the tissue loss can also extend to the brain's white matter, which is responsible for transmitting information between different regions of the brain. The corpus callosum and hippocampus are two specific brain structures that are often affected by Alzheimer's disease. The corpus callosum is a large bundle of nerve fibers that connects the left and right halves of the brain, while the hippocampus is involved in the formation of new memories. The loss of tissue in these structures can lead to a decline in cognitive function and memory loss [2]. Consequently,

DOI: 10.1201/9781003366249-14

the early stages of Alzheimer's disease may be identified and discovered by studying the alterations in the brain's unique structures. Individuals with mild cognitive impairment (MCI) are more likely to advance to the last stage of irreversible brain illness [3]. MCI is a condition that is characterized by a decline in cognitive function, but not to the same extent as in Alzheimer's disease. MCI may be classified as stable MCI (sMCI) or progressive MCI (pMCI) to predict the early stages of Alzheimer's disease. People with sMCI tend to remain at a stable level of cognitive function, while those with pMCI are at a higher risk of developing Alzheimer's disease. The stages of Alzheimer's disease-related dementia are typically classified as normal cognitive (NC) function, sMCI, pMCI, and eventually Alzheimer's disease (AD). These stages represent a gradual decline in cognitive function and increasing difficulty with activities of daily living.

Magnetic resonance imaging (MRI) is the main medical imaging technique used to study the anatomical changes associated with Alzheimer's disease. MRI uses magnetic fields and radio waves to create detailed images of the body's organs and tissues. There are two main types of MRI: structural MRI (sMRI) and functional MRI (fMRI). sMRI shows the size, shape, and location of different organs and tissues, while fMRI measures brain activity. MRI can be used to identify changes in the brain that may be associated with Alzheimer's disease, such as atrophy or shrinkage of the hippocampus. This information can help doctors diagnose and monitor the progression of Alzheimer's disease [4]. MRI is a crucial tool for doctors to diagnose Alzheimer's disease, and it also plays a key role in research on Alzheimer's disease detection. The use of cognitive assessment data from patients over time (including those with normal cognitive function, mild cognitive impairment, and Alzheimer's disease) can help in identifying the disease at an early stage [5]. This data typically covers a period of 6 to 12 months and consists of various medical exams and assessments, such as the Assessment Scale Cognitive Subscale (ADAS-Cog 13), the Rey Auditory Verbal Learning Test (RAVLT), and Mini-Mental State Examination (MMSE).

The goal of AD prediction is to categorize several phases of dementia progression, such as NC, MCI, and AD, therefore early prediction becomes a pattern classification challenge. Many modeling strategies, such as statistical models, and algorithms for machine learning have been investigated using handmade characteristics to increase the model's capacity to grasp increasingly complex health problems.

In recent years, there has been a significant amount of research on the use of deep learning algorithms for early detection of AD due to their ability to automatically extract and represent data. Previous studies have primarily utilized convolutional neural networks (CNNs) for predicting AD, but more recent research has focused on using more complex multichannel CNN models and integrating both CNN and RNN (recurrent neural network) models to improve performance. The rapid advancement of deep learning technology has enabled more precise forecasting of the early stages of AD.

In this chapter, we review the latest published research on AD early detection using deep learning technology. Our focus is on the applied technologies rather than the technical details of the underlying models. We discuss the benefits of using deep learning algorithms for AD detection, as well as the challenges and limitations of this approach. Our review shows that deep learning algorithms have the potential to significantly improve the accuracy and speed of AD detection and can provide valuable insights into the progression of the disease. However, further research is needed to fully understand the potential of these algorithms and to overcome the challenges and limitations.

The review begins by discussing the use of CNNs in the early detection of AD. CNNs are a type of deep learning algorithm that is highly effective in tasks related to computer vision. They have been used to classify AD and normal cases, and auto-encoders with CNNs as their backbone have been used to generate low-dimensional representations of MRIs and PETs. The review highlights the benefits of using CNNs for AD detection, as well as the challenges and limitations of this approach. Overall, the review suggests that CNNs have the potential to improve the accuracy and speed of AD detection, but further research is needed to fully understand their capabilities and limitations [6]. The review also discusses the use of CNNs for semantic segmentation, which is a technique that involves highlighting specific regions of the brain from MRI scans that are related to AD progression. The review notes that the transfer learning strategy, which involves using pretrained neural network weights to predict or localize AD-related dementia, has been shown to improve the performance of CNNs. To further decrease prediction variance, the ensemble modeling approach can be used, which involves combining the outputs of multiple classifiers using an aggregation method such as majority or weighted majority voting. Overall, the review suggests that these techniques can be effective in improving the accuracy and reliability of AD detection using CNNs.

In this chapter, we review the use of deep learning algorithms for early detection of AD. We discuss the various deep learning methods that have been applied in this context, including CNNs, transfer learning, and ensemble modeling. We compare the advantages and disadvantages of each method and discuss the challenges and limitations that need to be addressed in order to improve their performance. In our conclusion, we summarize the key findings of this review and discuss the potential of deep learning algorithms for enhancing early detection of Alzheimer's disease. We also provide our perspective on future directions for research in this area, including the need for larger and more diverse datasets, and the development of more sophisticated deep learning models. Overall, we believe that deep learning algorithms have the potential to significantly improve the accuracy and speed of AD detection and can provide valuable insights into the progression of the disease.

14.2 LITERATURE REVIEW

14.2.1 CONVOLUTIONAL NEURAL NETWORK FOR EARLY DETECTION OF ALZHEIMER'S DISEASE

H. Li et al. proposed a new approach for classifying AD and normal cognitive function using CNNs. The study used CNN feature maps to develop a time-to-event predictive model, which was combined with other clinical characteristics associated with AD dementia. This model was able to predict patients' progression to AD with high accuracy. This research suggests that CNNs can be a valuable tool for early detection and treatment of AD. Further research is needed to fully understand the potential of this approach and to identify ways to improve its performance [3]. In this study, MRI scans from the ADNI1 and AIBL2 datasets were used to train a CNN for early detection of AD. The hippocampus region was extracted from 3D MRIs using a local label learning technique, and the resulting 3D volume was used to create the training dataset. The CNN model used both left- and right-extracted hippocampus images as inputs for label categorization. The trained CNN feature maps were then used in conjunction with clinical variables to construct a LASSO regularized Cox regression model. One limitation of this approach is that the CNN and regression models were trained independently, making it difficult to combine them into a single framework. Additionally, the use of two separate models may have reduced the overall performance of the system. Further research is needed to develop more integrated approaches that can better capture the relationship between CNN feature maps and clinical variables in predicting the progression of AD.

- X. Gao et al. proposed a new CNN design for identifying AD and healthy cognitive function [6]. The study combined 2D and 3D CNNs into two separate models, which shared feature maps during the computation process. The final layer of the model predicted outcomes by averaging the output feature maps of both models. This approach allowed the use of both 2D and 3D MRI data in the CNN model, but it was dependent on a balanced dataset and a sufficient number of MRI images.

One potential limitation of this approach is its reliance on a balanced dataset. In real-world scenarios, the availability of MRI data may be uneven, and the performance of the model may be affected by imbalanced data. Future research could explore ways to improve the robustness of this approach to imbalanced data, such as using data augmentation or weighting the loss function. Overall, this study demonstrates the potential of combining 2D and 3D CNNs for identifying AD and healthy cognitive function and highlights the need for further research in this area.

Jo et al. proposed a deep learning algorithm for predicting individual diagnosis of AD and MCI based on a single cross-sectional brain structural MRI scan [7]. The study used data augmentation techniques, such as picture rotation and translation, to prevent overfitting and achieved good performance. One potential limitation of this approach is its reliance on a single MRI scan. In real-world scenarios, multiple MRI scans may be available for each patient, and incorporating this additional information may improve the accuracy of the model. Future research could explore ways to incorporate multiple MRI scans into the model, such as using RNNs or other time series models. Overall, this study demonstrates the potential of deep learning algorithms for predicting AD and MCI and highlights the importance of data augmentation in preventing overfitting.

Duc et al. proposed a model that combined a classifier and a regressor to predict AD [8]. The training data included patches of multiple anatomical landmarks and handcrafted features, such as clinical scores and demographic factors. The model used a three-channel CNN trained on the landmark patches, and the final layer combined the CNN feature maps with the handcrafted features to form a multiclassifier (labels: AD, pMCI, sMCI, and NC) and a regressor to predict clinical scores. The limitation of this approach is its reliance on handcrafted features. While these features may be useful in predicting AD, they may not capture all of the relevant information present in the MRI data. Future research could explore ways to incorporate more comprehensive features extracted from the MRI data, such as using more sophisticated CNNs or integrating other types of data, such as positron-emission tomography (PET) images or genetic information. Overall, this study demonstrates the potential of combining a classifier and regressor in a single model for predicting AD and highlights the importance of incorporating both MRI data and clinical variables in the model.

Based on brain MRI, Yang et al. suggested an upgraded inception network to forecast the early stages of AD [9]. To highlight AD's vulnerable brain areas, image preparation was comprised of histogram equalization and subthreshold segmentation. The improved inception model had one extra branch made of two convolution layers (3×3 kernel) with sigmoid activation, and the output of this branch was multiplied by the output of the base inception. This additional branch broadened the image's receptive area. It created the matching attention heat map with all values between [0, 1], highlighting the attention region of MRIs such as the hippocampus region. However, this improved model lacks a detailed mathematical explanation of how the model identifies certain MRI areas.

M. Amin-Naji et al. used MRI scans to categorize AD and NC patients using the Siamese CNN (SCNN) [10]. The suggested SCNN utilized three ResNet-34 branches to create three vectors, which were then used to construct the output feature maps for AD early prediction. This approach randomly picked MRI pictures from either the AD or NC datasets to feed SCNN on the anchor and positive branches for two vectors (anchor vector, positive vector). One positive pairwise distance was calculated using these two vectors. The photos of the negative branch, on the other hand, contain labels against the positive and anchor branches to form the negative vector. The negative pairwise distance, on the other hand, was determined using both the negative vector and the anchor vector. For example, the negative branch selects photographs of NC subjects, whereas both the positive and anchor branches select images of AD people. The loss function employed both positive and negative pairwise distances. The goal of model training is to maximize the difference between pairwise distances, which implies that as the distance between the anchor and positive pictures reduces, so does the distance between the anchor and negative images. The suggested study aided in the use of the unsupervised learning approach to categorize AD and NC topics. The SCNN, on the other hand, was a binary classifier that could only predict AD versus NC versus MRI.

M. Liu et al. proposed a technique for predicting clinical ratings using MRI data [11]. The information was obtained using MRI landmark patches, but because the clinical scores in the dataset were partial, the proposed work focused on using deep learning algorithms to forecast the missing clinical scores. The regression accuracy was limited, however, because the missing clinic score update depended on the entire clinical score. A limitation of this approach is its reliance on partial clinical scores. In real-world scenarios, patients may have a complete set of clinical scores, and incorporating this additional information may improve the accuracy of the model. Future research could explore ways to incorporate complete clinical scores into the model, such as using more sophisticated deep learning models or integrating other types of data, such as PET images or genetic information. Overall, this study demonstrates the potential of deep learning algorithms for predicting missing clinical scores and highlights the importance of incorporating both MRI data and clinical variables in the model.

M. Kavitha et al. [12] studied a modified U-Net-like design for PET segmentation and classification. The method used a CNN with a bottleneck architecture and a multiclass logistic regression classifier at the final layer to predict AD, normal cognitive function, and MCI from PET images. This study highlights the potential of deep learning algorithms for PET segmentation and classification but also notes limitations such as reliance on PET images and the use of a logistic regression classifier.

In a recent study, the effects of various optimizers, overfitting approaches, and CNN model topologies on the classification of AD stages were investigated. A. M. Taqi et al. [13] used data augmentation and different optimizers to classify AD and normal cognitive function. L. Yue et al. [14] proposed a strategy for predicting AD using a custom CNN. Jarrett et al. [15] suggested a similar CNN design to forecast the early stages of AD using dense and residual block nets. A. Fedorov et al. developed a two-channel 1D CNN to predict AD using hand-engineered features. A. Fedorov et al. [16] used the Deep InfoMax (DIM) approach to build deep representations of MRIs. DIM is an unsupervised learning technique that maximizes the mutual information between the input and output of a deep neural network encoder [17]. These studies highlight the potential of deep learning algorithms for AD prediction but also highlight limitations such as the need for large, diverse datasets and the development of more advanced deep learning models.

In their study, Bhandari et al. [18] demonstrated the use of segmentation techniques to analyze brain subregions and predict early-stage AD. The MRI dataset used in the study included both AD and normal cognitive patients. The MRIs were processed using skull stripping and histogram equalization to improve the image quality. The multilevel thresholding algorithm was then applied to segment-specific regions, including white matter, corpus callosum, gray matter, and hippocampus regions on the MRI. The resulting segmented images were fed into a CNN for AD prediction. The proposed framework utilized multilevel thresholding to highlight AD-related brain regions on MRI, improving the performance of the CNN. However, the automatic thresholding algorithm relied on high contrast between the background and foreground on MRI slices, and the applied segmentation algorithm was not integrated with the CNN model training.

Choi et al. [19] proposed a deep learning approach for predicting AD using MRI data. The proposed method combines voxel-based, region-based, and patch-based approaches into a unified framework with a deep learning model. The method first segments three tissues – gray matter, white matter, and cerebrospinal fluid – on each MRI. Each region is then interpreted through a deep learning network to obtain a prediction score related to AD status. All scores are then averaged to determine the final output. This approach allows artificial intelligence (AI) models to segment regions of interest (ROIs) on the input images for both classification and regression. However, the method relies on the accuracy of the preprocessed segmented data, which must be inspected by professionals to ensure its accuracy.

14.2.2 THE ENSEMBLE LEARNING STRATEGY FOR ALZHEIMER'S DISEASE DETECTION

The proposed hybrid ensemble learning method by Jabason et al. [20] uses a combination of a CNN and an image optimization selection process to predict AD based on MRI images. The technique uses the image entropy method to improve the selection of MRI images and features three channels that accept MRI images in different planes. The final prediction is obtained through the use of a soft voting approach. This method expands the range of ensemble learning models, but the voting mechanism cannot adjust the weights of the predictions from the different channels in the final ensemble.

- X. Fang et al. proposed a method to combine three CNNs using the AdaBoost algorithm for the classification of AD using multimodality imaging [21]. The study used both MRI and PET images as input for the CNNs, with each channel comprising different CNN models (GoogLeNet, ResNet, and DenseNet). The final predictions from the individual CNNs were then input into the AdaBoost model to improve accuracy. This approach allowed for the combination of models trained on different imaging modalities, but the use of AdaBoost may bias the learning of the model toward data noise.

14.2.3 TRANSFER LEARNING STRATEGY FOR ALZHEIMER'S DISEASE PREDICTION

Chakraborty et al. [22] studied the use of transfer learning for early detection of AD. The study involved preprocessing structural MRI and diffusion tensor imaging data, including segmentation of the hippocampus, gray matter, and white matter. The preprocessed data was used to train a CNN model using transfer learning to improve model performance. The study showed that transfer learning can be effective for enhancing the diversity of data used for training, but the authors also noted that using old model structures may limit the potential of transfer learning.

Soufiene et al. [24] used transfer learning and VGG19 and Inception V4 to distinguish AD versus NC. Soufiene et al. [23] studied the identification of AD using MRIs using transfer learning algorithms. The proposed approach used the image entropy algorithm to optimize feature selection and evaluated several configurations of VGG pretrained models to overcome overfitting concerns. These studies show the potential of transfer learning for improving the performance of deep learning models for AD detection.

In summary, recent research has focused on using deep learning algorithms, specifically CNNs, for early detection of AD. Previous studies have used simple CNN models, while more recent research has explored the use of complex multichannel CNN models and the integration of both CNN and RNN models. These advances in deep learning technology have enabled more accurate forecasting of the early stages of AD. However, further research is needed to develop more integrated approaches that can better capture the relationship between CNN feature maps and clinical variables, as well as to address challenges such as overfitting and the need for larger and more diverse datasets.

14.3 DISCUSSION AND CONCLUSION

14.3.1 AI Technologies for Alzheimer's Disease Detection and Perspectives

There are pros and cons of each AI technology in terms of performance and complexity. CNNs are the most commonly used AI technology in AD prediction, and they have shown good performance in classification and regression tasks. Graph convolutional networks (GCNs), and RNNs are less commonly used, but they can capture the spatial and temporal relationships in brain imaging data, respectively. Ensemble learning methods are useful for improving the performance of individual classifiers but require a large amount of data and computational resources. Image segmentation can highlight specific brain regions related to AD, but it is dependent on the quality of the preprocessing steps. Transfer learning methods can reduce the amount of data and computational resources needed for training, but they rely on the quality of the pretrained model. Overall, AI technologies have the potential to significantly improve the accuracy and speed of AD detection, but their effectiveness can be limited by the quality of the data and the complexity of the algorithms.

For example, Choi et al. [19] used a CNN to segment three tissues from each MRI, including gray matter, white matter, and cerebrospinal fluid, and used a deep learning network to predict an AD status for each region. These scores were then averaged to determine the final output. This approach allows for the integration of voxel-based, region-based, and patch-based approaches into a single unified framework using deep learning. However, the segmentation relies on predefined hypotheses about target regions in the preprocessing stage, and the segmented data must be manually inspected by experts to ensure their accuracy.

Another approach is to use transfer learning, where pretrained models are finetuned on a new dataset. For example, Soufiene et al. [24] used transfer learning algorithms to identify AD using MRIs. The study used the image entropy algorithm for feature selection, and various configurations of VGG pretrained models were evaluated to address overfitting concerns. Transfer learning can improve both model training speed and performance, but the accuracy of the model depends heavily on preprocessing of the medical imaging data to highlight AD-related regions. Additionally, the large amount of data can lead to overfitting, which can weaken the pretrained model. Table 14.1 summarizes the contributions of the reviewed studies

TABLE 14.1

Categories of machine learning techniques for Alzheimer's disease detection

ML technique	Task	Reference	Contribution	Data
CNN	Regression	[3]	Lasso regularized cross regression model with CNN	MCI and NC (MRI) and clinical variables
	Classification	[6]	A novel Inception v3 architecture	AD and NC (MRI)
	Classification	[7]	Siamese convolutional neural network applied on 3 channel images	AD and NC (MRI)
	Classification and regression	[8]	CNN used for MRI classification and clinical score	AD and NC (MRI)
	Classification	[9]	Novel data processing and data augmentation methods	AD and NC (MRI)
	Classification	[10]	Jointly train CNN with 2-channel and 3-channel MRI scans	AD and NC (MRI)
	Segmentation and classification	[2]	Multilevel threshold segmentation that uses grey wolf optimization	AD and NC (MRI)
	Segmentation and classification	[12]	Integrate voxel-based with region-based and patch-based data into the CNN mode	AD and stable cognitive impairment and progressive mild cognitive impairment and NC
Ensemble learning	Classification	[20]	3D MRI image entropy and ensemble CNNs	AD and NC (MRI)
	Classification	[21]	Deep ensemble generalization loss function	AD and NC (MRI)
Transfer learning	Classification	[22]	Pretrained CNN model with long short-term memory trained with MRI on three planes	AD and NC
	Classification	[24]	Image entropy and VGG pretrained model	AD and NC

in the area of using AI technologies for AD prediction. These studies have explored various AI technologies, including CNNs, GCNs, ensemble learning methods, RNNs, image segmentation, and transfer learning methods. The studies have used these technologies to improve the accuracy of AD prediction by extracting essential features from MRI images, building regression models for AD score prediction, and training different classifiers. Some studies have also used image segmentation algorithms to highlight sensitive brain regions in MRI images and transfer learning to adapt pretrained models to new training data.

14.3.2 Preprocessing Techniques of Medical Imaging Dataset

Raw MRI or PET images do not provide high-quality results due to the various radiation and imaging equipment characteristics. Scanned images of Alzheimer's disease patients show a variety of changes in different brain regions. Previous research has found that certain sensitive regions, such as the hippocampal regions, gray matter, white matter, and cerebrospinal fluid, can more accurately reflect the symptoms of AD. One alternative method is to first take 2D images and then segment the gray matter, white matter, and cerebrospinal fluid on these images using medical imaging software or the MATLAB toolbox. Region segmentation can highlight image characteristics, improving the interpretability of AI models. In addition to the aforementioned brain areas, other tissues reflect the AD state to a certain extent, and it is difficult to segment all of them using ROI approaches. LPE (Learn Patch Extract) places landmarks on various sensitive regions of MRIs using specific algorithms to capture critical information, and small patches of landmarks are extracted to create the dataset for testing and training from MRIs. Both ROI and LPE methods require a strong hypothesis of brain areas and a skilled postprocessing check of data segmentation. If either fails to meet data quality control standards, the performance of the model in the real world will be unreliable. It is also challenging to obtain a large number of processed MRI images that have been reviewed by trained professionals. In all studies, RP (Return Patch) methods are used before ROI and LPE. However, when AI technologies are applied to large amounts of data, RP approaches are more feasible, and it is easier to incorporate preprocessing into the data pipeline of proposed methods.

14.3.3 Limitations and Future Directions

The use of traditional machine learning algorithms with handcrafted features has been extensively studied for predicting Alzheimer's disease. However, recent advances in AI technology, such as convolutional neural networks and recurrent neural networks, have shown even better performance through the automatic extraction of high-level features from datasets. The advantage of deep learning technology is that it can either combine handcrafted features with feature maps of input data, or directly extract specific patterns from input data for classification or regression tasks. This makes it possible to integrate AI technology into high-level applications without the need for manual extraction of features by trained professionals.

The use of deep learning technologies for AD prediction has certain limitations, including the lack of training data and the focus on supervised learning. Unsupervised learning techniques may be used to compress and cluster the dataset, but this can decrease the performance of clustering due to a lack of data embeddings. However, certain limitations when applying deep learning technologies in AD patients' classification as follows:

- One limitation is the focus on supervised learning in most of the reviewed methods. This means that MRIs or PETs without labels are discarded, reducing the available data for training the model. Some researchers have applied unsupervised learning techniques to compress and cluster the dataset, but this can lead to lower-dimensional data that is not interpretable and reduces the performance of the clustering.
- Another limitation of deep learning in AD prediction is the reliance on supervised learning, where MRIs or PETs with missing labels are discarded. While some researchers use unsupervised learning techniques to compress and cluster the data, low-dimension data is unable to accurately represent relationships between data points, leading to poor clustering performance.

REFERENCES

1. Alzheimer's Association, "2019 Alzheimer's disease facts and figures," *Alzheimer's & Dementia*, vol. 15, no. 3, pp. 321–387, Mar. 2019, doi: 10.1016/j.jalz.2019.01.010.
2. D. Chitradevi and S. Prabha, "Analysis of brain sub regions using optimization techniques and deep learning method in Alzheimer disease," *Applied Soft Computing*, vol. 86, p. 105857, Jan. 2020, doi: 10.1016/j.asoc.2019.105857.
3. H. Li, M. Habes, D. A. Wolk, Y. Fan, and Alzheimer's Disease Neuroimaging Initiative and the Australian Imaging Biomarkers and Lifestyle Study of Aging, "A deep learning model for early prediction of Alzheimer's disease dementia based on hippocampal magnetic resonance imaging data," *Alzheimer's & Dementia*, vol. 15, no. 8, pp. 1059–1070, Aug. 2019, doi: 10.1016/j.jalz.2019.02.007.
4. F. Li and M. Liu, "Alzheimer's disease diagnosis based on multiple cluster dense convolutional networks," *Computerized Medical Imaging and Graphics*, vol. 70, pp. 101–110, Dec. 2018, doi: 10.1016/j.compmedimag.2018.09.009.
5. H. Li and Y. Fan, "Early prediction of Alzheimer's disease dementia based on baseline Hippocampal MRI and 1-year follow-up cognitive measures using deep recurrent neural networks," in 2019 IEEE 16th International Symposium on Biomedical Imaging (ISBI 2019), Venice, Italy, Apr. 2019, pp. 368–371. doi: 10.1109/ISBI.2019.8759397.
6. X. W. Gao, R. Hui, and Z. Tian, "Classification of CT brain images based on deep learning networks," *Computer Methods and Programs in Biomedicine*, vol. 138, pp. 49–56, Jan. 2017, doi: 10.1016/j.cmpb.2016.10.007.
7. T. Jo, K. Nho, and A. J. Saykin, "Deep learning in Alzheimer's disease: Diagnostic classification and prognostic prediction using neuroimaging data," *Frontiers in Aging Neuroscience*, vol. 11, p. 220, Aug. 2019, doi: 10.3389/fnagi.2019.00220.
8. N. T. Duc, S. Ryu, M. N. I. Qureshi, M. Choi, K. H. Lee, and B. Lee, "3D-deep learning based automatic diagnosis of Alzheimer's disease with joint MMSE prediction using resting-state fMRI," *Neuroinform*, vol. 18, no. 1, pp. 71–86, Jan. 2020, doi: 10.1007/s12021-019-09419-w.
9. K. Yang, E. A. Mohammed, and B. H. Far, "Detection of Alzheimer's disease using graph-regularized convolutional neural network based on structural similarity learning of brain magnetic resonance images," in *IEEE 22nd International Conference on Information Reuse and Integration for Data Science (IRI)*, Aug. 2021, pp. 326–333.
10. M. Amin-Naji, H. Mahdavinataj, and A. Aghagolzadeh, "Alzheimer's disease diagnosis from structural MRI using Siamese convolutional neural network," in *4th International Conference* on *Pattern Recognition* and *Image Analysis (IPRIA)*, Tehran, Iran, Mar. 2019, pp. 75–79.

11. M. Liu, J. Zhang, C. Lian, and D. Shen, "Weakly supervised deep learning for brain disease prognosis using MRI and incomplete clinical scores," *IEEE Trans. Cybern.*, vol. 50, no. 7, pp. 3381–3392, 2020, doi: 10.1109/TCYB.2019.2904186.

12. M. Kavitha, N. Yudistira, and T. Kurita, "Multi-instance learning via deep CNN for multi-class recognition of Alzheimer's disease," in *IEEE 11th International Workshop on Computational Intelligence and Applications (IWCIA)*, Hiroshima, Japan, Nov. 2019, pp. 89–94.

13. A. M. Taqi, A. Awad, F. Al-Azzo, and M. Milanova, "The impact of multi-optimizers and data augmentation on TensorFlow convolutional neural network performance," in *IEEE Conference on Multimedia Information Processing and Retrieval (MIPR)*, Miami, FL, Apr. 2018, pp. 140–145.

14. L. Yue et al., "Auto-detection of Alzheimer's disease using deep convolutional neural networks," in *14th International Conference on Natural Computation, Fuzzy Systems and Knowledge Discovery (ICNC-FSKD)*, Huangshan, China, Jul. 2018, pp. 228–234.

15. D. Jarrett, J. Yoon, and M. van der Schaar, "Dynamic prediction in clinical survival analysis using temporal convolutional networks," *IEEE Journal of Biomedical and Health Informatics*, vol. 24, no. 2, pp. 424–436, Feb. 2020, doi: 10.1109/JBHI.2019.2929264.

16. A. Fedorov et al., "Prediction of Progression to Alzheimer's disease with Deep InfoMax," in *IEEE EMBS International Conference on Biomedical & Health Informatics (BHI)*, Chicago, IL, May 2019, pp. 1–5.

17. R. D. Hjelm et al., "Learning deep representations by mutual information estimation and maximization." arXiv, Feb. 22, 2019. Accessed: Nov. 24, 2022. [Online]. Available: http://arxiv.org/abs/1808.06670

18. A. K. Bhandari, V. K. Singh, A. Kumar, and G. K. Singh, "Cuckoo search algorithm and wind driven optimization-based study of satellite image segmentation for multilevel thresholding using Kapur's entropy," *Expert Systems with Applications*, vol. 41, no. 7, pp. 3538–3560, Jun. 2014, doi: 10.1016/j.eswa.2013.10.059.

19. J.-S. Choi, E. Lee, and H.-I. Suk, "Regional abnormality representation learning in structural MRI for AD/MCI diagnosis," in *Machine Learning in Medical Imaging*, vol. 11046, Y. Shi, H.-I. Suk, and M. Liu, Eds. Cham: Springer International Publishing, 2018, pp. 64–72.

20. E. Jabason, M. O. Ahmad, and M. N. S. Swamy, "Classification of Alzheimer's disease from MRI data using an ensemble of hybrid deep convolutional neural networks," in *IEEE 62nd International Midwest Symposium on Circuits and Systems (MWSCAS)*, Dallas, TX, Aug. 2019, pp. 481–484.

21. X. Fang, Z. Liu, and M. Xu, "Ensemble of deep convolutional neural networks based multi-modality images for Alzheimer's disease diagnosis," *IET Image Processing*, vol. 14, no. 2, pp. 318–326, Feb. 2020, doi: 10.1049/iet-ipr.2019.0617.

22. C. Chakraborty, S.B. Othman, F.A. Almalki et al. FC-SEEDA: Fog computing-based secure and energy efficient data aggregation scheme for Internet of healthcare things. *Neural Computing & Applications* , (2023). doi: 10.1007/s00521-023-08270-0

23. Soufiene Ben Othman, Abdullah Ali Bahattab, Abdelbasset Trad and Habib Youssef, "PEERP: A priority-based energy-efficient routing protocol for reliable data transmission in healthcare using the IoT", in *The 15th International Conference on Future Networks and Communications (FNC)* August 9–12, 2020, Leuven, Belgium, 2020.

24. Soufiene Ben Othman, Faris A. Almalki, Chinmay Chakraborty, Hedi Sakli, "Privacy-preserving aware data aggregation for IoT-based healthcare with green computing technologies", *Computers and Electrical Engineering*, vol. 101, p. 108025, 2022.

Index

For Product Safety Concerns and Information please contact our EU
representative GPSR@taylorandfrancis.com
Taylor & Francis Verlag GmbH, Kaufingerstraße 24, 80331 München, Germany

www.ingramcontent.com/pod-product-compliance
Lightning Source LLC
Chambersburg PA
CBHW060351220326
41598CB00023B/2874